Nursing Knowledge Development and Clinical Practice

Sister Callista L. Roy, PhD, RN, FAAN, is a Professor and Nurse Theorist at the William F. Connell School of Nursing at Boston College, where she teaches doctoral, master's, and undergraduate students. Dr. Roy is best known for her work on the Roy adaptation model of nursing. Her current clinical research is an intervention study to involve families in cognitive recovery of patients with mild head injury. Her other scholarly work includes conceptualizing and measuring coping and developing the philosophical basis for the adaptation model and for the epistemology of nursing. Roy has numerous publications, including books and journal articles, on nursing theory and other professional topics. Her works have been translated into many languages all over the world. With her colleagues of the Roy Adaptation Association, she has critiqued and synthesized the first 230 research projects published in English based on her adaptation model. Dr. Roy also has delivered invited papers, lectures, and workshops throughout North America and 30 other countries over the past 30 years on topics related to nursing theory, research, curriculum, clinical practice, and professional trends for the future. She began her education at Mount Saint Mary's College, located in Los Angeles, the city where she was born. Dr. Roy has master's degrees in pediatric nursing and sociology from the University of California at Los Angeles, where she also earned her PhD. She holds honorary doctorates from four other institutions. Her postdoctoral studies in neuroscience nursing were at the University of California at San Francisco.

Dorothy A. Jones, EdD, RNC, ANP, FAAN, is a Professor of Adult Health at the William F. Connell School of Nursing at Boston College, where she formerly served as Chair of the Adult Health Department from 1995 to 1999. She is a Senior Nurse Scientist at the Massachusetts General Hospital in Boston, Massachusetts, and formerly a President of the Eastern Nursing Research Society. She has been involved in nursing language development serving as past President of the North American Nursing Diagnosis Association. Jones' research includes a NIH-funded study focusing on patients' recovery at home following ambulatory surgery, theory development related to Margaret Newman's Health as Expanding Consciousness, evaluation research, and instrument development. Her many awards include Boston College's Teaching Excellence Award in 2005, Partners Award for Excellence in Practice in 1998 and 2003, the Indiana University School of Nursing Outstanding Alumni Award, and the Sigma Theta Tau International Founders Award in 2000. Jones has a strong record of curriculum development and mentorship with graduate students, as evidenced by their scholarship nationally and internationally. She received her BSN from Long Island University and Brooklyn Hospital School of Nursing in Brooklyn, New York, and earned graduate degrees from Indiana University and Boston University.

Nursing Knowledge Development and Clinical Practice

Editors

Sister Callista Roy, PhD, RN, FAAN
Dorothy A. Jones, EdD, RNC, ANP, FAAN

SPRINGER PUBLISHING COMPANY

New York

Springer Publishing Company, LLC
11 West 42nd Street, 15th Floor
New York, NY 10036-8002

Acquisitions Editor: Sally J. Barhydt
Managing Editor: Mary Ann McLaughlin
Production Editor: Matthew Byrd
Cover Design: Joanne E. Honigman
Composition: Techbooks

07 08 09 10/5 4 3 2 1

Library of Congress Cataloging-in-Publication Data

Nursing knowledge development and clinical practice/editors, Sister Callista Roy, Dorothy A. Jones.
    p. ; cm.
  Includes bibliographical references and index.
  ISBN 0-8261-0299-9
1. Nursing—Philosophy. 2. Knowledge, Theory of. 3. Clinical medicine. 4. Nursing—Practice.
  I. Roy, Callista. II. Jones, Dorothy A.
  [DNLM: 1. Nursing Theory. 2. Philosophy, Nursing. 3. Knowledge. 4. Models, Nursing. WY 86 N9736 2007]
RT84.5.N87 2007
610.73—dc22

2006022207

Printed in the United States of America by Bang Printing

Contents

Part I: State of the Art of Nursing Knowledge: Visions and Issues

Part II: Philosophical Basis for Knowledge

Part III: Integrated Knowledge for Nursing Practice

Part IV: Impact on Health and Patient Care—Exemplars for the Future

Contributors

Sr. Callista Roy, PhD, RN, FAAN
Boston College
William F. Connell School of Nursing
Chestnut Hill, MA

Dorothy A. Jones, EdD, RNC, ANP, FAAN
Boston College
William F. Connell School of Nursing
Chestnut Hill, MA
Massachusetts General Hospital
Boston, MA

Anne-Marie Barron, PhD, APRN
Simmons College
Massachusetts General Hospital
Boston, MA

Diane Berry, PhD, RN, ANP
University of North Carolina at Chapel Hill
Chapel Hill, NC

Peggy Chinn, PhD, RN, FAAN
Univeristy of Connecticut (Emerita)
Emeryville, CA

Marga Coler, EdD, RN, CS, CTN, FAAN
Federal University of Paraiba
Brazil

Matthew Coler-Thayer, BA
Vrije Universiteit Amsterdam
The Netherlands

Maria Miriam Lima da Nóbrega, DNSc, MN, RN
Federal University of Paraiba—Health
  Sciences Center
Brazil

Nancy Dluhy, PhD, RN
University of Massachusetts—Dartmouth
Dartmouth, MA

Joanne Dochterman, PhD, RN, FAAN
University of Iowa
Swisher, IA

Jane Flanagan, PhD, RN, ANP
Boston College
William F. Connell School of Nursing
Chestnut Hill, MA

Telma Ribeiro Garcia, DNSc, MN, RN
Federal University of Paraiba
Brazil

Judith R. Graves
Indiana University School of Nursing
Indianapolis, IN

Katherine Gregory, PhD, RN
Boston College
William F. Connell School of Nursing
Chestnut Hill, MA

Debra Hanna, PhD, RN
New York Presbyterian Hospital
Columbia University Medical Center
New York, NY

Marcelline Harris, PhD, RN
Mayo Clinic
Rochester, MN

Hesook Suzie Kim, PhD, RN
University of Rhode Island
   (Emerita)
Haymarket, VA
Buskerud University College
Kongsberg, Norway

Elizabeth R. Lenz, PhD, RN, FAAN
Ohio State University
Columbus, Ohio

Yi-Hui Liu, RN, MS
Boston College
William F. Connell School of
   Nursing
Chestnut Hill, MA

Ruth Palan Lopez, PhD, RN
Sharon, MA

Theresa Meehan, PhD, RGT, RNT
University of Dublin
School of Nursing, Midwifery
   & Health Systems
Dublin, Ireland

Margaret Newman, PhD, RN, FAAN
University of Minnesota (Emerita)
Memphis, TN

Carolyn Padovano, PhD, RN
MITRE Corporation
McLean, VA

Donna Perry, RN
Massachusetts General Hospital
Boston, MA

Beth Rodgers, PhD, RN, FAAN
University of Wisconsin
Milwaukee, WI

Janice Thompson, PhD, RN
University of Southern Maine
College of Nursing
Portland, ME

This book had its origins in the paradox of the rich growth in nursing knowledge at the beginning of the 21st century and, at the same time, unresolved concerns with health care delivery systems and with care. One vehicle for the growth of knowledge has been conferences that address nursing knowledge on multiple levels. A series of such conferences was conducted in the northeastern United States between 1984 and 2001. The cycle of conferences (see the Appendix, History of New England Knowledge Conferences) brought nursing scholars together with developing scholars to dialogue about the links of philosophy, theory, and research as the basis of outcomes for practice. As co-chairs of the last five conferences, the editors envisioned bringing the best of the deliberations about knowledge together in a volume that would address care delivery issues, identify major paradigmatic perspectives, and use those perspectives to create new approaches to practice. Some chapters originally were presented at the conferences; others were solicited to complete the total vision of providing exemplars that link paradigmatic perspectives to practice outcomes.

As the project developed and time passed, the goals and approaches seemed to gain more urgency. Nursing knowledge can have an impact on practice issues today. However, that knowledge needs to be focused and articulated in a way that meets the needs of practice. Examining the range of paradigmatic perspectives, we focused early in our thinking on the classical problem-solving and process-oriented approaches and added a third perspective aimed at a future vision of integrated knowledge based on the thinking of several scholars, including knowledge as universal cosmic imperative.

The scholars whose papers are included have provided thoughtful approaches to nursing knowledge that we believe will be helpful to the whole field of nursing. A wide audience of nurses today are accepting increasing accountability for quality of patient care and seeking articulation of the science of nursing. Masters and doctoral students and faculty are primary groups immersed in increasing levels of responsibility in advanced practice and clinical research. In addition, we hope to speak to nurses holding responsibility for patients from the level of vice-presidents for patient care services and chief nurses to those providing primary care across the health care spectrum in both in-patient and out-patient settings. We aim to stimulate a dialogue of how nursing knowledge is envisioned and how these perspectives can affect practice. Further, this dialogue will include involvement in health care policy as a way of handling the increasing complexity and inadequacy of the systems. The text provides both principles and exemplars for improving practice based on nursing knowledge. The hope is that readers can draw on the depth and breadth of the presentations in this volume to help shape the future of nursing.

We organized the book into four parts, each with an introduction. In Part I we look at the state of the art of nursing knowledge and some of the issues and visions of the contemporary scene of knowledge and practice. It begins with a chapter laying out the many factors influencing knowledge development in nursing and documenting some of our achievements, along with the challenges for practice. This section closes with a chapter that presents a call to action. Part II examines the philosophical basis for knowledge and provides a synthesis of problem-solving and process perspectives and examines how a synthesis of these perspectives provides insight into nursing knowledge development, utilization, and evaluation in clinical and academic settings for the future. The chapters in Part III are focused on specific approaches to integrated knowledge and the effects these can have on practice on both the individual and systems level. Part IV provides six exemplars to provide future impact on health care systems and patient care.

The authors, and our editors, have been very patient while we shaped and re-shaped this text, updated material, and synchronized the various chapters into a whole. We admit that sometimes the work had to wait while ongoing commitments took priority. However, our urgency to bring these insights about nursing knowledge to the nursing readership did not waver and we are happy to have this opportunity to present them to you.

In a time of change within health care as well as nursing education, it is hoped that this text celebrates the nursing knowledge developments to date and those to come as well as their impacts on patient care and most importantly the unique focus nursing has on the human experience. It is in fact this knowledge that can demonstrate nursing's complementarity with other health care providers, be shared within interdisciplinary forums addressing health issues on a global level, infuse curriculum, and shape clinical investigations. Having found the Knowledge Conferences so effective a channel for our developing field, we end our remarks with both hopes and plans for the next sequence of conferences on nursing knowledge to be initiated in the near future.

Sister Callista Roy
Dorothy A. Jones

Part

State of the Art of Nursing Knowledge: Visions and Issues

Introduction

The end of the 20th century saw unprecedented growth in nursing knowledge. An understanding of the nature and focus of nursing knowledge finally had been articulated. Programs of research were contributing to an accumulated knowledge base for practice. Yet this era also saw a time of great turmoil and seemingly ineffective efforts to improve the quality of health care. When market-driven principles ruled health care reform, nursing knowledge failed to provide transformed nursing care systems. This text explores this paradox and then provides a link to an alternative preferred future where nursing knowledge offers opportunities and new directions for clinical practice.

Nursing knowledge is positioning itself to provide visions that can create effective responses to the issues facing health care. The need for cost containment ushered in an era of health care reform during the 21st century. Serious cost containment strategies have been in effect since the mid-1990s; still, the United States far exceeds all other nations in per capita health care spending. Technological advances, including genomic science, have also created unique issues for health care providers. In general, ethical and public policy debates have not kept up with these advances.

Larger social trends raise equally complex issues for nursing knowledge to address. Information technology brings concerns for confidentiality, privacy, and security for an increasingly enlightened public. Changing demographics including an aging population, increasing ethnic diversity, poverty and other disparities are creating challenges to accessing care. Attendant issues involve ethical concerns about quality of life in both chronic and end-of-life care; culturally competent care and marginality; and the paradox of lack of health care insurance in a land of plenty. The vision that nursing knowledge brings to the challenging issues of nursing practice are based on principles and values for creating effective practice systems. Nursing is a human practice discipline that facilitates well-being of individuals, families, and communities using a scientific knowledge base within caring relationships. As a discipline with a social mandate, nurses are eager to take responsibility for social transformation. Possibly there is no time in history when this need was deeper and more far reaching. So, too, nursing has never been more ready to respond to the challenge. This text provides direction for relating nursing knowledge development to clinical practice.

Part I outlines the vision that nursing knowledge can bring to contemporary health care issues and how that vision can create a better reality for the future. In chapter 1 advances in nursing knowledge and the challenges in health care delivery are described together with a Consensus Statement that provides the basis for transforming practice. The author of chapter 2 focuses on the specific vision of careful nursing, a unique tradition that Irish nurses bring to contemporary issues. The crucial role of terminology in nursing as a practice discipline is addressed in chapter 3. Chapter 4 addresses the impact of mid-range theory on knowledge development and practice. Chapter 5 presents a call for more universal language from nurses in Brazil. Finally, in chapter 6, the author sounds a clear challenge to action and a movement toward unity around disciplinary purpose and articulation of goals true to an agreed upon mission.

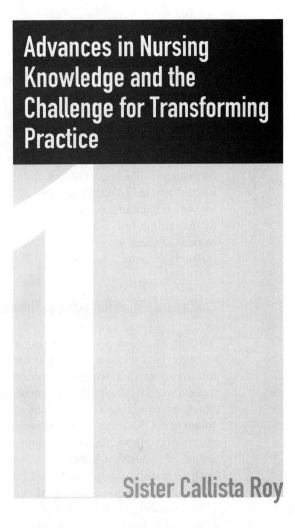

Advances in Nursing Knowledge and the Challenge for Transforming Practice

Sister Callista Roy

T he rich growth in nursing knowledge at the beginning of the 21st century was marked by increased understanding of conceptual nursing knowledge and how to create knowledge for practice. The depth and breadth of these developments is noted in the nursing literature, in the development of doctoral education in nursing, and in the content of nursing conferences. These advances in knowledge are explored in this chapter along with the recognition of unresolved concerns with health care systems and care delivery. From the juxtaposition of these developments and challenges, the assumptions that set the stage for change are derived. Finally, the basis for transformation of nursing care is provided in a Consensus Statement.

Advances in Knowledge

In nursing literature, doctoral education, and professional conferences, we note the maturing of the discipline, particularly in conceptual focus, philosophical perspectives, methodologic inquiry, and sociopolitical commitments. As with the development of any discipline, the manifestations of progress in different arenas are interactive and iterative. Advances in one area stimulate movement in another area, and each time the spiral evolves to higher levels. This interrelatedness is particularly so for nursing as a professional practice discipline. The profession utilizes specialized knowledge to contribute to the needs of society from nursing's specific perspective of promoting health and well-being. Practice, then, is the unifying factor for all of knowledge development. For example, nurses often enter doctoral education with burning issues from advanced practice. In these programs modes of thinking are exercised that produce new insights to pose challenging questions for research. The results of this thought and research are presented at conferences and in journal articles. Likewise, seminal articles in the literature both stem from and stimulate innovative thinking about practice. Scholars and developing scholars in practice and academic settings build on these insights to further knowledge for practice. Developments in each of these interrelated spheres depict the maturing focus of nursing knowledge, methods of inquiry, and potential for relating knowledge to practice.

Conceptual Focus Reflected in Theoretical Literature

Nursing literature at the beginning of this century, whether textbooks or journals, basic or advanced, reflects a view of knowledge as holistic and rooted in a broad perspective of human persons and their environment as related to health. The movement toward focusing nursing knowledge development within an understanding of the nature of nursing practice was advocated in the literature of the last three decades of the 20th century. Johnson (1974) articulated this perspective in a seminal article in which she described alternative approaches for developing nursing as a primary health profession. The medical model and laissez-faire approaches to describing nursing knowledge were contrasted with the possibilities of nursing describing the nature of its practice as the basis for developing knowledge. In a related influential article of this period, Donaldson and Crowley (1978) identified the commonalities of nursing to include concern with principles and laws of life processes, patterns of human behavior in interaction with the environment, and positive changes in health status.

Concurrently the 1970s saw the publication of several major conceptual approaches to nursing that continue to influence the discipline and have provided theoretical bases for nursing knowledge development. Orem (1971) viewed the person as a *self care system* and nursing as fulfilling one of three roles relative to meeting self care needs, that is, wholly compensatory, partially compensatory, and supportive-educative. Roy (1970, 1976) conceptualized the person as an *adaptive system* and the goal of nursing practice as promoting adaptation. Rogers (1970) described the person as a *unitary energy field* identified by pattern and organization that is coextensive with the environment. She viewed nursing as strengthening the human-environment energy field.

These authors, and other nurse theorists, continued to write in the 1980s and 1990s. They and their colleagues contributed to the depth of the discipline's philosophical perspective, particularly in relation to an understanding of the human person. Orem (1997) explored the person as a free agent and the significance of human choice. Roy (1997) emphasized the common purposefulness of human existence in a universe that is creative. Newman (1994) expanded upon Roger's concept of unitary human-energy fields and replaced the dichotomy between health and disease with a synthesis of health expressed as the pattern of the whole person-environment that encompasses disease and nondisease. Orem, Rogers, and Roy had the largest number of nursing publications based on their work from 1982 to 2000 as reported by one survey (Alligood, 2002, p. 645). Their conceptual work has continued to influence the profession through education and research, as well as through ongoing organizations and conferences devoted to knowledge development within each perspective.

Another major thrust of theoretical writing in nursing, beginning in the past century and continuing to influence nursing knowledge development, is the work on caring and cultural care. Leininger, a nurse anthropologist, developed the concept of *cultural care* over four decades from 1950 to 1990 and challenged nurses worldwide to reflect on care as the essence and central focus of nursing. Leininger (1991) noted that human care is a universal phenomenon because care acts and processes are necessary for human birth, development, growth, survival, and peaceful death. Cultural care, however, according to Leininger, involves both universality and diversity. Diversity is the variability and differences in meanings, patterns, values, lifeways, or symbols of care within and among social groups. Universality includes the common, similar, or dominant care patterns and symbols that are noted among many cultures.

Other nurse authors, notably Watson (1979, 1985) and Benner (Benner & Wrubel, 1989) also focused on care as the central concept of nursing. Watson regarded caring as the essence of nursing practice and as a moral ideal rather than a task-oriented behavior. She proposed that caring was intrinsically related to healing and focused on the authentic caring relationship between the nurse and the patient. Initially Benner's work examined the relationships among caring, stress, coping, and health. She noted that caring is primary as a basic way of being in the world. Further, what is stressful and what coping options are available are determined by caring. In later work with other colleagues, Benner has expanded upon the development of caring practices of the nurse, particularly in critical care (Benner, Tanner, & Chesla, 1996; Benner, Hooper-Kyriakidis, & Stannard, 1999).

Morse, Solberg, Neander, Bottorff, and Johnson (1990) published an analysis of 35 authors' works on the concept of caring. The purpose of the analysis was to identify various conceptualizations, evaluate their use and applicability to nursing practice, and identify trends and gaps in caring research. Five perspectives on caring—a human trait, affect, moral imperative, interpersonal interaction, and therapeutic intervention—were identified, as well as outcomes related to the patient's subjective experience and the patient's physiological response. The authors made two major recommendations for knowledge development: first, that further conceptual development and refinement of the concept is needed and second, that the focus of theory and research shift to incorporate a focus on the patient and the difference caring makes.

Other scholars have used research to derive theories related to caring. For example, McCance (2003) used a hermeneutic approach with narrative method to develop a conceptual framework based on caring in nursing practice. In this study, 24 patients were interviewed shortly after discharge from the hospital. Categories of the experience of caring were derived and placed into a framework using the three constructs. For *structure*, the author identified the nurses' attributes, such as professional competence and commitment, and organizational issues, for example, time and skill mix. *Process* included variables such as providing information and reassurance and showing concern. Feelings of well-being and patient satisfaction were among the *outcomes* identified.

Metatheory and Philosophical Perspectives

The decades following the formal introduction of nursing theory into the literature saw increasing discussion at the metatheoretical level. Dialogue on epistemology raised issues about the nature of knowledge and how one knows in nursing. Ontological questions looked at the nature of person and the nature of nursing. A major setting for the discussion of these issues and the philosophical roots of nursing knowledge was journals specifically dedicated to the integration of theory, research, and practice. Development over time is noted by looking at the founding of some of these journals and their current mission.

Image, as the journal of the Sigma Theta Tau National Honor Society, was first published in 1967 in response to a need for communication between the organization's National Council and the local chapters and individuals. A major purpose was to publish selected articles to communicate ideas of interest to nursing and in particular to establish a column known as a Forum. The *Forum* was to be a medium for reaction to "issues that are of particular concern to nurses who have a collegiate education, who strive for high professional standards, who practice nursing in leadership roles, who are committed to the ideals and purposes of the profession and who engage in creative work" (Goodwin, 1967, p. 10). The journal's role as a vehicle for communication on building knowledge for practice grew in the nearly 40-year history of the journal, as did its international focus. The renaming of the publication as the *Journal of Nursing Scholarship* reflects this growth. Currently, major sections are dedicated to world health, genomics for health, clinical scholarship, profession and society, and health policy and systems. In one rating of characteristics and database coverage of journals, this publication scored 10 out of a possible 10 points (Allen, 2001). The content of the journal, reputation, and citations were considered in the ratings.

Advances in Nursing Science (*ANS*) was founded in 1978 by Chinn. In her first editorial, Chinn noted that the premise for initiating the journal was that "for far too long, the wealth and diversity of nursing literature have suffered a lack of timely and creative reporting of the efforts of nurses concerned with the development of nursing science" and therefore the new journal would "focus on articles that address the full range of activities involved in the development of science, including empirical research, theory construction, concept analysis, practical application of research and theory, and investigation of the values and ethics that influence the practice and research activities of nursing science" (Chinn, 1978, n.p.). Currently, the primary purposes of the journal are

> to contribute to the development of nursing science and to promote the applica-
> tion of emerging theories and research findings to practice. Articles deal with any
> of the processes of science, including research, theory development, concept anal-
> ysis, practical application of research and theory, and investigation of the values
> and ethics that influence the practice and research endeavors of nursing sciences.
> (http:/www.nursing.uconn.edu/~plchinn/ANSathgd.htm)

In the nursing journal ratings noted earlier, ANS scored 8 out of 10 possible points, having lost points only on percent of research articles, but scoring high in reputation and citation, highlighting the wider contribution to scholarly dialogue.

In 1987, *Scholarly Inquiry for Nursing Practice* was designed by faculty at Adelphi University as a forum for dialogue on the development and testing of theory and research relevant to nursing practice. The editors used the additional strategy of having invited response papers to articles. This journal was retitled *Research and Theory for Nursing Practice: An International Journal*. Ketefian (2002) noted that the evolutionary changes of the journal meant the embrace of articles that address knowledge development in its broadest sense and that reflect research using a variety of methodologic approaches and that combine several methods. In addition, a fully international journal was envisioned whereby nurses on all continents would find articles relevant to their practice and find a voice to address concerns not specific to the Western social environment and context.

Parse initiated *Nursing Science Quarterly* in 1988 with a focus on "the publication of original works related to theory development, research, and practice, which tie directly to the knowledge base as articulated in the extant nursing theories." After 18 years, the journal continues to be devoted to the enhancement of nursing knowledge. The focus on existing nursing frameworks has been maintained. The last two journals discussed score 4 and 5, respectively, on the rating scale noted earlier.

Two important journals published abroad that make contributions to the metatheory and philosophical dialogue in nursing are the *Journal of Advanced Nursing* and *Australia Journal of Advanced Nursing*. The former was founded in the United Kingdom in 1976 "to become an international medium for the publication of scholarly papers and a means of documenting the ever growing body of nursing knowledge" (Smith, 1976, p. 1). The intent was that the journal become a means toward improving the effectiveness of practice, of enhancing standards of education and service management, and of fostering research-mindedness. The editor urged nurses to document and to share their scientific, theoretical, and philosophical information. Currently, under Alison Tierney as editor, the aim of the journal remains the same while the scope has expanded widely. Papers reflect the diversity, quality, and internationalism of nursing and particularly deal with areas such as: issues and innovations in nursing practice, education, and management; nursing theory and conceptual development and analysis; philosophical and ethical issues; integrative literature reviews; methodological issues in nursing research; health and nursing policy; and health management issues.

The Australian journal was founded in 1983 to extend the scope of writers in the nursing discipline beyond that provided in the all-purpose journal of the professional organization. Papers with a scholarly approach, that is, objective and analytical base, in every area of nursing were invited. In the 20th year of publication, the editor noted that the journal has served as a mechanism for disseminating ideas about nursing and evidence from scholarly activities in practice, education, and research. In particular, the editorial policy notes that the journal publishes scholarly papers that recognize the eclectic nature of global nursing, midwifery, and health care, and that contribute to their development and advancement. The editors urge that papers submitted have a sound scientific, theoretical, or philosophical base and reflect the diversity, quality, and internationalism of nursing. The British journal scores a strong 9 out of 10 in the review reported and the Australian journal scores 4 out of 10.

Among the many contributions of these journals and others like them, collectively the published papers reflect the rising the level of debate on the philosophical perspectives in nursing. The scope of perspectives has expanded to include papers on middle-range theory, nursing practice theory, and cultural theories in *Journal of Nursing Scholarship* (1998, 1999, 2005); studies of gaining meaning and environmental paradigms in *Advances in Nursing Science* (1996); spirituality and hermeneutic–phenomenology in *Journal of Advanced Nursing* (2000); and positivism and qualitative research in *Scholarly Inquiry for Nursing Practice* (2001). In one landmark paper in the inaugural issue of *ANS*, Carper challenged the reluctance of nurses to extend the term *knowledge* beyond the "empirical, factual, objectively descriptive, and general" (Carper, 1978, p. 35). She described four ways of knowing: the empiric, personal, ethical, and aesthetic. This articulation of extended ways of knowing was influential in generating both philosophical and methodologic debate.

Paradigmatic Positions

Nurse authors in the last two decades of the 20th century addressed a central issue about knowledge, that is, how do we know, which led us to consider our paradigmatic stance. Empirical science, from Aristotle's detailed observations of the development of the chick embryo in ancient Greece to Bacon's articulation of experimental design in medieval Europe to Crick's discoveries related to DNA in 20th-century United States, assumes that knowledge is developed from observations of the external world. This approach is based on the belief of Greek philosophers, reemphasized by later thinkers, that knowledge is obtained through the senses. Hegel and other German philosophers of the later 19th century suggested that the only reality that exists is in the mind and therefore knowledge is obtained only through intuited meanings. These two views of reality provide the basis of two distinct paradigms for how knowledge is developed.

Hardy (1978) introduced the term *paradigm* to the nursing literature. Using Kuhn's (1962) discussion of how science works and how it changes, Hardy questioned whether nursing was in a pre-paradigmatic stage. The rapid development of theoretical literature in the three decades that followed seemed to be a response of clarifying the general schools of thought in nursing, that is, to establish its paradigms. Thus the developing literature refuted the position of pre-paradigm status for nursing. However, what followed was also a vigorous dialogue of the deeper issues about the paradigms used for nursing knowledge development. Initially, the discussion centered on the demise of logical positivism and the rise of postmodernism (Stevenson & Woods, 1986; Suppe & Jacox, 1985).

Several strong voices in the literature argued against the dangers of overemphasizing one approach or the other, or making them mutually exclusive and incompatible (Gortner & Schultz, 1988; Norbeck, 1987). By the end of the 20th century, nurse authors identified several categorizations of paradigms from the nursing literature such as those by Parse (1987), Newman (1992), and Fawcett (1993). However, it seems reasonable to continue the discussion within the classic distinctions about knowledge as "discovered in the world," that is, problem solving, empiric, or "created in the mind," that is, process-oriented, interpretive.

The several schools of thought in nursing that emerged from these distinctions are articulated in the literature and summarized from both a knowledge perspective and philosophical basis, as well as related to research and practice in Table 1.1. The approach we take is that it is timely to summarize two paradigmatic positions on knowledge for practice as problem solving and process-oriented. A third perspective, the universal cosmic imperative, is introduced in chapter 11. It builds on Roy's philosophical assumption of veritivity (Roy, 1988; Roy & Andrews, 1999) and assumes a purposeful universe implying a broad use of research traditions.

Other scholars continue to work toward creating a synthesis of the first two approaches that can be called integrative. The fragmentation resulting from dichotomizing approaches to nursing knowledge development was noted by Leddy (2000). She promoted

Table 1.1	Paradigms: Linking Philosophy, Research, and Practice Theory			
Knowledge Perspective	Philosophical Basis	Research Tradition	Practice Theory	Related Terms
Problem solving	Empiricism Rationalism Positivism Postpositivism Normal science Contemporary empiricism	Received view Observation Experimentation Confirmation or refutation Deductive theory Explanatory laws	Descriptive Predictive Prescriptive	Functionalism Instumentalism Reductionism Causal teleology Particulate-deterministic
Process-oriented	Idealism Postmodernism Phenomenology Existentialism Humanism Hermeneutic Relativity Dialectic	Perceived view Interpretive science Inductive theory Grounded theory	Contextual Perception of meaning Discovering patterns Feminism Caring praxis Dialogue Choice and action Personal transformation	Constructivism Deconstructivism Social meaning Ethnography Historicism Interactive-integrative
Universal cosmic imperative	Veritivity Humanism Purposefulness Shared meaningful destiny Spirit & matter Cosmic view of creation Person-environment self-organization	Discover truth Discern meaning Methaphysical and ethical inquiry Evolutionary creativity Critical analysis	Reflection on truth Choosing good Primacy of common good rooted in value of person Unity, diversity, subjectivity Colloboration Social transformation	Consilience Moderate realism Unitary-transformative

the notion of the two worldviews as complementary in nature, rather than competitive. Further, Kikuchi (2003) proposed that conceptualizations of nursing and nursing inquiry be placed in the philosophical view of moderate realism that obviates the dichotomies of the two worldviews, empiricism and idealism (see Liu, chapter 13 of this text). Similarly, Roy's view of a universal cosmic imperative perspective on nursing knowledge is a way of bridging current debates and provides a basis for new insights and multiple approaches to developing knowledge for nursing practice.

Use of Paradigms to Advance Knowledge

Advances in knowledge for practice have been made using the major paradigms. The stances taken by scholars at given academic and practice institutions reflect varying ways to expand upon the problem-solving, empiric approach, to expand upon the process-oriented, interpretive perspectives, or to provide for integration of the two. From the view of problem-solving empirics, two examples of developments include work on knowledge as symptom management and focus on a physiologic knowledge base for nursing practice. In symptom management studies, for example, Dodd and colleagues (1988) examined nursing interventions related to patient management of given symptoms, such as nausea, vomiting and retching, and mucositis resulting from the effects of chemotherapy and radiation. Similarly, a focus on the physiologic basis of nursing is a problem-based approach. Carrieri-Kohlman, Lindsey, and West (1993) developed a text on pathophysiological phenomena in nursing as human responses to illness. A number of programs of research also are problem solving for physiologic phenomena. Mitchell studied intracranial adaptive capacity and related nursing interventions (Mitchell 1999, 2001; Mitchell & Ackerman, 1992; Mitchell, Johnson, & Habermann-Little, 1986). Larson, Covey, and Corbridge (2002) focused their research on the effects of inspiratory muscle training and cycle ergometry training on strength and endurance of the respiratory muscles and pulmonary rehabilitation of people with chronic obstructive lung disease.

The nursing diagnosis movement begun in the United States in 1973 provides another example of knowledge development strategies based on the belief that knowledge exists in the external world to be discovered and in this case classified. Interestingly, some nurses developing ethical knowledge also use an approach based on Laudan's (1977, 1984) articulation of knowledge as problem solving (see, for example, Fry, 1994). The founding of the National Institute of Nursing Research, beginning with the National Center for Nursing Research in 1986, also was based on the premise of the need for a strong empiric base for nursing science.

Contributions from an interpretive perspective have grown significantly in recent years. The Holistic Nursing Society has published a journal for more than two decades. An important text by Blattner (1981) 25 years ago introduced holistic nursing concepts, including self-responsibility, caring, and life styling. The book was well-documented and cited many nurses making contributions to holistic understanding of people and their health. Nurses also made significant contributions to holistic knowledge from human experience by using or adapting qualitative methods. Perspectives used to develop such knowledge included grounded theory (Benoliel, 1996; Quint, 1967; Schreiber & Stern, 2001), ethnography (Maggs-Rapport, 2000; Sorrell & Redmond, 1995), phenomenology (Oiler, 1982; Omery, 1983; Lopez & Willis, 2004), and historical research (Donahue, 1996; Hughes, 1990; Sarnecky, 1990).

Summary of Conceptual Focus and Paradigmatic Contributions

The expanding nursing literature reflected a focus on the substance of knowledge for practice as the philosophical and scientific principles concerning the processes and patterns of persons in interaction with the environment to promote health. The third paradigmatic distinction may well prove most fruitful as the basis for visions of the future for nursing knowledge. Although it was apparent in the nursing literature in the last two decades of the 20th century, it is only now being identified and debated. Implied or explicated by some authors is the philosophical distinction between a relativistic universe and a purposeful and ordered universe as the basis for understanding person and environment. This distinction is explored further in this book.

Methodologic Inquiry and Advancing Knowledge

In addition to clarifying the conceptual and philosophical basis of knowledge development, scholars in nursing were also making advances in the methods that nurses use to develop knowledge. Thus parallel to the maturing theoretical nursing literature, authors in nursing were demonstrating advances in metholodologic inquiry. Research approaches to create and test theories for practice were increasing in breadth and depth from empiric, interpretive, and integrated perspectives.

Gortner (2000) described a shift in thinking in nursing knowledge development when nursing *research* became nursing *science*. Nurses recognized that what we thought was science was really research, the tool of science. By the closing decades of the last century and into the 21st, Gortner noted that "nursing science was depicted as a human science that had the additional requirements of intervention or clinical therapy" (p. 64). She described the progress that had been made in identifying and documenting the phenomena of interest and related propositions through research. Accordingly, this research was based on the knowledge domains and syntax identified by Donaldson and Crowley (1978) and further clarified by Meleis (1980). Gortner concluded that nursing science came of age with an explosion of fundamental and clinical science activities in nursing. Gortner's analysis suggested factors that influenced this coming into maturity. These included a shift from discrete studies to aggregates of studies, nursing faculty with doctoral preparation that included excellent research preparation and interests that fit with concentrations of research at the schools, more colleagueship among faculty, external competition for research support, the waning of arguments over appropriate methods, and the science enterprise being enhanced in many settings when a number of scientists became deans.

Research Literature

Journals focusing on nursing research were significant in the development of nursing science. *Nursing Research* was launched in 1951 to serve two purposes, first to inform members of the nursing profession and allied professions of the results of scientific studies in nursing and second to stimulate research in nursing. More than 50 years later rankings by the Institute for Scientific Information (ISI) Journal Citation Report (Journal Citation Reports, 2004) ranked the journal number 2 of 32 ranked and noted that it also has the second highest impact factor. This factor is based on the average number of times the articles from the journal published in the past 2 years have been cited in the review year. In the rating system noted earlier, the journal scores 10 and includes points for being listed high in other ratings.

It was 25 years before nurses in the United States, specifically those in the Midwest, identified the need to establish another such journal, *Research in Nursing and Health*. Harriet Werley, the journal's first editor, noted that the purpose, as for any scientific journal, was to "communicate newly discovered knowledge that was verified and deemed significant" (Werley, 1978, p. 3). Besides original research, the journal invited manuscripts on health issues relevant to nursing and investigations of implementation of research findings in clinical settings, as well as theoretical and methodological papers and integrated and critical reviews. This journal scores 9 out of 10 in the Allen rating (2001).

Werley was responsible for another major contribution to the publication of nursing research and to review and critique of cumulative knowledge. Working consistently from the late 1960s, first informally, then through nursing organizations, Werley with coeditor Joyce Fitzpatrick launched the *Annual Review of Nursing Research* in 1983. The preface of the first volume noted that as most disciplines mature, they develop media to review critically the work that leads the discipline forward. This provides the opportunity on a regular basis to evaluate advances made, existing gaps, and areas for further work. Werley envisioned that the review would result in a systematic assessment of knowledge development and provide nursing with an appropriate data-based foundation. Initially the annual volume of the *Annual Review* contained four parts: research on nursing practice, on nursing care delivery, on nursing education, and on the profession of nursing. After two decades, Fitzpatrick, the editor, noted that the series "has reflected the development of nursing science from infancy to its present maturity" (Fitzpatrick, 2002, p. ix). The first 14 reviews included chapters in the four key areas. Later, several volumes included research review chapters in clinical nursing and nursing care delivery, emphasizing the focus on clinical nursing research. Recent volumes have been topically focused including chronic illness, women's health, geriatric nursing care, the state of the science in nursing, health disparities among racial and ethnic minorities, and alcohol use and abuse.

Publication of Qualitative and Quantitative Research

Nursing literature in the latter half of the 20th century reflected to a representative degree the quantitative versus qualitative debate in relation to strategies for nursing research. However, this dialogue did not seem to produce significant insights beyond those identified in the discussions of the paradigmatic schools of thought discussed in the philosophical literature. What is apparent is the preferences of editorial boards at given times for one approach over another. A review of articles from the first few decades of *Nursing Research* showed a preponderance of quantitative research. It may be true that most research of the era was quantitative in nature, but it seems that the publication of qualitative research lagged behind the development of the use of these methods.

Although qualitative research seemed at times to be unwelcome by the editors of research journals, some journals had a greater receptivity. For example, the *Western Journal of Nursing Research* was founded in 1978 by Pamela Brink, a nurse prepared in anthropology and known for promoting qualitative methods. The journal had a stated three-pronged editorial philosophy with the following functions: publish completed research papers; disseminate information about research conferences, research grants available, and developing research projects; and provide practical "how-to" columns on the research process and its functions. In 2002, Brink continued her open editorial policy and promoted discussion of issues in research methodology. The Allen rating of this journal is 8 out of 10.

Two other journals that have a history of publishing qualitative research are the *Journal of Advanced Nursing* in the UK and the *Australia Journal of Advanced Nursing*.

Their role in philosophical discussions from varying paradigmatic views has been noted. Likewise, the publication of research using multiple approaches has been significant. Just as an example, it was noted that a recent issue of *Journal of Advanced Nursing* included articles on ethical debate, an ethnographic study, patient narrative as method, an observational study using discourse analysis, and a mixed methods study.

It can be noted that qualitative research by nurses is also published in journals edited by one or more other disciplines. Further, the editor of the widely esteemed journal *Qualitative Health Research*, Janice Morse, holds the PhD degree in both nursing and anthropology. What seems clear is that nurse scholars, and nurse editors included, are recognizing multiple ways of developing knowledge for nursing and thus the research literature is enriched.

Programs of Research

Other advances in research for practice, as noted by Gortner (2000), included focused programs of research. Investigators develop cumulative knowledge that includes integrated biobehavior foci and multiple methods. Johnson (1972) and colleagues conducted one of the early programs of research on sensory information, coping strategies, and recovery. These investigators used laboratory research and several clinical situations as well as descriptive, correlational, and intervention strategies.

Mishel's (1981 and 1997) program of research focuses on uncertainty in illness and interventions to prevent and manage chronic illness. Using multiple qualitative and quantitative research strategies, Mishel and her colleagues have theoretically and clinically derived and tested relationships among the antecedents of uncertainty, stimuli frame and structure providers, outcomes of uncertainty, and the mediating roles of appraisal and coping. Continually funded by the National Institutes of Health since 1984, Mishel has been cited as an exemplar of nursing intervention studies, for example, presenting her research for a Congressional Breakfast in 1999. Mishel has maintained a strong link of her theory and research to practice and her work has been foundational for research of other scholars (Stiegelis et al., 2004; Wineman, Schwetz, Zeller, & Cyphert, 2003).

Morse developed a program of research in the areas of comfort and comforting, enduring, and suffering from a qualitative perspective (University of Alberta Web site http://www.u.ualberta.ca, last accessed August 23, 2006). These studies also have included instrument development derived from qualitative strategies and tested empirically. This work has been funded by federal grants from both the United States and Canada. Morse has focused on the nurse-patient interaction and relationship, experience of illness and major trauma, the cross-cultural aspect of health care, patient falls and use of restraints, and women's health.

Given the theme of this text on nursing knowledge development and clinical practice, one final observation may be noted about methodologic inquiry reflected in the nursing literature. Highly rated specialty journals, based of the rating system noted earlier, increasingly publish nursing research. A total of nine clinical specialty journals were rated either 7, 8, or 9 out of 10 based on content, reputations, and citations, and the same journals had 37 to 84% of the content rated as research. For example, *Cancer Nursing* rated 9 out of 10 and had 84% of the content considered research articles in the period rated, and *Public Health Nursing* was rated 7 on the same scale with 78% of the content research articles.

Sociopolitical Commitments Basic to Nursing Knowledge

As a profession, nursing has a social mandate to contribute to the good of society. Just as the focus and methods of nursing knowledge development have "come of age" so too we identify an increasingly mature development of sociopolitical knowledge and of social responsibility. White (1995) noted that Carper's patterns of knowing in nursing were consistently cited in the literature for nearly 20 years. In her critique, the author makes a major modification by adding a fifth way of knowing, the sociopolitical, to better represent nursing knowledge in the last decade of the 20th century. White stated that Carper's patterns addressed the "who," the "how," and the "what" of the practice of nursing. However, the "wherein" of nursing practice is addressed by sociopolitical knowing. Specifically, she stated that "it lifts the gaze of the nurse from the introspective nurse–patient relationship and situates it within the broader context in which nursing and health care take place. Understandings of both the sociopolitical context for the nurse and patient and of nursing as a practice profession are needed" (pp. 83). Particularly in the 21st century, nursing needs this understanding to have a voice in bringing about alternative conceptualizations of health and health care. This need is emphasized by the fact that health care has become driven primarily by economics. White draws upon a model developed by Jacobs-Kramer and Chinn (1987) to facilitate Carper's patterns of knowing into clinical practice in nursing.

Later Chinn and Kramer (1999) further explicated the ways of knowing in the 5th edition of *Theory and Nursing: Integrated Knowledge Development*. The authors presented a model that provided an overview of the patterns, their interrelationship, and usefulness to conceptualize the broad scope of holistic practice. The model identified questions for knowledge development and processes related to knowing. *Empirics* related to the questions *What is this?* and *How does it work?* and used processes of replication and validation. *Personal* knowing asked, *Do I know what I do?* and *Do I do what I know?* and used response and reflection. *Aesthetics* focused on questions such as *What does it mean?* and *How is it significant?* used processes of envisioning and rehearsing. *Ethics* asks, *Is it right?* and *Is it responsible?* and relied upon valuing and clarifying. By the 6th edition in 2004, the authors renamed the text *Integrated Knowledge Development in Nursing*.

In addition, Chinn (1995) articulated an approach to nurses' accountability for helping to deal with imbalances of power in society. She used the acronym PEACE as both an intent and process rooted in women's ancient wisdom. PEACE was valued, and the skills, actions, and abilities that go with the value were articulated. Again, a series of questions, this time about the congruence of intent and actions, was used to identify how to work effectively with empowering all members of a group. Praxis asked, *Do I know what I do?* and *Do I do what I know?* Empowerment questioned: *Am I expressing my own will in the context of love and respect for others? A*wareness focused on *Am I fully aware of myself and others?* Consensus added the question *Do I face conflicts openly and integrate differences in forming solutions?* Finally, the skill and ability of *E*mpowerment questioned: *Do I value growth and change for myself, others, and the group?*

Early nursing publications on the concept of oppression discussed the characteristics of oppressed groups and how oppression is maintained, often based on the work of Freire (1968). For example, Roberts (1983) developed such a description from literature on groups, including Latin Americans, American blacks, and Jews. Roberts noted Friere's insight that the major characteristics of oppressed behavior stem from the ability of dominant groups to identify their norms and values as the right ones in the society and from their power to enforce their norms and values. Roberts then analogously applied the model to nurses as an oppressed group.

A later paper by Kendall (1992) outlined a theory of emancipatory nursing actions derived from the work of Freire, as well as the critical theory of Habermas (1988) and R. Katz's (1984) description of synergistic community. The author noted that the proposed theory is a practice theory that advocates for oppressed groups. Further emancipatory nursing actions "are those that increase the potential for oppressed groups to take power from those who oppress them, whether that be fighting for a national health insurance policy, and increase in funding for the homeless, or a change in the political power base of an organization" (Kendall, 1992, p. 9). Because poverty, education, and social problems are linked to health concerns, Kendall, and many others, noted that they cannot be addressed in isolation. To respond to the challenge to care for clients who are socially, politically, and economically disadvantaged, nurses must develop knowledge that addresses health within the social context of their clients' lives.

The sociopolitical approach to knowledge has been given impetus by concerns related to health disparities. The Institute of Medicine (IOM, 2003) published a report showing clearly that members of racial and ethnic minorities receive lower quality of health care than whites even when income and health insurance are comparable. The range of health conditions for which care is substandard is broad, including cardiovascular disease, cancer, and diabetes. The causes are seen as multifaceted. The National Center on Minority Health and Health Disparities was established within NIH in 2000 and since that time all the Institutes, Centers, and Offices, including the National Institute for Nursing Research, have included reducing health disparities in their goals and funding priorities. Nurse scholars are making significant contributions to understanding health disparities and developing effective strategies toward the goal of eliminating them (Anderko, Bartz, & Lundeen, 2005; Giddings, 2005).

Meleis (1997; Meleis & Im, 1999) proposed that an important goal for nursing research is to develop knowledge about the nature and consequences of marginalization. The authors defined marginalization as the process through which persons are peripheralized on the basis of their identities, associations, experiences, and environments. As noted in the IOM report, people are marginalized by the inequities that they experience in the societies where they are living and this process leads to depriving them of quality care. Meleis makes an appeal for researchers in nursing to passionately "bring public attention to the needs, the voices, the suffering, the dehumanization, and the strategies to provide quality care for the marginalized such as the poor, the homeless, the lesbians, the gays, the immigrants, the home workers, the domestic workers, the commercial sex workers, the confused elderly and the disabled" (Meleis & Im, 1999, p. 101).

Summary of Advances in Knowledge

In summary, the developments of the latter part of the last century and at the beginning of the 21st century reflect nursing as a maturing practice discipline with a clear focus for knowledge, multiple philosophical perspectives, strong methodologic inquiry, and increasing sociopolitical commitments. These developments are also reflected in and received impetus from doctoral education and professional conferences.

Doctoral Education and Professional Conferences

The maturing of nursing as an academic and practice discipline relates to doctoral education and professional conferences because both serve key roles in socialization, dialogue, debate, and emerging trends. Again, these influences are interactive with developments in the focus for knowledge, philosophical perspectives, research methods, and sociopolitical involvement.

The Role of Doctoral Education

The focus of doctoral education in nursing currently is "to prepare students to pursue intellectual inquiry and conduct independent research for the purpose of extending knowledge" (American Association of Colleges of Nursing [AACN], 2001, p. 10). The first doctoral program for nurses was established at Teachers College, Columbia University, in 1933 and led to the EdD degree. New York University initiated a doctoral degree program in 1934. The PhD degree was first offered at the University of Pittsburgh in 1954. DNSc programs were initiated in 1964 at the University of California at San Francisco (UCSF) and in 1967 at the Catholic University of America. According to the AACN, since 1970 most new programs in nursing have offered the PhD degree and many DNS programs have been converted to PhD programs. Thirty new programs were added in the decade of the 1980s and 26 in the 1990s. The total institutions offering doctoral programs in nursing as of February 2006 was 101. Ten programs offered the Nursing Doctorate (ND), which prepares individuals for practice and is not a research-focused degree. Discussions continue on alternative forms of a practice doctorate.

Indicators of quality in research-focused doctoral programs in nursing (AACN, 2001) noted that the program of study is influenced by the faculty's areas of expertise and scholarship, the mission of the parent institution, and the discipline of nursing. The core and related course content is described as including historical and philosophical foundations to the development of nursing knowledge; existing and evolving substantive nursing knowledge; methods and processes of theory/knowledge development; research methods and scholarship appropriate to inquiry; and development related to roles in academic, research, practice, or policy environments.

Some doctoral programs in nursing take a given perspective on knowledge development and are known for related contributions. A few examples can be cited. The problem-solving approaches of Dodd (1988) and Carrieri-Kohlman and colleagues (1993) described earlier and originating with faculty at UCSF have resulted in large numbers of doctoral graduates prepared in physiologic and symptom-management research. At the same time, other doctoral and postdoctoral students studying at UCSF with Benner contributed to knowledge development from a process perspective, particularly hermeneutic-phenomenologic. Similarly, humanistic transpersonal caring, under the leadership of Watson, has provided a paradigm for knowledge development by students at the University of Colorado.

Practice level theory and empiric research is a main focus for doctoral and postdoctoral studies at the University of Michigan, particularly in health promotion and risk reduction. Faculty mentors involved in this work have included Nola Pender, studying interventions to promote physical activity among youth; Carol Loveland-Cherry, who is looking at school and family interventions to decrease adolescent substance abuse; and Susan Boehm, whose work includes behavioral interventions as they relate to health promotion, illness prevention, and screening and detection. Boston College selected ethical reasoning as one foci for the PhD program started in 1988. In the first 15 years of the 120 graduates, many conducted research in this area and significant papers were published (Hanna, 2004, 2005; Olson, 1991).

Meleis and Im (1999) identified the effect of developments in doctoral education as part of the tremendous changes in nursing as a discipline. They noted that nursing has better graduate programs "designed to educate scholars and graduates who are well-prepared, well-mentored and well-supported individuals as agents for knowledge development" (p. 94). This trend of strong doctoral programs leading to varying paradigmatic perspectives that yield knowledge for practice can be expected to continue in the first decades of this century. One contribution to this effort is the rapid growth of doctoral programs globally. The International Network of Doctoral Education in Nursing (INDEN) listed 273 doctoral programs located in every region of the globe by 2003.

Conferences

The historical role played by conferences in the theoretical development of nursing is often acknowledged (Alligood & Tomey, 2006; Moody, 1990; Walker & Avant, 2005). One important series of conferences were those held as part of the nurse–scientist program. The topic for an early conference held under the auspices of Frances Payne Bolton School of Nursing in 1966 was "Research—How Will Nursing Define It?" Papers by nurse investigators about research from varying approaches were used to discuss the kinds of questions that could be conceived to be nursing questions and how methods and designs could be constructed for systematic study. The following year the title was "Symposium on Theory Development in Nursing." The role of theory related to research was addressed. Significant papers from the conference were published in *Nursing Research* in 1968 and included those by Dickoff and James, Johnson, and Ellis that contributed greatly to ongoing theoretical dialogue for many years following. The conference in 1968, under the auspices of the School of Nursing at the University of Colorado, was called "Conference on the Nature of Science and Nursing." Focus of the panel discussion was on the position of the pure and applied scientist (Simon, 1968). Notably in 1969 the topic changed to "The Nature of Science in Nursing" and again University of Colorado was the sponsor. Leininger, the conference chair, noted that 70 participants from 21 universities attended. Important papers published included "The Nature of Nursing Science" (Abdellah, 1969) and "Theories, Models, and Systems for Nursing" (McKay, 1969).

The University of Kansas Medical Center, Department of Nursing Education, held three conferences funded by the Division of Nursing on nursing theory, two in 1969 and one 1970. Catherine Norris, chair of the conferences, noted in the introduction to the published proceedings, "Intelligent and effective clinical practice in nursing requires the rationale and guidelines provided by the scientific base. In a rapidly changing society which has a rapidly expanding technology, the nursing profession is ever more dependent on this scientific or theoretical framework if fragmentation of patient care and nursing services are to be avoided," and she emphasized communities of scholars who created "dialogues on critical nursing issues and which stimulate nursing research that has the potential for improving the quality of nursing care offered to patients" (Norris, 1969, n.p.). General systems theory and implications for nursing emerged as an important topic. Diers and Dye (1969) presented a paper on "Situation Producing Theory." It is notable that at the 1970 conference, Loretta Zderad talked about empathy from a humanistic perspective.

Also as part of the nurse–scientist program, a symposium entitled "Approaches to the Study of Nursing Questions and the Development of Nursing Science" was held in 1972. Rozella Schlotfeldt chaired the symposium at Frances Payne Bolton School of Nursing and highlighted the issue that nursing is a practice discipline and may use knowledge contributed by basic science. She noted that, "A time arrives, however, when each profession spawns practitioner-inquirers who seek answers to important questions that no basic scientist has asked and those which none will ever ask" (Schlotfeldt, 1972, p. 484). Most nurses presenting papers had been prepared in other disciplines and all addressed approaches to the study of nursing questions.

Conferences to discuss and derive nursing diagnosis began in 1973 (Gebbie & Lavin, 1975). A nurse theorist group was convened by Sr. Callista Roy to contribute to the theoretical basis for the nursing diagnosis. The group met with the national conferences and as a working subgroup about twice a year from 1976 to 1980. The stated goals were to develop a theoretical framework for nursing diagnosis and to make recommendations regarding the levels of generality of the diagnostic categories. However, in retrospect speaking at the 25th anniversary of NANDA, Roy noted that a major contribution of the project was the face-to-face working of the theoretical thinkers of the time, including Margaret Hardy, Rosemarie Ellis, Joyce Fitzpatrick, Martha Rogers, Margaret Newman, Rosemary Parse, Marjorie Gordon, Imogene King, Dorothea Orem, and Callista Roy.

The professional nursing organizations also presented conferences that contributed to the development of nursing knowledge. For a number of years, the American Nurses Association (ANA) included the organizational unit of the Council of Nurse Researchers, which sponsored semiannual research conferences. Later, this work was continued by the Council for the Advancement of Nursing Science (CANS) whose mission is to better health through nursing science. In addition, the ANA convened groups of nurse scholars to develop and publish the first *Nursing's Social Policy Statement* in 1980, which defined nursing as, "the diagnosis and treatment of human responses to actual or potential health problems" (ANA, 1980, p. 6). The revision published by ANA in 2003 emphasized essential features of professional nursing including: the provision of a caring relationship that facilitates health and healing, advancement of professional nursing knowledge through scholarly inquiry, and influence on social and public policy to promote social justice.

The National League for Nursing conducted a workshop on theory development in Kansas City in 1977 entitled "Theory Development: What, Why, and How?" The published papers presented different viewpoints on nursing theory development by nursing leaders most actively involved at the time, including Johnson, King, Fawcett, Zderad, Paterson, Rinehart, and Hardy. The content was significant, but reportedly the attendance was small. In contrast, conferences of the same era sponsored by a nursing journal attracted large numbers of participants and became very theory focused. Alligood (2002) noted that the Nurse Educator Conferences in Chicago (1977) and New York (1978) indicated a shift of emphasis from research to theory at the national level. The first conference did not have a theory theme, but 800 nurses attended the breakout session in which Sister Callista Roy presented how to use the Roy Adaptation Model as a guide for nursing practice. Thus the second conference was planned around nursing theory and brought a large group of nurse theorists to the same stage to speak to an audience of 2,000 nurses. Alligood noted that this second conference underscored a growing awareness that the nature of knowledge needed for nursing practice was theoretical knowledge. The conference served as a vehicle for this awareness but not necessarily as a vehicle for the forward movement of knowledge development in nursing.

From that point forward, it seemed that the potential for conferences was not fully utilized in the struggle nurses face to bring knowledge to bear on the multiple problems of providing adequate health care. In the 1980s, one important contribution for growing perspectives on knowledge was the publication of *Setting the Agenda for the Year 2000: Knowledge Development in Nursing* (Sorensen, 1986), the results of the 1985 annual meeting of the American Academy of Nursing. The format of advisory group sessions, a scientific session, and forums was planned to enable fellows to exchange ideas to begin using the academy as a think tank. An important paper by Stevenson and Woods (1986) addressed "Nursing Science and Contemporary Science: Emerging Paradigms." Simulated by this analysis, the Academy Fellows brought their wealth of knowledge and experience to eight forum groups that addressed issues surrounding the content and process of nursing knowledge development. A synthesis of a common perspective was presented as "The Future of Nursing Science: Response of the Academy."

Deliberations about the content of future nursing science described the phenomena of nursing as "human-environment interactions enhancing health" and further as

> the organized diversity of theory, research, and practice is the basis for conceptualizing our phenomena. Explaining the philosophical foundation, practice heritage, and current social mandate of nursing enables us to decisively articulate our agenda. In the process the pragmatic concerns of language and political relevance will be balanced with the focused growth of our science. (Roy, 1986, p. 25)

Issues related to the process of knowledge development raised by the Academy forum groups included the plurality of methods to deal with holism, specialization and collaboration, and the need for longitudinal studies and replication.

Nursing Knowledge Conferences

At the same time that the American Academy of Nursing was dealing with these issues, the basis for a resurgence of the potential of conferences was laid by a group of doctoral students with the assistance of Margaret Hardy who initiated a series called the "Annual Nursing Science Colloquia" at Boston University from 1984 to 1987 (see Appendix). Conferences focused on strategies for theory development and included presentations by nursing leaders such as Ada Sue Hinshaw, Glenys Hamilton, Shake Ketefian, Hesook Suzie Kim, Jean Johnson, Donna Swartz-Barcott, and Jeanne Quint Benoliel. Besides the forum to discuss the development of knowledge for nursing science, the colloquia were an important opportunity for doctoral students to be socialized into the discipline and associate with leaders in the field in a way reminiscent of the nurse–scientist conferences of the 1960s and early 1970s.

From 1990 to 1994, the University of Rhode Island (University of Rhode Island College of Nursing, 1993 & 1994) continued the impetus and ran a series of five symposia devoted to knowledge development in nursing. The emphasis was on the interconnectedness among philosophy, theory, research, and practice and the influence on the development of nursing knowledge. Linkages among philosophy, theory, methods of inquiry, and practice were explored as were the philosophies of realism, relativism, interpretivism, humanism, and praxis. Nursing practice theories and pluralism in theories for practice were the focus of one symposium. Speakers throughout the series included Susan Gortner, Frederick Suppe, Margaret Newman, Marilyn Rawnsley, David Allen, Nancy Woods, Sr. Callista Roy, Hesook Suzie Kim, John Phillips, Lorraine Walker, Sue Donaldson, and Nancy Dluhy. Dialogue among all participants remained an important strategy for these conferences.

In the later 1990s, the Boston College School of Nursing (Boston College School of Nursing, 1996 & 1997), in conjunction with Eastern Nursing Research Society and Sigma Theta Tau, Alphi Chi Chapter, initiated a series of five conferences on nursing knowledge impact. Speakers included Beth Rogers, Margaret Newman, Sr. Callista Roy, Lorraine Walker, Hesook Suzie Kim, Janice Thompson, Peggy Chinn, Jean Watson, Dorothy Jones, Marjory Gordon, and Jacqueline Fawcett. A feature of the series was the Knowledge Consensus Conference in 1998 that used a participatory process to generate a value-based position paper linking nursing knowledge and practice outcomes signed by more than 90 participants. (The Consensus Statement appears at the end of this chapter.) Responses to the consensus paper were featured at the "Emerging Nursing Knowledge 2000" International Conference held in collaboration with the School of Nursing and Midwifery, University College Dublin, Ireland, and the Institute of Nursing Science at the University of Oslo, Norway. Eight invited international papers were presented as well as 26 concurrent sessions and posters by scholars from 6 countries and 12 states in the United States. Time was also planned for dialogue, refinement of the emerging consensus, and movement of the collective wisdom to an action plan for the impact of nursing knowledge on critical needs in practice. The Knowledge Conference in 2001 in Boston featured exemplars for knowledge-based changes in practice.

Concerns With Health Care Systems and Delivery

The recent era of significant development in knowledge for nursing practice has coincided with a time of drastic challenges in the health care delivery system. The unparalleled growth of health care costs precipitated an era of health care reform. Serious cost containment strategies have been in effect in the United States since the mid-1990s and still the spending per capita in this country for health care far exceeds all other nations. Market-driven principles have ruled health care reform. Problems with health care systems and care delivery go beyond economic concerns. The juxtaposition of the developments in nursing knowledge for practice and turmoil in health care represent a great paradox for nursing; this time of growth is a time of great challenge.

Health Care Challenges

Health care was dramatically impacted by major scientific and sociopolitical movements of the late 20th century. The wave-particle duality of quantum physics made it possible to move from simple x-rays to magnetic resonance imaging and countless other diagnostic and treatment options. The human genome project was launched in 1990 with the goal of mapping the entire human genome sequence. With participation from numerous laboratories in more than a dozen countries, in February 2001 headlines proclaimed that the code of life had been mapped and findings published in the journals of *Science* and *Nature*. This and other potentially powerful information was accumulating more rapidly than it could be analyzed, understood, and thoroughly evaluated. It has been estimated that 20 million people were enrolled in health care research studies in the United States in 2001. Ethics and public policy have not necessarily kept pace with the advances in science and technology.

Information replaced energy as the most important resource. The information age brought with it issues related to confidentiality, privacy, and security. For example, as new regulations were put in place related to the patient's medical record, many questions remain of who can have access to what information and how it can be transmitted securely. With the almost infinity of data in cyberspace on the World Wide Web, any patient can have immediate access to an array of information on medical conditions and their treatments. Massive availability of health-related information that is not analyzed, understood, and evaluated raises similar difficulties as noted with rapidly advancing science. The result is a more informed, but not entirely knowledgeable nor an empowered, public.

Sociopolitical Influences

Some sociopolitical developments greatly influencing health care include the increasing age of the population, income gaps, and diversity with attendant health disparities. In the 20th century, the number of Americans over 65 years grew from 3 million in 1900 to 36.3 million in 2004. The U.S. Census Bureau predicts that the number will increase to 86.7 million by 2050 (DeNavas-Walt, Proctor, & Lee, 2005). The significant effects on health care are highlighted in a comment from a report on aging that "the hospital is becoming the intensive care unit, the nursing home is becoming the hospital, and the home is becoming the nursing home" (Martin, 2001, p. 25).

The income gaps in the United States provide similar profound health care challenges. It is commonly reported that the wealthiest 20% of the population control as much wealth as the bottom 80%. In fact, between 2002 and 2003, the income of the lowest 20% of the population declined 1.9%, from $18,326 to $17,984, while the income of the top 80% increased 1.1%, from $85,941 to $86,867. The poverty rate and the number of poor rose in 2003 to 12.5% or 35.9 million. The depth of poverty within this group is striking: 40.8% (13.4 million) of the poor population are listed as severely poor; that is, their family incomes are below one-half the poverty threshold (U.S. Census Bureau report, 2004). One child in 6 is born poor and 1 in 3 will be poor at some point in his or her childhood. *Time* magazine (quoted by National Council of Churches USA on their Web site, http://www.ncccusa.org, last accessed February 5, 2003) noted that the national assets in the United States have not been so unevenly distributed since just before the stock market crash in 1929.

Demographic changes have profound implications for health care. For example, the number of persons without health insurance is continually rising and in 2004 was at 45.8 million, 8 out of 10 of whom were in working families. One reporter (Lazarus, 2004) expanded on the problem, quoting public surveys showing that 5 million fewer jobs now provide health insurance than just 3 years before, and for jobs that do provide coverage, insurance premiums climbed 11.2% in 1 year or four times faster than both inflation and average U.S. workers' wages. Most companies noted that in the near future it was very likely that they would raise employee contributions to health coverage.

Related figures showed that already 8.4 million children were without health insurance or 11.4% of all children under age 18 (DeNavas-Walt, Proctor, & Lee, 2005). A report on data assembled and analyzed by Physicians for a National Health Program was entitled "US Health Care Crisis Facts: Uninsured, Access, Quality, Cost, Superprofits, Market-Driven Chaos." The generalization is made that "Managed Care Companies are abandoning America's seniors and disabled (from Medicare Managed Care and Plus-Choice), contending costs and losses are forcing their hand. At the same time, their top executives take home millions." Some of the facts they provide are (a) The top executives in these companies received an average of $2.4 million per year in compensation, exclusive of unexercised stock options in 1997. (b) Sixty-one of the 90 health maintenance organizations (HMOs) that are pulling out of the Medicare market are owned by 9 for-profit, publicly traded insurance companies. (c) The number of Americans without health insurance, nearly 1 in every 6 persons, constitutes a higher proportion than at any time since Medicare and Medicaid were passed in 1965. (d) Medicaid enrollment has fallen by 1.8 million, apparently as a result of welfare cutbacks. (e) Forty-three percent of the uninsured had a problem paying their medical bills last year and yet 16.5% of people with insurance also had problems paying medical bills, because they had only partial coverage.

Another challenge for health care delivery is the increasing diversity of the population of the United States, primarily reflected in the changing trends in international migration. Historically the foreign-born residents of this country increased each decade until 1930 and then declined until 1970 (Immigration and Naturalization Service Web site, http://www.ins.usdoj.gov/graphics/index.htm, February 15, 2006). From 1970 to 2005, there has been a rapid increase from 9.6 million to 35 million foreign-born residents. The increase of 7.5 million since 2000 makes this the highest 5-year period of immigration in American history. Further the percent of immigrants to the total population increased from 7.9% in 1990 to 12.4% in 2005 (Center for Immigration Studies Web site, www.cis.org, February 15, 2006). One in 20 persons in the United States is foreign born or has one or both parents who are foreign born. High concentrations of immigrants are found in major metropolitan areas such as New York and Los Angeles, with 4.7 million each. In other areas, the percentage foreign-born to native population is high; for example, Miami has 42.7% foreign born. Trends in countries of birth have also changed. Historically, European countries and Canada were leading countries of birth for the foreign-born population; however, in 1999–2000, the eight countries with the highest numbers were Mexico, China, Philippines, India, Cuba, Vietnam, El Salvador, and Korea.

An additional fact affecting health care is that in 2000 there were 72.1 million foreign-born children living in the United States. Births to foreign-born women in 1970 were 6% of the total but 20.2% in 1999. Poverty status for immigrants and their U.S.-born children is 18.4% compared with 11.7% for native born. As for education, one-fifth of the foreign born have less than a 5th-grade education as compared with 1 in 20 of the native born. Although the percent participating in the labor force for both groups is about the same, 44.5% of the foreign born in 1999 had employment-based health insurance compared with 54.6% of the native born. Among immigrants one-third lack health insurance, which is two and a half times the rate for native born. The extensive diversity of languages, cultures, and resources presents challenges to health systems and individual nurses in practice.

Problems of Access and Quality

Advances in science, medicine, and public health have not translated into better health care for all. Gulzar (1999) demonstrated that the gap between health care services available and the health care needs of people exist in the richest countries such as the United States and Canada and in the poorest such as Pakistan. The author defined access to health care conceptually as "the fit among personal, sociocultural, economic, and system-related factors that enable individuals, families, and communities to have timely, needed, necessary, continuous, and satisfactory health services" (p. 17). In Gulzar's analysis, the operational definition of access to health care is related to its several dimensions. This means that "the ability of people to access health care is influenced by health care system and user-related aspatial characteristics including need for services, sociocultural, psychological, financial, and attitudinal variables and geographic or spatial characteristics such as distance, architectural, and transportational variables which may be barriers or facilitators" (p. 17).

The burgeoning literature on health care disparities was referred to earlier in the discussion of the contributions of nurses to social political knowledge. Problems of both access and quality are noted in this literature. In summarizing the issue of racial health care disparities, Katz (2001) noted key examples of specific treatments that Whites are more likely to receive than Blacks such as cardiorevascularization even when judged necessary rather than discretionary cerebrovascular surgery, total hip and knee replacement, and renal transplantation. Hispanics were less likely to receive many interventions, including total hip replacement, cardiac procedures, and preventive measures. Recognizing the significant problem of racial health disparities, other scholars have argued for taking seriously the influence of geography in medical practice for both the statistical measurement of the incidence of disparities and for the design of reforms to reduce disparities (Chandra & Skinner, 2003).

Examples of problems of adequate access are found daily in nursing practice. Patients were sent home after same day surgery with instructions that may fall short in meeting their needs (Jones, Flanagan, & Coakley, 2000). An emergency department nurse may be dealing with the family of a child with a spinal cord injury and is acutely aware that there is no rehabilitation service in the state for children who have such injuries. Systemwide, one can easily infer the issues of access from the major demographic changes discussed. Increasing numbers of elderly living with multiple chronic illnesses raise questions of the physical capacity of the health system to deal with needs. At the same time, the elderly may have transportation and architectural barriers to what care is available. The continuity of care of the elderly is and will continue to be a major challenge. The significant income gaps noted and the rising numbers of persons without health insurance presents financial barriers to equal access. Financial and geographic barriers are intensified for the diverse populations who also have sociocultural barriers, such as differences in language and beliefs about health and health care.

The issue of quality of health care is tied to the issue of access. If access means timely, needed, necessary, continuous, and satisfactory health services, then quality health care means the level to which all persons receive care that meets these criteria. In particular, the beliefs about health care and its place in the economic system affect quality. Throughout the industrialized world all countries except the United States have some kind of national health system that considers health care a right and provides for basic level care to all citizens. Several attempts have failed to establish this right with an organized system to implement at least basic care for everyone in the United States. Federal legislation in 1965 established Medicare as a form of health insurance for persons over 65 and Medicaid administered by individual states as coverage for welfare recipients.

In the 1970s and 1980s, a number of factors, including advancing science and technology, caused health care costs in the United States to rise dramatically. At the same time, the public expected to benefit from such advances regardless of the cost (Schaag & Phipps, 1999). However, by 2004 the National Coalition on Health Care reported that premiums for employer-based health insurance rose by 11.2% and that this was the fourth consecutive year of double-digit increases. Further, this involved all types of health plans including HMOs, preferred provider organizations (PPOs), and point-of-service plans (POS). By early 2006, debates arose about shifting health care expenses and whether to mandate employer health benefits. When employers do not provide health care coverage, the individual states struggle to handle health care costs for citizens with the burden placed on the taxpayers. At the same time, businesses buckle under the rising cost of heath insurance. Many labor contract disputes focus on health care coverage. In the climate of increasing costs, managed care, which had been evolving gradually, soon took over the health care system in what one author called "a de facto reform that was carried out by the private health insurance market" (Newbergh, 2002, p. 31).

Influence of Managed Care

Managed care is a system of health insurance that offers health care coverage but limits the choice of providers and self-referrals. The two major types of managed care plans are HMOs and PPOs. The promise of this approach was cost containment strategies such as capitation, that is, a fixed sum of money for a patient's overall care. This arrangement was meant to create an incentive to do only what was necessary for good care and not waste resources. Managed care was expected to reduce overuse of the system such as costly referrals to specialists and lengthy hospital stays. It was also expected to improve preventive care. Insurance companies and fee-for-service physicians have rapidly developed PPOs as an alternative to HMOs. Physicians and hospitals are now contracted to the insurance companies. Gage (1998) reported that in barely a decade managed care came to dominate health care insurance and delivery systems. In some cases, it is the only option offered by an employer. By 1995 nearly three-fourths of all employees with health insurance were enrolled in some form of managed care. In 1998, Gage reported that the expected cost containment had not been realized and that the research on quality of care is inconclusive.

In other words, the HMOs have not been the answer to access to affordable and high quality health care. One study (Nathanson, Ramirez-Garnica, & Wiltrout, 2005) noted that children with cystic fibrosis (CF) using managed care attended CF centers significantly less frequently than those with nonmanaged care. The authors noted that their findings suggest that under managed care children with CF may not have equal access to experts in CF. Another study (Simonet, 2005) reported that most surveys indicated that a lack of choice of a provider is a major source of discontent for patients under HMOs. In a broad study of psychiatric patients, authors concluded that managed care delayed rather than prevented return visits to the psychiatric emergency service and that increasing numbers of patients with mental illness in need of treatment were coming to the attention of law enforcement officials after managed care was implemented (Claassen, Michael-Kashner, Gilfillan, Larkin, & John-Rush, 2005).

Historically health care professions have been strategic in efforts to improve quality of health care. For example, in 1918 the American College of Surgeons aimed to improve medical care in hospitals by establishing a standardization program and the Joint Commission on Accreditation of Hospitals was formed in 1952, later becoming known as the Joint Commission on Accreditation of Health Care Organizations. With the federally funded programs in place and the insurance companies managed care, quality assurance activities proliferated. For example, the Health Care Finance Administration requires managed care plans contracted to Medicare to complete a quality report called *Health Plan Employer Data and Information Set*. The National Committee for Quality Assurance accredits HMOs. Most hospitals have utilization review programs and case management programs. Total quality management (QM) and continuous quality improvement (CQI) are widely marketed approaches that focus on patient outcomes and the systems that support attaining these outcomes.

Still the media report the numbers of patients who die each year in hospitals because of errors, large numbers of patients enter the system by using emergency departments, patients are befuddled by rejected claims for health care reimbursement, and debates are set off about the number of days of hospital care that should be paid for, for example, after giving birth. At the same time, the health care providers are overburdened with unreasonable amounts of paperwork to document eligibility and provide rationale why a patient needed more than the amount of care covered in the plan. Nurses in other countries can identify how concerns about access and quality have developed and are manifested in the health care systems of their own countries.

Challenge for the Future

In the 21st century, the unresolved concerns with the health care system and care delivery present a challenge. Nurses are keenly aware of the changing demographics and issues of access and quality of health care. The late-20th-century developments of a clear focus of nursing knowledge and effective methods to develop knowledge are highly relevant to the current health care challenge. These advances in knowledge are the basis for dealing effectively with the challenge to transform the future of nursing practice. Four ways of thinking about the future have been outlined (Roy, 2000; Sullivan, 1999). *Possible futures* are unlikely and are referred to as wildcards because they have low probability, but high impact, such as the fall of the Berlin Wall. *Plausible futures* are based on trends and deal with what could happen based on a range of scenarios and one example could be increasing environmental consciousness. A *probable future* is one that will happen as an extension of the present, often in a direction one does not want such as spiraling health care costs. The final type of future is a *preferred future*, that is, what one would want to happen, such as adequate health care for all.

One can use the vision of development in nursing knowledge to create a future for practice that does not exist yet and is not likely to unfold without changes in the present. Nurse scholars creating knowledge are called upon to provide visions for a possible future that is also preferred. The Nursing Knowledge Consensus Paper, featured in this chapter (see the following section), provides the assumptions and principles that are basic for transformation of practice. This book explores these possibilities.

Consensus Statement on
Emerging Nursing Knowledge
A Value-Based Position Paper Linking Nursing Knowledge and Practice Outcomes
USA Nursing Knowledge Consensus Conference, 1998
Boston, Massachusetts

INTRODUCTION: A Series of conferences was held in the Northeastern area of the USA during the 1980s and 1990s and were well attended by nurses from throughout the USA and representatives of other countries. This series was followed by the historic convening of Knowledge Consensus Conference 1998 in Boston, Massachusetts, from October 22–24, 1998. The focus of the conference was to build on previous presentations and perspectives on developments within nursing science using a participatory process. The goal for the 140 conference participants, consensus builders, and facilitators was to discuss and synthesize various perspectives on knowledge development related to (1) the nature of the human person, (2) the nature of nursing, (3) the role of nursing theory, and (4) the links of each of these understandings to nursing practice. This document summarized the key assumptions, scientific principles, and values for each issue that had the greatest amount of consensus.

I. ONTOLOGY OF THE PERSON
   A. <u>Assumption:</u> Understanding the human person, as individuals, families, communities, and groups, is the focal point of knowledge development and nursing.
   B. <u>Scientific Principles and Values:</u>
      1. The person is characterized by wholeness, complexity and consciousness. Personhood can be considered on individual, family and community levels. The person is sentient with multiple dimensions including individuality and embodiment. A human being is evolving, in process, fluid, and changing. Each person or social group has purpose, promise, and potential for continuing transformations. The social and cultural environment for the person, family, or community reflects multiple values and social-political perspectives. Nurses recognize both the commonalities and differences of people. Humankind is moving from an ethnocentric to global perspective.
      2. The person is capable of choice and has free will tempered by the context of one's past, present, and future. The individual is inherently good, has rights, and is self-directed. At the same time, each person recognizes the rights of others and works toward increasing freedom and emancipation for self and

other persons. Conflicting rights are to be resolved, resulting in balance and harmony. Such balance and harmony are sought at all levels for individuals and groups, from electrolytes to the cosmos.

3. The person is interdependent and lives in reciprocity, connection, affiliation and relationship. Through dialogue and exchange, together with self-reflection, the person makes meaning. Through such meaning, the person understands self, and other persons, particularly within family and community, as well as the larger world. Personal meanings and knowledge are shared through distributed cognition.

4. The person in both Eastern and Western traditions has a yearning beyond the human. This characteristic has been termed spirituality and involves seeking a common destiny. Spiritual beliefs may be spoken or unspoken and are particularly rooted in family and social traditions. For some, the soul of the person is viewed as the energy of the universe and an existential reality.

II. ONTOLOGY OF NURSING

A. <u>Assumption:</u> Nursing is a human practice discipline that facilitates well-being using a scientific knowledge base and values in a caring relationship.

B. <u>Scientific Principles and Values:</u>

1. The essence of nursing lies in modes of being, including the nurse's true presence of his or the whole self. The nurse uses the mode of being with and being for, in the process of human to human engagement. Other terms used to describe this fundamental aspect of nursing include interaction, mutuality, and encounter. The engagement is mutual, an iterative process that includes giving and receiving and being humble. Nursing provides a presence with others derived from the soul or spirit of the nurse that interfaces with the soul and spirit of the other. This relationship includes respect and acceptance of where the person is and the nurse's openness to another person's reality. The nurse appreciates the patient and the space between the nurse and the patient. An empathetic presence requires reflection by the nurse and engaging persons in the process of their journey. It also includes intimacy, trust, and authenticity. Further, commitment, responsibility, and accountability are terms used to characterize the nature of nursing. Caring is described as including presence, feeling empathy, and nurturing that is oriented to promotion of health and well-being. Caring takes place within the context of a therapeutic relationship and is considered a moral imperative of nursing. Caring relationships occur with individuals, family, community, and societies as a whole.

2. Nursing by its nature brings intentionality to the therapeutic process. In addition to being for the other, the nurse acts for the other. Actions of the nurse focus on health. Health involves fulfilling human potential and enabling well being for individuals, families, communities, and groups. Some nurses refer to the goal of nursing action as movement on the health–illness continuum. For the nurse, the human encounter is purposeful and focuses on building and bridging human possibilities. The nurse uses both philosophic and scientific knowledge to empower others. Nursing knowledge is based on understandings and values related to the nature of persons. The science of nursing involves complex ways of knowing, including clinical wisdom. Nurses strive to be competent and recognize their limitations. Nurses' work is with

humans and includes the role of raising consciousness about the sacredness of human beings. Helping people to make healthy choices requires knowledge, integrity, and accountability. Nurses are responsible for their actions and put the patient, family, or community first. Ethical and moral principles are used in respecting the autonomy of persons.

3. Cultural competence is a core element of nursing. Caring by the nurse is transcultural. To be transcultural is more than a value; it is a demand for action. Cultural competence and scientific competence are not hierarchical but integrated in nursing action. Nurses have a special accountability to transcend ethnocentrism. A nurse cannot be effective if he or she is confined in the narrowness of one's own culture. The knowledge base of nursing is meaningful to the patient and the patient's needs and to the needs of the family and community. Such needs occur within a given social context. Nurses value cultural differences and strive to individualize knowledge for care. Nurses recognize the real and strive for the ideal. At the same time, nurses acknowledge the complexity in the world. They question how privilege may blind the nurse to the wisdom of ordinary people and thus how the needs of some people may not be recognized by nursing.

4. As a discipline with a social mandate, nurses take responsibility for social transformation. Political activism is one form of valuing and acting within the discipline. Nurses are altruistic and strive to do what is morally right in the service of human beings and society. Nurses are proactive in engaging health promotion and prevention of ill health. They advocate for others and work to provide access to health care for all. Nurses examine the constraints of modern organizations and work to create systemic change that is more responsive to the needs of the global population. Nurses strive to return the face of humanity to health care systems. Nurses are open to change, anticipate change, and respond to the challenge of change. Current challenges include changes in economic and technologic realities at national and international levels. A goal for nursing knowledge and action is to empower communities. Commitment to empowerment of others requires a fierce compassion from nurses.

III. NURSING THEORY
    A. <u>Assumption</u>: Nursing theory expresses the values and beliefs of the discipline, helps to frame the human experience, and guides the caring process.
    B. <u>Scientific Principles and Values:</u>
        1. Nursing theory is the vehicle used to operationalize a disciplinary perspective. It embraces a wholistic view of what it means to be human and helps frame the nurse–patient experience. Theory is respective of personal meaning, human diversity, the uniqueness of the individual, and spiritual expression. It provides the context from which nurses come to understand personal responses to a dynamic and changing health care environment.
        2. In nursing theory, the discipline articulates core beliefs and common assumptions. Guided by these universal philosophical links, multiple epistemological views emerge to help understand the complex, dynamic, interactive and transforming caring experience that occurs between the nurse and patient, family, community, or other social group. The result is knowledge (content and

language) that depicts how nurses think and what they think about. Nursing theory creates a way to link the disciplinary ontology with a unique perspective about the dynamic person/environment interaction. It is useful in providing an approach to guide nursing practice, education and research.

3. Theory creates a way to organize knowledge. It allows for the integration of knowledge from other disciplines that can inform and expand the sphere of understanding from a nursing perspective. Theory is not static. Rather, it is iterative, dynamic, and evolving. It must be continually updated and informed by practice and research. Theory helps to clarify existing knowledge and direct new discoveries. Through synthesis and reflection, nurses are able to develop the content of the discipline and create the bridge between theory and practice.

4. Theory helps to illuminate practice. It creates the disciplinary knowledge needed to guide clinical judgments, actions, and articulate clinical outcomes that acknowledge a disciplinary contribution to global health. Theory should reflect reality. It is only then that it is clinically useful. Theory directs the nurse to uncover new knowledge about the human experience in a unique way. The testing and refinement of theory helps to generate information that can be used to fill the existing knowledge gaps needed to describe and explain the human experience of individuals, families, communities, and groups.

IV. LINKING THE NATURE OF PERSON, THE NATURE OF NURSING, AND NURSING THEORY TO NURSING PRACTICE

A. <u>Assumption:</u> The essence of nursing practice is the nurse–patient relationship that embodies beliefs about the nature of person and the nature of nursing.

B. <u>Scientific Principles and Values:</u>

1. Nursing practice manifests a unique understanding of the person from a disciplinary perspective. The connection between the nurse and the patient fosters human health and supports self-discovery. The nurse uses problem solving and process skills, such as reflection, to come to know the person, family, community, or social group. This knowing results in actions that guide patients and groups in making choices and decisions that promote personal and group growth. Knowledge and creative artistry are used to tailor nursing care to an individual or group's unique responses and behaviors across the health care experience.

2. The nurse-patient relationship is a dynamic, evolving, and transforming partnership, grounded in trust and truth. It flourishes in an environment that is sensitive to the uniqueness of the person or group and includes attention to biophysical, cultural, and spiritual dimensions of both. The intentional presence of the nurse is essential for coming to know and understand what it means to be human and humans in relationships. This knowledge provides the basis for the mutual selection of interventions that can promote health and self-determination.

3. Nursing practice occurs within a sociopolitical environment. As a discipline, nursing continues to make visible the role it plays in problem solving and decision making. Nursing demonstrates the effectiveness for the health of

a society of a practice that achieves outcomes of personal growth for individuals and groups, promotion and evaluation of change, self-knowing, and personal and social transformation. It is essential that the contributions of nursing be described within the framework of quality and cost-effectiveness. Nurses use language that has collaborative acceptance in order to justify contributions to care that are recognized by sources of funding for health care. Nursing knowledge, both theory and research, are used to inform health care policy and provide the basis for nurses' voice for change and social reform.

4. Nursing practice uses knowledge, both theory and research based, to guide care and promote change. The patient, as individuals, families, communities, and groups, is the central focus of nursing care. Nursing education, practice, and research assist in optimizing the patient experience within a caring environment. Nursing education reflects the reality of practice while providing students with the knowledge needed to reform and direct health care across settings. Nurse mentors are essential to professional development and optimal patient care. Nursing theory provides a framework for understanding the nurse–patient interaction and helps direct patient care. The continued preparation of nurses who can define the discipline to the public and other health care providers is critical to the advancement of the discipline. Nursing practice creates environments that optimize and differentiate the unique contributions of nurses to patient care and the health of the society.

Signed by:

Joan Agretellis
Steve L. Alves
Patricia Arcari
Marilyn Asselin
Barbara Banfield
Anne-Marie Barron
Diane Berry
Rita F. Braun
Suellen Breakey
Janice M. Brencick
Suzanne H. Brouse
Margaret R. Brown
Nancy Burns
Christine Callahan
Genevieve Chandler
Hsiao-Chuan Chao
Lenny Chiang
Jean Chiasson
Mandy Coakley
Mary Jane Costa
Joanne M. Dalton

Deborah D'Avolio
Nancy M. Dluhy
Marjorie Dobratz
Mary Ellen Doherty
Ann Dylis
Laurel Eisenhauer
Patsy Fasnacht
Kelly Fisher
Jane Flanagan
Cheryl Gibson
Marjory Gordon
Kathy Gramling
Rosemary Hall
Debra R. Hanna
Patricia Hanrahan
Carolyn Hayes
Kathryn S. Hegadus
June Horowitz
Marjorie A. Isenberg
Barbara Bennett Jacobs
Dorothy A. Jones

Hesook Suzie Kim
Jan-Louise Leonard
Anners Lerdal
Pay-Fan Lin
Paula Lusardi
Barbara Madden
Anne Manton
Colette Matarese
Anne M. Mayo
Ellen McCarty
Ditsapelo McFarland
Cynthia Medich
Michele Mendes
Brenda Millette
Sheila L. Molony
Karen H. Morin
Sandra Mott
Laura Mylott
Margaret Newman
Hollie Noveletsky
Anna Omery

Susan A. Orshan
Paulette Osterman
Carolyn Padovano
Barbara Patterson
Carole Pearce
Karen Vincent Pounds
Laurel E. Radwin
Fran Reeder
Joan Roche
Beth Rodgers

Sr. Callista Roy
Susan Ruka
Josephine Ryan
Donna Schwartz-
  Barcott
Mary Margaret
  Seagraves
Beth Shannon
Hrafn Oli Sigurosson
Bjorn Sjostrom

Vincent J.
  Stankiewicz
Sharon Stark
Janice Stecci
Rosemary Theroux
Janice L. Thompson
Angela E. Vicenzi
Glenn Webster
Joyce Wright
Donna Zucker

REFERENCES

Abdellah, F. G. (1969). The nature of nursing science. In *Conference on the Nature of Science in Nursing* (pp. 390–393). Boulder: University of Colorado, School of Nursing.

Allen, M. (2001). *Key and Electronic Nursing Journals Final 2001 Edition*. Retrieved July 5, 2005, from http://nahrs.library.kent.edu/resource/reports/keyjrnls_chart2001ed.pdf.

Alligood, M. R. (2002). The state of the art and science of nursing theory. In A. M. Tomey & M. R. Alligood (Eds.), *Nursing theorists and their work* (5th ed., pp. 634–649). St. Louis, MO: Mosby.

Alligood, M. R. & Tomey, A. M. (2006). *Nursing theory: Utilization and application.* St. Louis, MO: Mosby.

American Association of Colleges of Nursing (AACN). (2001). *Indicators of quality in research-focused doctoral programs in nursing.* Washington, DC: American Association of Colleges of Nursing.

American Nurses Association. (1980). *Nursing: A social policy statement.* Washington, DC: American Nurses Association.

American Nurses Association. (2003). *Nursing's social policy statement.* Kansas City, MO: American Nurses Association.

Anderko, L., Bartz, C., & Lundeen, S. (2005). Practice-based research networks: Nursing centers and communities working collaboratively to reduce health disparities. *Nursing Clinics of North America, 40*(4), 747–758.

Benner, P., Hooper-Kyriakidis, P., & Stannard, D. (1999). *Clinical wisdom in critical care: A thinking-in-action approach.* Philadelphia: W. B. Saunders.

Benner, P., Tanner, C., & Chesla, C. (1996). *Expertise in nursing practice: Caring, clinical judgment, and ethics.* New York: Springer.

Benner, P., & Wrubel, J. (1989). *The primacy of caring: Stress and coping in health and illness.* Menlo Park, CA: Addison-Wesley.

Benoliel, J. (1996). Grounded theory and nursing knowledge. *Qualitative Health Research, 6*(3), 406–28.

Blattner, B. (1981). *Holistic nursing.* Englewood Cliffs, NJ: Prentice-Hall.

Boston College. (1996). *Knowledge Conference 1996: Proceedings.* In C. Roy & D. Jones (Eds.). Chestnut Hill, MA: BC Press.

Boston College (1997). *Knowledge Impact Conference II: 1997 Proceedings.* In C. Roy & D. Jones. (Eds.). Chestnut Hill, MA: BC Press.

Carper, B. A. (1978). *Advances in Nursing Science, 1*(1), 35.

Carrieri-Kohlman, V., Lindsey, A. M., & West, C. M. (1993). *Pathophysiological phenomena in nursing: Human responses to illness.* Philadelphia: W. B. Saunders.

Chandra, A., & Skinner, J. (2003). *Geography and racial health disparities* (Working Paper). Cambridge, MA: National Bureau of Economic Research.

Chinn, P. L. (1978). Editorial. *Advances in Nursing Science, 1*(1), n.p.

Chinn, P. L. (1995). *Peace and power: Building communities for the future* (4th ed.). New York: National League for Nursing.

Chinn, P. L., & Kramer, M. K. (1999). *Theory and nursing: Integrated knowledge development* (5th ed.). St. Louis, MO: Mosby.

Claassen, C. A., Michael-Kashner, T., Gilfillan, S. K., Larkin, G. L., & John-Rush, A. (2005). Psychiatric emergency service use after implementation of managed care in a public mental health system. *Psychiatric Services, 56*(6), 691–698.

DeNavas-Walt, C., Proctor, B., & Lee, C. (2005). Income, Poverty and Health Insurance Coverage in the United States: 2004. *U.S. Census Bureau, Current Populations Reports.* Washington, DC: U.S. Government Printing Office. (pp. 60–229).

Diers, D., & Dye, M. C. (1969). Situation producing theory. *Proceeding Nursing Theory Conference.* Lawrence, KS: University of Kansas.

Dodd, M. (1988). Efficacy of proactive information on self-care in chemotherapy patients. *Patient Education and Counseling, 11*, 215–225.

Donahue, M. P. (1996). *Nursing, the finest art: An illustrated history* (2nd ed.). St. Louis, MO: Mosby.

Donaldson, S. K., & Crowley, D. M. (1978). The discipline of nursing. *Nursing Outlook 26*, 113–120.

Fawcett, J. (1993). From a plethora of paradigms to parsimony in worldviews. *Nursing Science Quarterly, 6*(2), 56–58.

Fitzpatrick, J. J. (2002). Preface. *Review of Nursing Research, 20*, ix–x.

Friere, P. (1968). *Pedagogy of the oppressed.* New York: Herder and Herder.

Fry, S. T. (1994). Ethical implications of health care reform. *American Nurse, 26*(3), 5.

Gage, B. (1998). The history and growth of medicare managed care. *Generations, 22*(2), 11–18.

Gebbie, K. M., & Lavin, M. A. (1975). Utilization of a classification of nursing diagnoses. *Proceedings of the First National Conference* (pp. 21–36). St. Louis, MO: Mosby.

Giddings, L. S. (2005). Health disparities, social injustice, and the culture of nursing. *Nursing Research, 54*(5), 304–312.

Goodwin, B. (Ed.). (1967). Forum. *Image: Sigma Theta Tau National Honor Society of Nursing, 1*(1), 10.

Gortner, S. R. (2000). Knowledge development in nursing: our historical roots and future opportunities. *Nursing Outlook, 48*(2), 60–67.

Gortner, S. R., & Schultz, P. R. (1988). Approaches to nursing science methods. *Image: Journal of Nursing Scholarship, 20*(1), 22–24.

Gulzar, L. (1999). Health policy: Access to health care. *Image: Journal of Nursing Scholarship, 31*(1), 13–19.

Habermas, J. (1988). *On the logic of the social sciences.* Cambridge, MA: MIT Press.

Hanna, D. (2004). Moral distress: The state of science. *Research and Theory for Nursing Practice, 18*(1), 73–93.

Hanna, D. (2005). The lived experience of moral distress: Nurses who assisted with elective abortions. *Research and Theory for Nursing Practice, 19*(1).

Hardy, M. E. (1978). Perspectives on nursing theory. *Advances in Nursing Science, 1,* 37–48.

Hughes, L. (1990). Professionalizing domesticity: A synthesis of selected nursing historiography. *Advances in Nursing Science, 12*(4), 25–31.

Institute of Medicine. (2003). *Unequal treatment: What healthcare providers need to know about racial and ethnic disparities in health care.* Washington, DC: National Academies Press.

Jacobs-Kramer, M. L., & Chinn, P. L. (1987). *Theory and nursing: A systematic approach.* St. Louis, MO: Mosby.

Johnson, D. E. (1974). Development of theory: A requisite for nursing as a primary health profession. *Nursing Research, 23,* 372–377.

Johnson, J. E. (1972). Effects of structuring patients' expectations on their reactions to the threatening events. In R. M. Schlotfeldt (Ed.), *Symposium on Approaches to the Study of Nursing Questions and the Development of Nursing Science. Nursing Research, 21*(6), 499.

Jones, D., Flanagan, J., & Coakley, A. (2000). Nursing diagnosis at 24 and 72 hours following same day surgery with general anesthesia. In M. Rantz & P. LeMore (Eds.), *Proceedings of the 13th North American Nursing Diagnoses.* Glendale, CA: CINAHL Information Systems.

Journal Citation Reports. (2004). *ISI web of knowledge.* The Thompson Corporation. Boston College, Boston. 15 Feb. 2006.

Katz, J. (2001, Sept. 26). Patient preferences and health disparities. *Journal of the American Medical Association, 286,* 1506–1509. Retrieved February 2, 2006, from http://jama.ama-assn.org.

Katz, R. (1984). *Empowerment and synergy: Expanding the community's healing resources.* New York: Hayworth Press.

Kendall, J. (1992). Fighting back: Promoting emancipatory nursing actions. *Advances in Nursing Science, 15*(2), 1–15.

Ketefian, S. (2002). Editorial. *Research and Theory in Nursing Practice, 16*(1), 3–4.

Kikuchi, J. (2003). Nursing knowledge and the problem of worldviews. *Research and Theory for Nursing Practice, 17*(1), 7–17.

Kuhn, T. S. (1962). *The structure of scientific revolutions.* Chicago: University of Chicago Press.

Larson, J. L., Covey, M. K., & Corbridge, S. (2002). Inspiratory muscle strength in chronic obstructive pulmonary disease. *AACN Clinical Issues: Advanced Practice in Acute and Critical Care, 13*(2), 320–332.

Laudan, L. (1977). *Progress and its problems: Towards a theory of scientific growth.* Berkeley: University of California Press.

Laudan, L. (1984). Science and values: The aims of science and their role in scientific debate. Berkeley: University of California Press.

Lazarus, D. (2004, Sept. 10). Healthcare's reality. *San Francisco Chronicle.* Retrieved February 2, 2006, from http://www.sfgate.com/cgi-bin/article.cgi?file=/chronicle/archive/2004/09/10/BUGU58MFDG1.DTL.

Leddy, S. K. (2000). Toward a complimentary perspective on worldviews. *Nursing Science Quarterly, 13*, 225–233.

Leininger, M. (1991). Cultural care theory and uses in nursing administration. In M. Leininger (Ed.), *Culture care diversity and universality: A theory of nursing* (pp. 373–390). New York: National League for Nursing.

Lopez, K. A., & Willis, D. G. (2004). Descriptive versus interpretive phenomenology: Their contributions to nursing knowledge. *Qualitative Health Research, 14*(5), 726–735.

Maggs-Rapport, F. (2000). Combining methodological approaches in research: ethnography and interpretive phenomenology. *Journal of Advanced Nursing, 31*(1), 219–225.

Martin, L. (2001). *Who will care for each of us? America's coming health care labor crisis.* Chicago: University of Illinois at Chicago, College of Nursing, Nursing Institute.

McCance, T. (2003). Caring in nursing practice: The development of a conceptual framework. *Research and Theory for Nursing Practice, 17*(2).

McKay, R. (1969). Theories, models, and systems for nursing. In *Conference on the Nature of Science in Nursing* (pp. 393–400). Boulder: University of Colorado, School of Nursing.

Meleis, A. I. (1980). Toward scholarliness in doctoral dissertations: An analytical method. *Research in Nursing and Health, 3*, 115–124.

Meleis, A. I. (1997). *Theoretical nursing: Development and progress* (3rd ed.). Philadelphia: Lippincott Raven.

Meleis, A. I., & Im, E. (1999). Transcending marginalization in knowledge development. *Nursing Inquiry, 6*, 94–102.

Merx, K. (2006, Jan. 31). Business groups fight mandates that could benefit taxpayers. *Detroit Free Press.* Retrieved February 3, 2006.

Mishel, M. H. (1981). The measurement of uncertainty in illness. *Nursing Research, 30*, 258–263.

Mishel, M. H. (1997). Uncertainty in acute illness. *Annual Review of Nursing Research, 15*, 89–91.

Mitchell, P. H. (1999). Decreased adaptive capacity: Intracranial. In B. J. Ackley & G. B. Ludwig (Eds.), *Nursing diagnosis handbook* (4th ed., pp. 395–400). St. Louis, MO: Mosby.

Mitchell, P. H. (2001). Decreased behavioral arousal. In C. Stewart-Amidei & J. A. Kunkel (Eds.), *AANN's neuroscience nursing: Human responses to neurologic dysfunction* (2nd ed., pp. 93–118). Philadelphia: W. B. Saunders.

Mitchell, P. H., & Ackerman, L. (1992). Secondary brain injury reduction. In G. M. Bulecheck & J. C. McCloskey (Eds.), *Nursing interventions* (2nd ed., pp. 558–573). Philadelphia: W. B. Saunders.

Mitchell, P. H., Johnson, F. B., & Habermann-Little, B. (1986). Promoting physiologic stability: Touch and ICP. *Community Nursing Research, 18*, 93.

Moody, L. E. (1990). *Advancing nursing science through research: Vol. 1.* Newbury Park, CA: Sage.

Nathanson, I., Ramirez-Garnica, G., & Wiltrout, S. A. (2005). Decreased attendance at cystic fibrosis centers by children covered by managed care insurance. *American Journal of Public Health, 95*(11), 1958–1963.

Newbergh, C. (2002). The health tracking initiative. In S. L. Isaacs & J. R. Knickman (Eds.), *To improve health care: Vol. 4* (pp. 29–49). San Francisco: Jossey-Bass.

Newman, M. A. (1992). Nightingale's vision of nursing theory and health. In F. Nightin-gale (Ed.), *Notes on nursing: What it is, and what is not* (Commemorative ed., pp. 44–47). Philadelphia: Lippincott.

Newman, M. A. (1994). *Health as expanding consciousness.* New York: National League for Nursing Press.

Norbeck, J. S. (1987). In defense of empiricism . . . in nursing research. *Image: Journal of Nursing Scholarship, 19*(1), 28–30.

Norris, C. M. (1969, Mar.). *Proceedings of the First Nursing Theory Conference* (pp. 254–483). Kansas City: University of Kansas Medical Center, Department of Nursing.

Oiler, C. (1982). The phenomenological approach in nursing research. *Nursing Research, 31*(3), 178–181.

Olson, D. (1991). Empathy as an ethical and philosophical basis for nursing. *Advances in Nursing Science, 14*(1), 62–75.

Omery, A. (1983). Phenomenology: A method for nursing science. In J. Paley (Ed.), *Positivism and qualitative nursing research* (pp. 371–387). *Scholarly Inquiry for Nursing Practice: An International Journal, 14*(2). New York: Springer.

Orem, D. E. (1971). *Nursing: Concepts of practice.* New York: McGraw-Hill.

Orem, D. E. (1997). Views of human beings specific to nursing. *Nursing Science Quarterly, 10*(1), 26–31.

Parse, R. R. (1987). *Nursing science: Major paradigms, theories, and critiques.* Philadelphia: W. B. Saunders.

Quint, J. C. (1967). The case for theories generated from empirical data. *Nursing Re-search,16,* 109–114.

Roberts, S. J. (1983). Oppressed group behavior: Implications for nursing. *Advances in Nursing Science,* 21–30.

Rogers, M. E. (1970). *An introduction to the theoretical basis of nursing.* Philadelphia: F. A. Davis.

Roy, C. (1970). Adaptation: A conceptual framework in nursing. *Nursing Outlook, 18,* 42–45.

Roy, C. (1976). *Introduction to nursing: An adaptation model.* Englewood Cliffs, NJ: Prentice-Hall.

Roy, C. (1986). The future of nursing science: Response and the Academy. In G. E. Sorensen (Ed.), *Setting the agenda for the year 2000: Knowledge development in nursing* (pp. 21–28). Kansas City, MO: American Academy of Nursing.

Roy, C. (1988). An explication of the philosophical assumptions of the Roy adaptation model. *Nursing Science Quarterly, 1*(1), 26–34.

Roy, C. (1997). Future of the Roy adaptation model: Challenge to redefine adaptation. *Nursing Science Quarterly, 10*(1), 42–48.

Roy, C. (1999). NANDA and the nurse theorists: The truth of theory. In M. J. Rantz & P. LeMone (Eds.), *Classification of nursing diagnoses: Proceedings of the thirteenth conference* (pp. 59–67). Glendale, CA: Cinahl Information Systems.

Roy, C. (2000). The visible and invisible fields that shape the future of the nursing care system. *Nursing Administration Quarterly, 25,* 119–131.

Roy, C. & Andrews, H. (1999). The Roy Adaptation Model. Stamford, CT: Appleton & Lange.

Sarnecky, M. T. (1990). Historiography: A legitimate research methodology for nursing. *Advances in Nursing Science 12*(4), 1–10.

Schaag, H. A., & Phipps, W. J. (1999). Issues affecting adult health care. In W. J. Phipps, J. K. Sands, & J. Mark (Eds.), *Medical surgical nursing: Concepts & clinical practice* (6th ed., pp. 1–24). St. Louis, MO: Mosby.

Schlotfeldt, R. M. (1972). Approaches to the study of nursing questions and the development of nursing science. *Nursing Research, 21*(6), 484–486.

Schreiber, R. S., & Stern, P. N. (2001). *Using grounded theory in nursing.* New York: Springer.

Simon, H. M. (1968). Panel discussion: The position of the pure and applied scientist. In M. Leininger (Ed.), *Conference on the nature of science and nursing. Nursing Research, 17*(6), 507.

Simonet, D. (2005). Patient satisfaction under managed care. *International Journal of Health Care Quality Assurance, 18*(6–7), 424–440.

Smith, J. P. (1976). Editorial. *Journal of Advanced Nursing, 1*(1), 1.

Sorensen, B. E. (1986). *Setting the agenda for the year 2000: Knowledge development in nursing.* Kansas City, MO: American Academy of Nursing.

Sorrell, J. M., & Redmond, G. M. (1995). Interviews in qualitative nursing research: Differing approaches for ethnographic and phenomenological studies. *Journal of Advanced Nursing, 21*(6), 1117–1122.

Stevenson, J. S., & Woods, N. F. (1986). Nursing science and contemporary science: Emerging paradigms. In G. E. Sorensen (Ed.), *Setting the agenda for the year 2000: Knowledge development in nursing* (pp. 6–20). Kansas City, MO: American Academy of Nursing.

Stiegelis, H. E., Hagedoorn, M., Sanderman, R., Bennenbroek, F. T. C., Buunk, B. P., van den Bergh, A. C. M., et al. (2004). The impact of an informational self-management intervention on the association between control and illness uncertainty before and psychological distress after radiotherapy *Psycho-Oncology, 13*(4), 248–259.

Sullivan, E. J. (1999). *Creating nursing's future: Issues, opportunities and challenges.* St. Louis, MO: Mosby.

Suppe, F., & Jacox, A. K. (1985). Philosophy of science and the development of nursing theory. In H. Werley & J. Fitzpatrick (Eds.), *Annual review of nursing research: Vol. 3* (pp. 241–267). New York: Springer.

Thinking Qualitative Faculty. (2006). "Janice M. Morse Bio." *International Institute for Qualitative Methodology.* http://www.uofaweb.ualberta.ca/TQfaculty.cfm. 23 Aug. 2006.

University of Rhode Island College of Nursing. (1993 & 1994). Building a cumulative knowledge base for nursing from fragmentation to congruence of philosophy, theory, methods of inquiry and practice. In *Invited Papers of the 4th and 5th Symposia of the Knowledge Development Series.* Kingston: University of Rhode Island College of Nursing.

Walker, L. O., & Avant, K. C. (1995). *Strategies for theory construction in nursing.* Upper Saddle River, NJ: Pearson Prentice Hall.

Watson, J. (1979). *Nursing: The philosophy and science of care.* Boston: Little, Brown.

Watson, J. (1985). *Nursing: Human science and human care—A theory of nursing.* Norwalk, CT: Appleton-Century-Crofts.

Werley, H. (1978). Editorial. *Research in Nursing & Health, 1*(1), 3.

White, J. (1995). Patterns of knowing: Review, critique, and update. *Advances in Nursing Science, 17*(4), 73–86.

Wineman, N. M., Schwetz, K. M., Zeller, R., & Cyphert, J. (2003). Longitudinal analysis of illness uncertainty, coping, hopefulness, and mood during participation in a clinical drug trial. *Journal of Neuroscience Nursing, 35*(2), 100–106.

WEB SITES VISITED

http://www.nursing.uconn.edu/~plchinn/ANSathgd.htm. *Advances in Nursing Science Author's Guide*, edited by P. Chinn. Retrieved August 13, 2002.

http://www.ncccusa.org/poverty/index.html. National Council of Churches, *Update on Poverty*. Retrieved February 5, 2003.

http://www.ins.usdoj.gov/graphics/index.htm. Immigration and Naturalization Service.

http://www.census.gov. U.S. Census Bureau, United States Department of Commerce. Retrieved February 19, 2002.

http://www.bc.edu/bc_org/avp/son/theorist/consensus2.html. Consensus paper.

http://www.cis.org. Center for Immigration Studies.

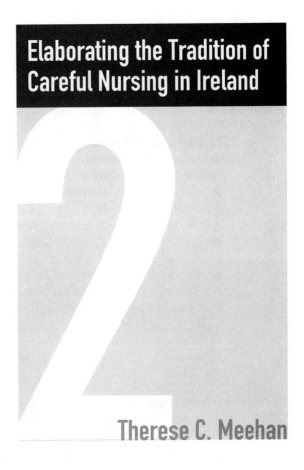

Elaborating the Tradition of Careful Nursing in Ireland

2

Therese C. Meehan

In 2000, Doona proposed "careful nursing" as Ireland's conceptual legacy to nursing. This concept has lain hidden in historical archives until Doona recently retrieved it in her historical research on the diaries of Irish nurses who helped nurse sick and wounded British soldiers during the Crimean war of 1854–1856. This is not to say that the sense of the concept has been dormant in the thinking and practice of Irish nurses. It has been and remains very much alive, although it is not much talked about.

The traditions of nursing have long acknowledged the significance of the nurse–patient relationship, and the term *care* is currently used, and sometimes overused, to describe the focus of nursing. But what is careful nursing? What did Irish nurses of the mid-19th century mean by the term? What does careful nursing mean for the profession today? What could it contribute to international nursing knowledge development and, in turn, to fostering best possible nursing practice? These are the questions being opened for debate.

In addition to the great debt owed to the historical research of Mary Ellen Doona (1995, 1999, 2000), the ideas presented are also drawn from other significant historical research on the topic (Bauman, 1958; Bolster, 1964; Gillgannon, 1962; Hammack, 1952; Hughes, 1948), from the writings of 19th-century Irish nurses (Bridgeman, 1854–1856; Carroll, 1883; Croke, 1854–1856a, 1854–1856b; Doyle, 1897; McAuley cited in Carroll,

1883), from an English nurse closely associated with them (Taylor, 1856), and from British government and military correspondence pertaining to nursing during the Crimean war.

Background

In 19th-century Ireland, there was a great need for nursing service, and those who felt drawn to it, mostly women, just went out and did it. One such woman in the 1820s was a Dublin heiress, Catherine McAuley. She put all her money and energy into her nursing service, and other women joined her. Initially, McAuley had no intention of forming a women's religious order. However, society at the time required that women operate either within the context of a marriage or a religious community. Thus, in 1831 she founded the Institute of Our Lady of Mercy, better known as the Sisters of Mercy. The order grew rapidly and established a home and hospital visiting nurse service. These nurses worked closely with prominent Dublin physicians and surgeons, notably Colles, Stokes, and Graves. McAuley was particularly drawn to working with Robert Graves because both were of the opinion that the standard fever treatments of the time, such as blistering, leeching, and a low diet, were harmful to patients (Walsh, 1907). They advocated for an alternative treatment including frequent feeding of fever patients whether they had an appetite or not. They shared a deeply felt view that the most important element in treating the sick is

> the conservation of the patient's strength with the preservation of his morale and that this can be best accomplished when the patient is constantly under the care of an experienced nurse, noting every symptom and averting every possible source of worry and every form of exhaustion of energy. (Walsh, 1907, p.172)

Nurses' work under McAuley was held in very high regard. During the cholera epidemic of 1832, the physician in charge of the cholera hospital in Dublin declared that the hospital could not be carried on without the nurses. He gave McAuley "fullest control [of the hospital], held long consultations with her, and attributed their small percentage of deaths (about 30 percent), in comparison with the usual high percentage [about 80 percent], to her wise administration" (Furlong circa 1832 as quoted in Bauman, 1958, pp. 58–59). Twenty-three years later, when the Crimean war was declared, these women had built up extensive nursing practice experience along with a highly ordered system of nursing management.

The term *careful nursing* first appeared in print in a letter written by Ellen Whitty (1854) to London officials. Whitty was responding to public outcry about the lack of nurses to care for the many soldiers in the British army suffering and dying from infections and wounds in the war between Turkey and Russia being fought on the Crimean peninsula. Approximately one-third of soldiers in the allied British army were Irish. Whitty expressed concern for their plight and offered nursing services. She wrote:

> Attendance on the sick is, as you are aware, part of our Institute; and sad experience amongst the poor has convinced us that, even with the advantage of medical aid, many valuable lives are lost for want of careful nursing. (Whitty, October 18, 1854)

This offer was accepted readily by the British Secretary at War. Fifteen sisters were engaged as part of a second group, following that of Nightingale, to nurse at the Crimea. These women were engaged as nurses rather than as religious sisters. The nurses sent to the Crimea included Margaret Alcock, Joanna Bridgeman (leader), Anne Butler, Isabella Croke, Julia Dixon, Kate Doyle, Elizabeth Hersey, Eliza Heyfron, Mary Hurley, Arabella Keane, Margaret Lalor, Joseph Lynch, Grace Rice, Winifred Sprey, and Anne Whitty.

Most ranged in age from about 30 to 40 years, although one was 22 and another 54. They tended to come from families of significant social standing and were well-educated. For example, Joanna Bridgeman was related to the great Irish liberator Daniel O'Connell, and as a young debutante had been acclaimed for her grace and charm. Although quiet in manner, these women were of definite and independent mind. All were highly competent nurses. Doona (2000) estimated that each had between 4 and 15 years of experience in nursing. Bridgeman had commenced her "nursing training" in 1832 under the guidance of an aunt who had established a center for the poor in Limerick. Bridgeman learned nursing knowledge and skill during years of periodic epidemics and famines. Through close observation of cholera symptoms, she had developed a system of stuping (application of moist heat) that had become well known and widely used (Bolster, 1964).

Two English women should also be considered part of the careful nursing group. Mary Stanley, sister of the Dean of Westminster, was appointed by the British Secretary at War to the overall leadership of this second group. Fanny Taylor was a devoted nurse who later published a graphic account of nursing practice at the Crimea (Taylor, 1856). It has been estimated that both women, as well as some of the Irish nurses, would have been at least equal to Florence Nightingale in social standing (Summers, 1988).

At the Crimea, the political and social context within which these nurses worked, and their relationship with Florence Nightingale, were rent with many difficult circumstances and issues that greatly affected them. These will not be addressed here, other than to say that they went to the Crimea at the behest of the British government with the complete understanding they would work under the direction of Nightingale. However, upon their arrival at Constantinople, Nightingale refused to employ them (Bridgeman, 1854–1856; Croke, 1854–1856a; Doyle, 1897). She considered that the government had gone over her head and not properly consulted her about their employment. She claimed that there was no need for more nurses, even in face of the fact the Scutari hospital was overflowing with approximately 5,000 sick and wounded soldiers, between 50 and 90 of them dying daily (Doona, 2000). Nightingale renounced any connection with them, and the Secretary at War advised the Irish nurses to try to find employment for themselves where they could (Bolster, 1964; Hughes, 1948).

The nurses found employment in three hospitals outside the jurisdiction of Nightingale. For the first 9 months, they were employed at the Barrack Hospital and the General Hospital at Koulali, about 3 miles from Scutari. Joanna Bridgeman served as superintendent at the General Hospital at Koulali. Later they were invited by the army inspector general of hospitals to the General and Hut Hospitals at Balaclava, about 2 days by ship across the Black Sea on the coast of the Crimean peninsula and close to the battlefield. Bridgeman was superintendent here as well. The nurses worked for 6 months until it was clear the war was ending.

Careful Nursing

Against this historical backdrop, the concept of careful nursing will be elaborated upon in terms of definitions of the generally accepted nursing metaparadigm concepts. This effort is a beginning step in the specific theoretical knowledge development that remains an ongoing process. The author advances this proposal, based on the nurses' thoughts and actions and observations of their practice as recorded in the literature (Bauman, 1958; Bolster, 1964; Bridgeman, 1854–1856; Carroll, 1883; Croke, 1854–1856a, 1854–1856b; Doyle, 1897; Gillgannon, 1962; Hammack, 1952; Hughes, 1948; McAuley cited in Carroll, 1883; Taylor, 1856). It is considered judicious at this beginning point to remain as true as possible to the thinking of the nurses. In taking this approach, however, terms are used that may not resonate well in today's mainly secular society. Ideas and examples of practice may seem simple and obvious to modern nurses, but they were of vital importance in the mid-19th century and some nursing innovations flew hard in the face of accepted practice. It is the philosophy and principles underlying their practice that may be most important for modern nurses to consider.

Metaparadigm Concepts

The following observations link careful nursing to what are today considered the meta-paradigm concepts of nursing: person, environment, health, and nursing.

Person

Within the concept of careful nursing, the human person is a spiritual, physical, emotional, and social being. The spiritual dimension is considered fundamental and unifying and gives form to the person as an expression of God's love and purpose in the world. At the same time, the physical, emotional, and social dimensions are considered just as important and are viewed as an inseparable expression of the person's spiritual nature. Human persons are in continuous communication with their environments – spiritually, physically, emotionally, and socially – establishing and maintaining individual and community relationships. Each human person possesses a unique combination of special abilities that may be consciously recognized and expressed in fulfilling a unique and meaningful purpose in life. Aside from any particular physical, emotional, or social characteristics, the human person possesses an inner sacredness, dignity, and beauty reflected in an intrinsic order, balance, strength, fortitude, and potential for good. At the same time, the human potential for maleficence is also clearly recognized.

Environment

The environment encompasses the physical, emotional, and social surroundings of the person embedded within a spiritual dimension. The spiritual is universal and gives rise to goodness, order, and beauty as expressions of God's creativity and purposefulness in the world. At the same time, the environment encompasses a myriad of actual and potential maleficent forces that may be of physical, emotional, or social origin.

Health

Health is a unitary experience of harmony, relative contentedness, and personal dignity. It arises from experiencing alignment with the spiritual origin of life and from the experience of fulfilling a unique and meaningful purpose in life. Healing is a natural restorative process. Promotion of health includes creating a restorative environment and mitigating to every extent possible maleficent physical, emotional, and social influences. Health may also include accepting with equanimity influences and circumstances that lie beyond the domain of justice but cannot be altered.

Nursing

Nursing is an intellectual endeavor and an art that has its impetus in the spiritual dimension of the nurse. It involves: (a) creating a restorative environment and removing or minimizing adverse environmental influences on the person, (b) nurturing human life and fostering the natural restorative process within the person, (c) supporting the intrinsic dignity of the person, and (d) acting with great tenderness and compassion, often in the face of human sadness. This latter aspect is encompassed in the Latin term *mater misericordiae*. Nursing is a way of sharing in God's love for humanity through fostering comfort and healing of the human person and striving for perfect knowledge and skill in the prevention of illness and care of the sick and wounded. The purpose of nursing is the prevention of illness and the promotion of health.

Characteristics of Careful Nursing

The key features that depict the concept of careful nursing in practice are listed in Table 2.1. The first feature is the nurses' *inner sense of calm*, even under the most adverse circumstances, and their ability to communicate this calmness to the patient environment. Observers of the Irish nurses commented frequently on the nurses' ability to maintain a

Table 2.1

Careful Nursing: Characteristics and Enabling Factors

Characteristics

1. inner sense of calm
2. creation of orderly environment
3. perfect skill in fostering physical comfort and healing
4. development and revision of intervention
5. attitude of disinterested love
6. sharing a common understanding of nursing practice

Enabling Factors

1. collaborative manner of attentiveness
2. management approach equally authoritative and participatory
3. authority derived from service
4. caring for themselves

sense of calm, even in the face of sudden stressors and when surrounded by agony and chaos. Their calm presence produced a sense of calm in their environment, especially in patients and fellow workers. As early as the 1830s, physicians in Dublin were commenting on the sense of calm associated with careful nursing and its beneficial influence on patients.

Another feature of careful nursing is the *creation of an orderly environment*, harmonious and restorative, as free as possible from influences adverse to comfort, healing, and healthy human development. Careful nursing emphasized the importance of establishing and maintaining, to every extent possible, physical order and cleanliness in the patient environment in order to ease distress of patients and staff and to comfort and protect patients from adverse environmental influences. The nurses established regular scrubbing of floors, beds, and equipment, and regular changing and washing of patients' bedclothes and linen. They stopped practices such as cutting up animal carcasses in close proximity to patients suffering from infectious diseases. Their ward kitchens, very important adjuncts to careful nursing at that time, were reported to be models of order and cleanliness. Great emphasis was placed on harnessing healing aspects of the natural environment such as fresh air, sunshine, and flower gardens.

Third, careful nursing involves *perfect skill in fostering physical comfort and healing* for patients, accomplished through close and continuous observation, meticulous attention to detail, and close supervision of nursing care delegated to assistants. The nurses worked tirelessly and meticulously in observing and attending to individual patient needs such as dressing wounds, washing, feeding, ensuring adequate fluids, repositioning, and providing exercise. Circumstances required that these responsibilities be frequently delegated to orderlies (nursing assistants) who were trained by instruction and example and who were required to be equally tireless and meticulous in their work. The nurses stressed the importance of responding quickly to patients' requests and not leaving food and fluids out of their reach. They tried always to stay with patients who were close to death and ensure that they were not taken to the "dead-house" before they were actually dead. Reverence for the care of the body and recognition of the influence upon it of emotions and mental powers were considered essential to careful nursing.

Development and revision of nursing interventions to relieve patients' symptoms and promote comfort and healing also is a defining feature of careful nursing. The nurses brought with them Bridgeman's specific method of stuping and ensured that it was provided for appropriate patients. They instituted "night watching" for fever patients and considered this especially essential for cholera patients. Doyle wrote that, "If a fever patient is not well nursed during the night no amount of care will bring back what he loses – some nourishment must be given every two hours or more frequently . . . in these cases nursing is everything. The doctors were often surprised in the morning to find their patients so well over the night" (1897, p. 73). They instituted the use of aromatic vinegar water to sponge patients for comfort. They saw to the careful preparation and frequent administration of fluids, mainly lemonade and barley water. They instituted "rice pudding reform" and revised the preparation of the commonly used arrowroot and wine mixture to enhance its palatability and effectiveness.

Another key feature is the nurses' *attitude of disinterested love* of patients, exemplified in attentiveness to patients, which is free of self-interest. This is an ideal that was cultivated by the nurses as a professional way of being that framed their interactions with patients. It was characterized by great tenderness in all things, affection, kindness, sympathy, humor, and a bright and joyous spirit. It was encompassed within their broader intent to be instruments of God's love for humanity. It did not, however, preclude the need to sometimes be severe and firm. Observers often commented upon this attitude. For example, the commander-in-chief of the British army remarked upon their "unfailing kindness" and "disinterested attention to patients" (Codrington, 1856, as quoted in Bolster, 1964, p. 256). The concept of disinterested love is an early Christian concept and ideal. It is associated in the literature with meditation and prayer, both of which are proposed to have restorative properties. McAuley observed that within the context of this attitude, characteristics such as tenderness, affection, kindness, and sympathy arise from the heart and reside in the will, not in feelings. There is abundant evidence that this attitude was therapeutic for patients.

Careful nursing includes nurses *sharing a common understanding* of the nature of nursing practice. It was often remarked that the nurses appeared to be of "one mind" in their work and that if one was called away from doing something another could pick up her work with barely a pause in the work. This contributed to an impression of harmony and unity in their work, which was in turn mirrored in the attitudes and actions of their coworkers.

Enabling Factors for Careful Nursing

In addition to the key characteristics, careful nursing is recognized by certain enabling factors (see Table 2.1). A *collaborative manner of "attentiveness,"* trustworthiness, confidence, and innovativeness was found among the Irish nurses in working with other health professionals and health care administrators. There is no getting away from the fact that a distinctive characteristic of careful nursing was obedience, especially to doctors' orders. However, it is very evident that these nurses were not docile and that they were quick to question anything they thought not to be in the patients' best interest. Bridgeman would "make a great fight" with the deputy purveyor or chief medical officer till she got what she wanted for her patients. It is possible that in the 19th century the term *obedience* was used a little differently than it is today. For example, army generals normally signed letters to one another "your obedient and humble servant," as a matter of courtesy.

Obedience in the nurses may have been more indicative of the manner in which they provided service, exemplified by graciousness and respectfulness, even when they were personally furious with injustices that occurred. It was possibly also related to their reputation for responding immediately to needs and being trustworthy. McAuley had placed great emphasis on the importance of social virtues, such as courtesy, gentleness, respectfulness, and consideration for others in all matters, in enhancing human relations (Bauman, 1958). There are many examples of the tactful logic and graciousness with which the nurses brought about reversal or revision of doctors' orders and purveyors' directives. The degree of trust and confidence placed in Joanna Bridgeman is indicated by the purveyor-in-chief's decision to place entirely at her discretion all stores, food, and clothing. She was to act as if the hospital were her own, and the chief medical officer's announcement indicated that Joanna Bridgeman's orders were to be considered as if his own.

It seems reasonable to substitute the term *attentiveness* for obedience. In today's world, this term may better convey the qualities formerly attached to the term obedience. Nurses and physicians appear to have a close collaborative relationship, and on a more or less equal footing, in planning care and developing new treatments for patients. For example, Bridgeman's stuping procedure was redesigned to include a new chloroform treatment that the physicians were eager to try.

A management approach that is in equal measures authoritative and participatory was an enabler of careful nursing that included teaching and close supervision of nursing associates and assistants. Because of their long experience, the Irish nurses were looked to for guidance and leadership. Taylor (1856) wrote that, "long experience in [nursing] gave them great superiority over us, and they were ever ready to show us their method and enter into our difficulties" (p. 28). Bridgeman was described as governing "more like a Sister than a Superior" (Doyle, 1897, p. 95). They took great trouble to teach others all they knew.

Each nurse was responsible for between about 20 and 50 patients, and sometimes many more. The orderlies who served as nursing assistants were of the utmost importance. At first the nurses found the assistants very much hardened by the horrors of their experiences. They were in the habit of drinking freely "to drown their grief" (Doyle, 1897, p. 40). Because there had previously been no supervision of the orderlies' administration of stimulants, patients often were found drunk in their beds. Assessing the situation, the Irish nurses placed the orderlies under strict supervision and gave them great scoldings. At first they were very unhappy with the new discipline. The nurses, working closely with the orderlies, never making any complaint against them, effected change "gently, and as it were, imperceptibly" (Bridgeman, 1854–1856, p. 93). As time went on, the orderlies became exemplary nursing assistants.

Authority derived from service rather than from power per sé added to the effectiveness of careful nursing. The Irish nurses were in many ways powerless in the system. Many in the army were predisposed to immense bias and prejudice against them. Yet it is evident that they had great authority in all matters related to health. Their advice and assistance was sought on many and varied occasions and was always speedily and attentively given. The nurses' authority derived from wide-ranging in all matters relating to health care. They had great authority resulting from the great service they provided.

A final enabling factor identified in careful nursing is *nurses caring for themselves* physically and emotionally, keeping alive within themselves the interior spirit that guided their practice. The nurse work was extremely demanding physically, but Bridgeman saw to it that each nurse had regular and substantial meals, had their clothes washed and ironed, and that nurses got sufficient sleep when possible. Normally, two nurses were assigned full time to look after the other 13. Every effort was made to include periods of quiet and prayer within daily schedules and nurses commented on the importance of preserving overall health. It is possible that their cultivation of an attitude of disinterested love helped buffer nurses from the anguish, terrible injuries, and death with which they were constantly surrounded. What they dealt with in giving nursing care was in addition to the constant influx of lice, the "light infantry" of fleas, frequent harassment by droves of huge rats, earthquakes, the fickle weather of the Russian winter, and at Balaclava being within range of the shelling.

In the midst of this devastation the nurses, according to historical reports (Bolster, 1964), seemed always to have had a joyful optimism. Isabella Croke had a lively and mischievous sense of humor. Her wonderful 240-verse poem illustrating key events of their "Eastern Mission" (Croke, 1854–1856b) shows her continual search for a silver lining in the many clouds that overshadowed their lives. The diaries and letters attest to their humor and quick wit, which are combined with selected examples of the military humor and wit of the orderlies. These documents make for some very funny reading. The reader is left with the sense that the laughter mixed with their tears probably saved them often from feelings of desperation. Although two died, one of cholera and one of typhus, and one was an invalid at home with recurrent fever, the others more or less maintained their health. This was in contrast to many other nurses engaged during this war. The reason the Irish nurses were alone with the orderlies and fatigue men at Balaclava was that most ladies and paid nurses had "sunk" under the work. There seems little indication that the Irish nurses suffered from what is now called burnout.

Outcomes

The effectiveness of careful nursing is clearly documented in what modern nurses might call outcomes. The standard of nursing was so high at the Koulali General Hospital that it was widely known in the army and the Constantinople area as "the model hospital of the East" (Doyle, 1897; Taylor, 1857). The Irish nurses were known to be the answer to just about any human crisis that occurred. The Sultan of Turkey held them in the highest esteem and at the end of the war insisted on sending them a gift of £230 (about £16,000 today or about $25,000).

At the General Hospital at Balaclava, the army conducted a comparative study, comparing the effectiveness of the previous nursing system with the careful nursing system. The findings of this study were conveyed in a confidential report to the British government and were significantly in favor of the careful nursing system (Doona, 1999). The report included the following summary:

> The superiority of an ordered system is beautifully illustrated ... One mind appears to move all and their intelligence, delicacy and contentiousness invest them with a halo of confidence extreme. The medical officer can safely assign his most critical cases to their hands. Stimulants or opiates ordered every five minutes, will be faithfully administered tho' the five minutes labor were repeated uninterruptedly for a week. ... A calm resigned contentedness sits on the features of all, and the soft cares of the female and the Lady breathes placidly throughout. (Fitzgerald, 1856, as quoted in Doona, 2000, p.21)

Summary and Implications for Modern Nursing

In modern terms, careful nursing can be summarized as follows: nursing is an intellectual endeavor and an art. Through intellectual endeavor, nurses seek to excel at knowing. A broad education in the liberal arts and sciences combined with close and continuous observation in practice serves as a foundation for developing and using nursing knowledge. As McAuley cautioned in the 1830s, there is little place in nursing for hard and fast rules. Rather, excellence in nursing is the product of a broad education, perfect discipline, discernment, forbearance, and good judgment.

The art of nursing is the thoughtful and creative use of knowledge in practice. Nursing practice is characterized by inseparable modes of acting and being that create a restorative environment, provide protection from harm, and foster comfort, healing, and health. The balance between intellectual endeavor in nursing and the art of nursing practice is reflected by frequent references to the nurses as ladies of intellect and refinement. It is abundantly evident that for all their constant engagement in practice and the exhausting physical labor of it, the Irish nurses' minds were ever active, ever-thinking and questioning, while at the same time maintaining their facility for great tenderness in all things, affection, kindness, and sympathy.

Florence Nightingale was not pleased that her nursing system had been found wanting in the confidential report of the comparative study at Balaclava. Nonetheless, on a visit to Balaclava before the war ended, she requested from Bridgeman information on the Irish nurses' system of nursing. Bridgeman's (1854–1856) diary records that "Miss N. took notes of our manner of nursing which Rev. Mother explained to her, as she hoped some one might profit of it" (as quoted in Hughes, 1948, p. 123). It is interesting to observe the extent to which the content of the book later written by Nightingale (1860), *Notes on Nursing*, corresponds to the system of careful nursing.

Because of circumstances of the time, the Irish nurses were, as one observer put it, "denied even the passing tribute of one generous word" (Wiseman, 1856, as quoted in Bolster, 1964, p. 237) outside their own country for their contribution to the nursing effort during the Crimean war. This, together with the Irish nurses' own view that it would be unbecoming of them to be broadcasting about their work (Bolster, 1964), served to eclipse their significant contribution to the founding of modern nursing.

There is one last point that it is important to add. Although careful nursing was developed in Ireland, it was not unique to Ireland. French nurses provided similar nursing during the Crimean war as they had in France since at least the 7th century. Nurses in other countries of Southern Europe were also known to practice a similar system of nursing, for example, the male nurses of St. John of God.

We are left with the question of what careful nursing may mean for nursing knowledge development and practice today. Two approaches to answering this question could be explored. One is the development of a conceptual model of nursing based on careful nursing. The other is to examine concepts and propositions of careful nursing and compare them with concepts and propositions of current conceptual models of nursing.

Consideration could be given to whether there is a need for the development of an additional conceptual model of nursing founded on the principles of careful nursing. Although careful nursing contains many similarities to modern conceptual models of nursing, it does have some differences and introduces new emphasis on some concepts. The spiritual dimension of life would be an essential feature of a careful nursing model. It would require in nurses a certain disposition to be present and to act – to be ever-present, ever-thinking, and exceptionally attentive to patients needs, and to act with great tenderness in all things. It would also require nurses to be attuned to one another in the sense of "one mind appearing to move all." It would prescribe patterns of nursing management and staffing that would not require a great number of professional nurses but would require them to work very closely with a large number of nursing assistants and ensure that they followed their guidance. Education of nurses would include the understanding and cultivation of the ideal of disinterested love. It would also include cultivation of social virtues, that is, considerable amplification of what modern nurses call communication skills.

In the second approach, different ways of understanding the spiritual dimension of life could be explored and compared. The concept of disinterested love could be compared with the concept of nonattachment as it is understood in Buddhism and used by nurses in Buddhist countries. The roles of prayer and meditation in nursing could be further explored and compared. The importance of the nature of the nurse–patient interaction and the idea of acting with great tenderness in all things could be compared with concepts from Peplau's model of psychodynamic nursing and with Travelbee's theory of nurses' therapeutic use of self. Modern views of nursing management could be compared with the management principles inherent in careful nursing, perhaps especially as they relate to the role and supervision of nursing assistants. Many other possibilities are inherent in the key features of careful nursing that have been identified.

Conclusion

Thanks to the work of Doona and the opportunity provided by the Emerging Nursing Knowledge 2000 conference, the system of careful nursing is being reclaimed and added to the treasury of nursing knowledge. We trust that, in keeping with the wishes of our Irish nurse forebears, we do not appear too unbecoming in broadcasting about our legacy. Rather, we hope and trust, following the example of Joanna Bridgeman, that from this description "some one might profit" and that it will contribute to promoting the best possible nursing practice.

REFERENCES

Bauman, M. B. (1958). *A way of mercy*. Burlingame, CA: The Sisters of Mercy.

Bolster, (1964). *The Sisters of Mercy in the Crimean War*. Cork, Ireland: Mercier Press, 1964.

Bridgeman, M. F. (1854–1856). An account of the mission of the Sisters of Mercy in the military hospitals of the East, beginning December 1854 and ending in May 1856. Unpublished manuscript, Archives of the Sisters of Mercy, Kinsale, Ireland.

Carroll, T. A. (Ed.). (1883). *Leaves from the annals of the Sisters of Mercy: Vol. 2*. New York: Catholic Publication Society Co.

Codrington, W. (1856). William Codrington to John Hall, April 1856. Unpublished manuscript, Archives of the Sisters of Mercy, Kinsale, Ireland.

Croke, M. J. (1854–1856a). *Diary of Sister M. Joseph Croke*. Catherine McAuley Archives Museum, Dublin.

Croke, M. J. (1854–1856b). *Lines on the Eastern mission of the Sisters of Mercy: From October 1854 to April 1856*. Catherine McAuley Archives Museum, Charleville, Ireland.

Doona, M. E. (1995). Sister Mary Joseph Croke: Another voice from the Crimean war, 1854–1856. *Nursing History Review*, 3, 3–41.

Doona, M. E. (1999). *The confidential report on Crimean nursing*. Paper presented at the International Council of Nursing Centennial Conference, London.

Doona, M. E. (2000). *"Careful Nursing": Ireland's legacy to nursing*. Paper presented at the Third Annual Public Lecture for Nurses, University College Dublin, Dublin.

Doyle, M. A. (1897). *Memories of the Crimea*. London: Burns & Oates.

Fitzgerald, D. (1856). *Confidential report on Crimean nursing*. Crimean Nursing Papers, Archives of the Sisters of Mercy, Kinsale, Ireland.

Gillgannon, M. M. (1962). *The Sisters of Mercy as Crimean war nurses*. Unpublished doctoral dissertation, University of Notre Dame, Notre Dame, IN.

Hammack, H. L. (1952). *The work of the Sisters of Mercy in the Crimea and its reference to modern nursing*. Unpublished master's thesis, San Francisco College for Women, San Francisco.

Hughes, M. J. (1948). *Crimean diary of Mother M. Francis Bridgeman, war companion of Florence Nightingale 1854–1856*. Unpublished master's thesis, Catholic University of America.

Nightingale, Florence. (1860). *Notes on Nursing: What it is, and what it is not*. New York: Dover Publications, Inc.

Summers, A. (1988). *Angles and citizens: British women as military nurses, 1854–1914*. London: Routledge & Kegan Paul.

Taylor F. (1856). *Eastern hospitals and English nurses: Vols. I & II*. London: Hurst & Blacket.

Taylor F. (1857). *Eastern hospitals and English nurses: The narrative of twelve months' experience in the hospitals of Koulali and Scutari*. London: Hurst and Blacket.

Walsh, J. (1907). *Makers of modern medicine*. New York: Fordham University Press.

Whitty, V. (1854). Mother Vincent Whitty to Rev. William Yore, October 18, 1854. Crimean War Papers, Archepiscopal Archives, Dublin.

Wiseman, N. (1856). *Lenten Pastoral quoted in Bolster E. (1962) The Sisters of Mercy in the Crimean war*. Cork, Ireland: Mercier Press.

The Role of Terminology in Identifying the Content of the Discipline

3

Marcelline R. Harris
Judith R. Graves

T his chapter focuses on the significance of terminology for the discipline of nursing, written from the perspective of researchers in nursing informatics. Our interests concern effective methods by which to encode the content of the discipline in computer-based systems. After a discussion of terminology and the content of the discipline, we use an example from the discharge planning research literature to examine terminology issues related to domain knowledge.

Terminology, the Content of the Discipline, and Domain Knowledge

Among the factors researchers in information technology consider are (a) developing language for informatics, that is, coding, and (b) knowledge as language related to the content of the discipline. In this regard, the term *domain knowledge* refers to the knowledge of a particular subject area within the broader discipline of nursing. We have described previously the challenges to representing nursing domain knowledge in relation to the embedded structures that organize knowledge from the perspective of various users (Harris, Graves, Solbrig, Elkin, & Chute, 2000). In this chapter, the challenges of representing the content for the discipline are presented in relation to the terms used to encode concepts and relationships within computer-based systems.

Unfortunately, nursing knowledge has proven very difficult to define. Within this book, a range of knowledge perspectives and strategies from philosophical perspectives to mid-range theory development are provided. The content of knowledge for nursing as a discipline also is guided by statements such as the Social Policy Statement (American Nurses Association [ANA], 2002) and the Standards of Practice (ANA, 2002). Given this range, it is important to understand the perspectives that we hold related to domain knowledge to understand the terminology issues we present.

Terminology Issues

First, domain knowledge is a prerequisite for specifying the content of the discipline. Like other disciplines, nursing is characterized by the perspectives or ways members of the discipline view and characterize phenomena within the discipline as well as relevant phenomena outside the discipline (Meleis, 1997). Approaches to knowledge development are one of the factors that characterize disciplinary perspectives and thereby direct the content of the discipline. As noted, informatics is primarily concerned with the types of knowledge that can be made explicit and therefore encoded.

Historically, nursing has not had methods by which to encode highly tacit knowledge, presenting an obvious limitation to the completeness with which the content of the discipline can be encoded in computer-based systems. Davenport and Prusak (1998) provided an extensive discussion of this topic. The following definition has become a standard in the field of nursing informatics: Knowledge is information that has been synthesized so that interrelationships are identified and formalized (Graves & Corcoran, 1988). Encoding the formal, organized corpus of data, information, and knowledge that are generated by, made explicit, and derived from research and applied in practice is the focus of this chapter.

It may be noted that recent, promising work in nursing language development and classification has been done by groups such as the North American Nursing Diagnosis Association (NANDA, 2001), Nursing Intervention Classification (NIC) (McCloskey & Bulechek, 2000), and the Nursing Outcomes Classification (NOC) (Johnson, Maas, & Moorhead, 2000). Efforts to promote harmonization and unity across the three tax-onomies have been published (Dochterman & Jones, 2003). Registration of languages from groups such as NANDA, NIC, and NOC in Health Level Seven (HL7) further ensures nursing's adherence to standards that promote inclusion of nursing languages in information systems used to document care across disciplines.

As this work is developing, nonetheless, a second issue remains. Specifying both the nature of concepts and also the relationships among concepts are central to encoding knowledge in computer-based knowledge representation systems. Briefly terminological knowledge concerns the logical representation of the relationships among the attributes of concepts. Attributes are how we define essential features of concepts. Rodgers and

Knafl (2000) provided an extensive discussion of concept analysis and development in relation to nursing knowledge development.

The importance of specifying concepts and the relationships between concepts is not unique to nursing informatics. Of particular importance to nursing is the discussion by Rodgers and Knafl (2000) around the cognitive nature of concepts and the use of language as a way to express concepts. Many writers on nursing theory, research, and knowledge development define concepts as terms. The difference between concepts and terms may appear to be a somewhat subtle. The implications are far reaching not just in building computer-based systems but also in developing the knowledge base of the discipline. Although there is general agreement that concepts and terms are related to describing and representing knowledge, there is less agreement about what that relationship is. Rodgers and Knafl (2000) argued that many problems confronting knowledge development in nursing are in fact conceptual in nature.

> Conceptual problems can be confronted in a variety of ways: confusing terminology or ambivalent word use in attempts to characterize certain situations or phenomena; difficulty synthesizing existing knowledge on a topic, particularly because key concepts have been defined in diverse ways and, often, arbitrarily; problems defining important concepts for research or theory development; problems or questions concerning the origin of a concept and potential change in definition over time; concerns about differences in existing concepts across disciplines that hinder knowledge synthesis, growth, and communication; potential conflicts between concepts and actual situations encountered in nursing; the need for new or more effective concepts to characterize experiences encountered in nursing; and the appropriateness of combining two or more concepts to generate a useful construct. (Rogers and Knafl, 2000, p. 31)

Terminological Knowledge

When encoding terminological knowledge, it is important to define concepts according to logical, subsumptive relationships such as "is_a." "LPN is_a nurse" and "RN is_a nurse." The more specific concepts of LPN and RN are subsumed under the more general concept of "nurse." In other words, the concept is nurse and the axis includes types. Similarly, one can say "Nurse is_a provider," therefore the concepts of LPN, RN, and nurse all inherit the characteristics or attributes of the still more general concept of "provider." Although the concepts of LPN and RN share some attributes, that is, those that enable us to classify both concepts under the more general concept of "nurse," there are other attributes that differentiate the concepts of LPN and RN. Sometimes it is important to retrieve computer-based data related to the more general concept of nurse, other times it will be more important to retrieve data on the more specific concept of LPN or RN. Encoding terminological knowledge enables computers to "know" how the concept of RN is different from the concept of provider. Methods by which to encode terminological, sometimes called definitional knowledge, are the focus of many current research and development initiatives. An example is encoding content of the discipline relevant to the domain knowledge associated with hospital discharge planning, as discussed later in this chapter.

Assertional Knowledge

Assertional knowledge concerns the type of relational statements typically expressed in concept maps and research questions, that is, those that reflect the direction, shape, strength, symmetry, sequencing, probability of occurrence, necessity, and sufficiency of a relationship. Philosophers since the time of Aristotle and Plato have struggled to define not only concepts and knowledge but also the relationships of concepts to knowledge. Reviewing this philosophical legacy in the context of cognitive science, Margolis and Laurence (2000) argued that concepts are mental representations and that the structure of a concept must be robust and theoretically significant. Not all philosophers or cognitive scientists agree with this perspective, but the notion of concepts as mental representations is central to encoding concepts in computer-based systems, as is the notion of expressing knowledge in both terminological and assertional dimensions.

In considering assertions further, for example, the statement that "A higher proportion of hours of nursing care provided by registered nurses and a greater number of hours of care by registered nurses per day are associated with better care for hospitalized patients" is a relational statement (Needleman, Buerhaus, Mattke, Stewart, & Zelevinsky, 2002). In the publication, the authors asserted both statistically and with text the nature of the relationships between the concepts of "better care for hospitalized patients" and "hours of nursing care provided by registered nurses." Both rule-based and statistical approaches to assertional knowledge are well described in the literature on decision support systems. However, the broad implementation of such systems has been limited in large part by the lack of encoded terminological knowledge.

Communicating the Discipline

The third perspective concerns the role of language as a primary mechanism by which we communicate the content of the discipline. Computers cannot process language in the same way as humans. The word *terminology* is used to refer to the specifications that direct how concepts, relationships, and corresponding terms are stored within a database. Taken together, the classification of concepts, logical relationships, and terms provide an ontology that gives direction for the database schema and for the encoding of the content within that database. The benefit of such an approach to structuring computer-based systems is that content of the domain can be expanded or modified within the system as domain knowledge changes. New concepts can be introduced by naming them, defining their attributes, specifying where they fit in the specialization/generalization concept hierarchy, and naming their relationships to other concepts. Standardizing such terminologies will enable data interchange across disparate computer-based systems and applications that are dependent on the indexing and retrieval of concepts.

The Example of Discharge Planning

To illustrate these problems, we will use our work with a discharge planning nurse. Uncovering knowledge embedded in the discharge planning process is critical prior to including it in a clinical information system. The question we were asking was, "What concepts and associated terms would be needed to encode the content of the discipline related to discharge planning so that it can be entered, stored, and retrieved in a computer based system?" How would the system "know it when it sees it"?

Initial Steps in Defining Content and Terminology

As a first step, we looked at the literature for a concept analysis on discharge planning to provide a referent definition of the concept as well as associated expressions, attributes of the concept, and a specification of relationships between discharge planning and other concepts. Despite the proliferation of literature related to discharge planning, we were unable to identify a published concept analysis. In the articles reviewed, discharge planning was inconsistently defined. Further, the definitions stated were rarely specific enough to allow for the identification of attributes of discharge planning as used in a particular article, let alone allow for comparison of whether similar attributes of discharge planning were relevant across articles. Similarly, as we looked for terms that might be associated with selected concepts that could serve as antecedents and consequences of discharge planning (namely, relationships required for expressing assertional knowledge), we encountered the same problem, that is, the use of inconsistent definitions and terminologies.

At this point, it would clearly have been desirable to step back and conduct a systematic, deliberate concept analysis. However, because our primary intent was to identify terms used to represent concepts within the domain of discharge planning knowledge (not just the single concept of discharge planning), we shifted our focus to literature reviews as a method by which we might harvest terms and concepts that would need to be encoded in our information system. Among the articles retrieved was a Cochrane review concerning effective discharge planning (Parkes & Shepperd, 2000). The review included seven English-language articles that became a test set of articles to examine the utility of literature review as a method for identifying terms and concepts within the domain of discharge planning.

Specific Approaches to Identifying Terms and Concepts

Four approaches were used to identify the concepts and terms related to the content domain of discharge planning. Each approach is illustrated.

Meta-analysis

The first type of literature review method considered was meta-analysis. Meta-analysis, is a statistical procedure designed to provide a summary of results across independent studies that address a related set of research questions. It is a central method for Cochrane reviews. Cochrane reviews typically include only randomized controlled trials, based on the perspective that such study designs provide more reliable information than other sources of evidence (www.cochrane.org). Parkes and Shepperd reported that of the 3,098 citations relevant to discharge planning identified at the time of their review, only 8 met the criteria of a randomized and controlled trial. Given the variation in defining discharge planning and outcome measures, only a meta-analysis for effects of discharge planning on length of hospital stay in elderly medical patients could be completed. An example of one result from this meta-analysis was hospital length of stay was slightly reduced for elderly medical patients allocated to discharge planning (weighted mean differences -1.01, 95% CI -2.06 to 0.05).

Based on the meta-analysis, the summary of domain knowledge is useful in understanding the strength of the relationship between an intervention and outcomes as reported across studies. However, this approach provides a different example to discuss identifying domain content that can be encoded in information systems. Meta-analyses only provide a statistical synthesis of domain knowledge. Note that terms from the research findings discussed earlier suggest that concepts relevant to the domain are represented by the phrases "hospital length of stay," "slightly reduced," "elderly medical patients," and "discharge planning." More specific terms and concepts identified by researchers have been classified into more generalized concepts; therefore, terms relevant to specifying the content of the domain are lost. For example, in one study, the discharge planning intervention was implemented by a social worker functioning under a tightly prescribed protocol. In another study, a broad discharge planning and home follow-up program was implemented by advanced practice nurses. However, both processes were subsumed by the Cochrane reviewers into the more general term *discharge planning*. Similarly, in meta-analysis information about attributes of concepts is not preserved nor are terms indicating whether relationships between concepts are antecedents or consequences of discharge planning.

Heuristic Approach to Domain Knowledge

The second approach applied to identify the terms and concepts relevant to the domain of discharge planning has been described by Holzemer and Reilly (1995) as a "heuristic outcomes model that can help one to think through many of the variables that might be related to variations of client, provider, and setting characteristics, as well as to interventions and outcomes" (p. 184). The authors described how a 3 × 3 table constructed with column headings of inputs, process, and outcomes and row headings of client, provider, and setting can serve as a framework for sorting data. It provided a heuristic for specifying variables for inclusion in information systems. By filling in the cells of the table, the authors suggested that designers and implementers of information systems are able to make explicit links within the information system infrastructure. In this way, variations research can be advanced.

The approach to specifying concepts and relationships that Holzemer and Reilly described seemed relevant to solving the problem of encoding the domain knowledge of the discharge planning process and including it in a clinical information system. The seven articles used in the Cochrane review served as a source of variables identification. The model by Holzemer and Reilly offered several advantages over meta-analysis. Terms and concepts identified by researchers were represented in lists and additionally were classified as structure, process, or outcome variables, giving enhanced meaning. Terms used by each researcher to represent concepts were all preserved with no loss of terms and concepts. If a term such as *social worker implementation* was used, it was recorded and was not subsumed under the broader term of *discharge planning*. Relationships among variables were suggested depending on the cell in which the variable was placed; however, the nature of those relationships was not preserved. As with meta-analysis, attributes of concepts are not specified in this approach. This leaves the issue of the concept being refined to have a given meaning.

Integrative Review

Another approach to synthesizing domain knowledge is integrative review. Stetler and colleagues (1998) described a method for conducting an integrative review that emphasizes evaluation of the literature for its utility in clinical practice. These authors argued that among the limitations of other literature review methods, including meta-analysis, are "lack of a cohesive organization of findings around applicable but distinctly separate aspects of a concept," "lack of sufficient operational detail," and "nonspecific implications for practice" (p. 196).

The method described by Stetler and colleagues requires that two tables be developed when conducting a literature review. The first table focuses on methodological factors and lists purpose plus hypotheses or questions, measurement/operational definition of independent and dependent variables, sampling, design, and level of evidence. A second table is created to include utilization factors such as findings, fit, unknown factors relevant to practice problem, feasibility: risk, and feasibility: resources/costs/readiness.

Stetler's approach to identifying relevant concepts and terms provided advantages over both meta-analysis and Holzemer and Reilly's framework. Specifically, Stetler addresses the nature of relationships between concepts as specified in a text format within the findings column of the table. The attributes of concepts can be suggested in the methodology table columns in which operational definitions of variables within the study were recorded. Using this approach, it became readily apparent whether two studies using the term discharge planning were actually referring to the same concept. The generalization was made that the operational definitions were the same, the concepts were the same.

Software Approach

The final approach to identifying terms and concepts relevant to representing the content of the domain was arcs©. This is a computer software program that provides a methodology for storing, retrieving, aggregating, and graphically modeling assertional knowledge (Graves, 1990). Similar to the integrative review method described by Stetler, this software enabled us to record the full complement of terms and relationships used by the researchers, as well as the statistical relationships reported in the study. In addition, a concept map can be generated that graphically displays the concepts and relationships among concepts as well as color coding the direction and strength of those relationships reflected in the statistical analyses reported within each study.

Because arcs© follows the logic and common representation of assertional knowledge in a discipline, it is useful for making explicit the gaps and conflicts in the domain knowledge. If fully populated, such a database could potentially serve as a real-time resource for evidence-based practice support within clinical information systems. Using arcs©, we were also able to build a classification (e.g., social worker protocol as a type of discharge planning) that begins to get at the type of subsumptive relationships that must be expressed in order to inference terminological knowledge.

Summary

Table 3.1 summarizes the four approaches used to analyze the literature in relation to the need for specified terms, concepts, attributes, and relationships required to encode domain knowledge. Using these strategies, five terms were used to represent the concepts associated with independent variables in the seven articles reviewed. That is, five types of discharge planning interventions were described. In addition, 42 terms were used to represent concepts associated with the dependent variables.

Only one of the terms, discharge planning, could be directly mapped to a nursing terminology; the Nursing Interventions Classification (McCloskey & Bulechek, 2000) includes a coded intervention label of "discharge planning." As in the meta-analysis example cited earlier, if only a classification of the five types of discharge planning interventions is included in an information system, important information will be lost. Aggregation of knowledge in a field is complementary to but different than preserving the detail required to integrate content into an information system. There is a need to systematically identify and encode the knowledge suggested in the research literature. The notion of a research terminology, constructed from variables, conditions of the study, and the terms used in the research processes, has been proposed and a prototype method by which to harvest terms associated with research is maintained by Sigma Theta Tau International (Graves, 1999).

The challenges presented around encoding knowledge using terminological data are not unique to nursing. Although the rapid development and deployment of newer computer-based technologies have made a national health information infrastructure a possibility, terminology is widely recognized as one of the most significant barriers

Table 3.1	A Comparison of Literature Review Approaches to Requirements for Representing Domain Knowledge		
	Terms Represent Concepts	Attributes Specified	Relationships Specified
Meta-analysis	Terms represent a classification of concepts used by researcher	No	Statistical
Outcomes framework	As specified by researcher	No	Implied based on location in framework, nature of relationship not retained
Utilization-focused integrative review	As specified by researcher	Yes	Textual and statistical reporting
arcs© knowledge modeling software	As specified by researcher and as reviewer chooses to classify	Yes	Textual and statistical reporting and graphically modeled

to the electronic exchange of data (National Committee on Vital and Health Statistics [NCVHS], 2001).

Conclusion

Encoding explicit domain knowledge in clinical information systems is essential if the perspectives and content of the discipline are to be evident in such systems. A limited example of issues arising around terminologies has been presented. The intent is not to provide an overview of existing clinical terminologies nor of the state of the research in discharge planning. Rather the example illustrates the need to bring together clinical coding schemes and the concepts and terms used in the research literature. Terminology provides a critical interface between two sources of domain knowledge: practice and research. Participation in terminology initiatives is a task that should engage all who have a stake in the discipline. Taxonomies used to practice can make explicit the concepts and relationships most relevant in given practice areas. In this way the content of the discipline can be encoded for use in information systems.

REFERENCES

American Nurses Association. (1995 & 2002, June). *Nursing: Scope and standards of practice*. Washington, DC: American Nurses Association.

American Nurses Association. (2002, June). *Standards of practice and performance*. Washington, DC: American Nurses Association.

Davenport, T. H., & Prusak, L. (1998). *Working knowledge*. Boston, MA: Harvard Business School Press.

Dochterman, J. M., & Jones, D. A. (Eds.). (2003). *Unifying nursing languages: The harmonization of NANDA, NIC and NOC*. Washington, DC: American Nurses Association.

Gordon, M. (1998, Sept. 30). Nursing nomenclature and classification system development. *Online Journal of Issues in Nursing*.

Graves, J. R. (1990). A research-knowledge system (ARKS) for storing, managing, and modeling knowledge from the scientific literature. *ANS–Advances in Nursing Science*, *13*(2), 34–45.

Graves, J. R. (1999). *Directory of nurse researchers and the new research vocabulary of nursing*. Retrieved September 21, 2002, from http://www.stti.iupui.edu/library/dnr.html.

Graves, J. R., & Corcoran, S. (1988). Design of nursing information systems: Conceptual and practice elements. *Journal of Professional Nursing, 4*, 168–177.

Harris, M. R., Graves, J. R., Solbrig, H. R., Elkin, P. L., & Chute, C. G. (2000). Embedded structures and representation of nursing knowledge. *JAMIA–Journal of the American Medical Informatics Association, 7*(6), 539–549.

Holzemer, W. L., & Reilly, C. A. (1995). Variables, variability, and variations research: Implications for medical informatics. *JAMIA–Journal of the American Medical Informatics Association, 2*(3), 183–190.

Johnson, M., Bulechek, G., Maas, M., McCloskey Dochterman, J., & Moorhead, S. (2001). *Linking nursing diagnosis, interventions and outcomes*. St. Louis, MO: Mosby.

Johnson, M., Maas, M., & Moorhead, S. (Eds.). (2000). *Nursing outcomes classification (NOC)* (2nd ed.). St. Louis, MO: Mosby.

Margolis, E., & Laurence, S. (2000). *Concepts: Core readings*. Cambridge, MA: MIT Press.

McCloskey, J. C., & Bulechek, G. M. (2000). *Nursing interventions classification* (3rd ed.). St. Louis, MO: Mosby.

Meleis, A. I. (1997). Theoretical perspectives. In A. I. Meleis (Ed.), *Theoretical nursing: Development and progress* (pp. 93–101). Philadelphia: Lippincott-Raven.

National Committee on Vital and Health Statistics (NCVHS). (2001). *Information for health, a strategy for building the national health information infrastructure*. Retrieved September 21, 2002, from http://www.health.gov/ncvhs-nhii/.

Needleman, J., Buerhaus, P., Mattke, S., Steward, M., & Zelevinsky, K. (2002). Nurse-staffing levels and the quality of care in hospitals. *New England Journal of Medicine, 346*(22), 1715–1722.

North American Nursing Diagnosis Association (NANDA), (2001). *Nursing diagnoses: Definitions and classification 2000–2001*. Philadelphia: NANDA.

Parkes, J., & Shepperd, S. (2000). Discharge planning from hospital to home. *The Cochrane Database of Systematic Reviews*, Issue 3. Retrieved September 5, 2002, from http://www.cochrane.org.

Rodgers, B. L., & Knafl, K. A. (2000). *Concept development in nursing* (2nd ed.). Philadelphia: W. B. Saunders.

Stetler, C. B., Morsi, D., Rucki, S., Broughton, S., Corrigan, B., Fitzgerald, J., et al. (1998). Utilization-focused integrative reviews in a nursing service. *Applied Nursing Research, 11*(4), 195–206.

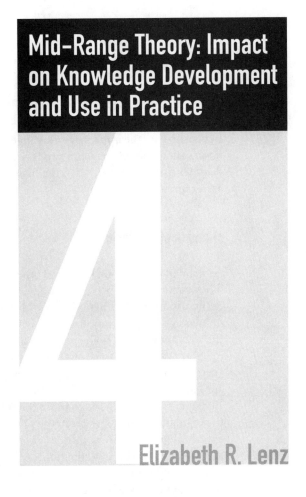

Mid-Range Theory: Impact on Knowledge Development and Use in Practice

Elizabeth R. Lenz

C. Wright Mills introduced the idea of middle-range theory to sociology in the 1940s, and Merton (1968) energized it in the 1960s. It was not until the 1980s that nursing gave substantial attention to middle-range theory. Dissatisfaction with the inability of nursing's grand theories to serve as useful guides to research and practice led a number of metatheorists to advocate using and/or developing theories that were less abstract and global. In 1992 at a doctoral forum, Suppe (1992) argued that nursing had matured beyond the need for its grand theories and should be focusing on theories of the middle range. He recommended that the grand theories be taught with emphasis on their contribution to the historical development of the discipline. Further, he recommended that the theoretical emphasis at the doctoral level should focus exclusively on mid-range theories as a useful basis for research and practice.

Since that time, nursing theory development has indeed shifted considerably in the direction Suppe recommended. Although we can point to a flurry of recent activity around mid-range theory in nursing, the jury is still out regarding the impact of that activity. In this chapter, I provide first a brief introduction to mid-range theories and their hypothetical roles in research and practice, then give an update about the generation

61

and use of mid-range theories, and finally offer a discussion of some of the challenges that face us in the coming decade if their potential is to be realized.

Background and Early Uses of Mid-Range Theory

In considering the impact of mid-range theory on knowledge development, some general observations can be made on two levels. First, the definitional concerns that nursing has dealt with are noted and then the historical role and use of mid-range theory in nursing are examined.

Meaning of the Term

As defined by Merton (1968) and others, middle-range theories are just that, mid-range. They stand midway between the all-encompassing global grand theories that address the entire discipline and hypotheses and theories that are very specific to a particular phenomenon or population. At least hypothetically, the scope and abstraction of mid-range theories should have some very real advantages. For example, they are sufficiently close to observable reality to be testable. In fact, a defining characteristic of mid-range theories, according to Suppe (1992), is that they postulate relationships between descriptors that are measurable or objectively codable. On the other hand, mid-range theories are sufficiently abstract and broad to fulfill the role of theory to allow us to identify and "capture" the regularities and patterns in the phenomena with which we deal, and to recognize and explain departures from those regularities. These theories allow us to stop reinventing the wheel with each investigation.

It is necessary to observe, however, that theories that are labeled middle-range by their developers and others often differ considerably from one another in scope and level of abstraction. Consider, for example, the differences among Polk's (1997) middle-range theory of resilience, Mishel's (1988, 1990) middle-range theory of uncertainty in illness, and Auvil-Novak's (1997) middle-range theory of chronotherapeutic intervention for postsurgical pain. The resilience theory is very abstract and applies to individuals who are facing any kind of disaster or catastrophic loss and are successfully transcending that adversity. It is not limited to illness situations. The uncertainty theory is sufficiently generic to be used in a variety of chronic and even acute illness situations and even to describe and to help design interventions for normal life changes, such as menopause. Both resilience and uncertainty theories are essentially descriptive. Although they suggest variables that may be important to consider in designing interventions, they are not prescriptive. On the other hand, the theory of chronotherapeutic intervention for postsurgical pain is much more specific, being applicable to pain in a particular context. It was developed as the basis for designing postoperative patient-controlled analgesia interventions and is essentially prescriptive. As a result, it has considerable potential for direct application in practice, whereas the other mid-range theories require some additional steps to develop applications.

The point is not to determine that one of these theories is any more valuable or useful than another, but simply to point out that there is considerable variability in what is labeled a mid-range theory. Liehr and Smith (1999) suggested that it may be useful to divide middle-range theory into three different levels (high middle, middle, and low middle). This kind of differential labeling may highlight differences among middle-range theories, but it accomplishes little unless it helps the potential user identify differences in the ways various theories can most appropriately be tested and used.

Liehr and Smith noted that as the last decade progressed, authors seemed more and more willing to label their theoretical products as middle range theories. This may place the term at risk for becoming a catch-all label. Conversely, some theories that would easily meet the criteria for mid-range have not necessarily been labeled as such. These terminological inconsistencies are problematic if they encourage us to ignore the contributions of some theoretical products or to treat as identical theories whose scope and function should be differentiated. Most scholars who write about middle-range theories have taken the easy way out and considered as middle range those works that are labeled as such by their authors. Given the inconsistencies, it may behoove us to be more discerning in the future and to apply accepted criteria.

With the exception of Meleis (Im & Meleis 1999), until very recently, few meta-theorists have acknowledged the existence of specific theories that are narrower in scope than middle range. In actuality, some theories labeled middle range might more appropriately be considered specific because they do not apply across clinical populations but are highly specific to a particular population or aspect of a phenomenon. Generally quite pragmatic, specific theories deserve more attention. This is the case because they are products that are intermediate in the development of more abstract and general theories and as guides to practice with specific clinical problems.

History of Mid-Range Theories in Research and Practice

Before considering the roles that mid-range theories are currently playing in nursing research and practice, it would be well to acknowledge what metatheorists believe these roles should be. Suppe (1996) has stated that middle range theories play three major roles in relation to research: (a) as frameworks to guide the nature of research to be conducted, including the questions that need to be answered and the design of the research needed to answer them; (b) as objects to be tested by research; and (c) as end products of theoretical thinking that serve to summarize and integrate nursing knowledge. The first two roles incorporate deductive thinking that moves from the theory to deduced hypotheses that are tested through empirical observation. The third role involves induction, that is, from observation to theory. In the first two roles, the theory is the starting point that drives the design of the research, and in the third instance, the theory is the product. Ultimately, the three roles are intertwined in a kind of circular relationship to one another. Observations are clustered together and similarities identified as empirical generalizations. These in turn are integrated into theories, from which are deduced hypotheses that can be tested by thorough empirical investigations.

The role of mid-range theories for practice has been less fully explicated. As with research, a reciprocal relationship is posited. Problems encountered and observations made in the practice arena give rise to the identification of themes and commonalities and generalizations, which may be summarized or explained theoretically. The theories or models so generated stimulate theoretical thinking and can serve as the starting point for what Kim (1996) termed the *theory primary approach to development*. Reciprocally, theories clearly have the potential to guide practice. They can provide either general approaches or more specific guidelines for practice, including the identification of at-risk populations or those that are particularly good candidates for particular therapies. Finally, theories can direct the design of specific preventive or therapeutic interventions.

Analysis of Use in Research

In a pair of papers published in 1998 (written in 1997), I examined the extent to which these hypothetical roles of mid-range theories in practice and research were being enacted at that time (Lenz, 1998a, 1998b). To summarize briefly, the theory-practice relationship was well established and receiving considerable attention in the literature. There was ample evidence then that mid-range theories were being produced as direct and indirect end products of research efforts. By direct end products I mean theories that are built on the basis of qualitative or quantitative research by the theory developer. The prime examples are theories that result from grounded theory studies, from empirically grounded concept development activities, and from integrating the results of several related studies into a synthetic model or theory. By indirect end products, I refer to theories that are built inductively from the published research of others, for example, a path model. However, it was apparent that some middle-range theories were being developed without any explicit reference to research. Rather the theorist used techniques such as deduction from a grand theory in nursing or another discipline, or derivation from a single or a combination of middle-range theories in nursing or another field.

In another analysis of the mid-range theories published by nurses between 1988 and 1998, Liehr and Smith (1999) found that the most common approach to mid-range theory building was induction through research (14 of 25) or from empirically based practice guidelines (3). Fewer of the theories were deduced from grand nursing theories (3) or derived from theories of other disciplines (4).

As for the role of theory in providing the basis for asking and answering research questions, I found that the results were mixed (see Lenz, 1998a, 1998b). It was clear that a few mid-range theories by prolific authors with many graduate students and productive research teams had exerted a major influence on nursing research. They spawned a variety of studies, the results of which then informed further work on the theory. More theories essentially stood alone as relatively isolated products; they were not cited as the basis for published research, even by their developers. A review of 3 ½ years of the journal *Nursing Research* was consistent with earlier analyses of the theoretical basis for nursing's research literature. More than half of the articles cited no theoretical basis. Where a theory was cited as foundational, it was most likely to be one generated outside of nursing, likely in a behavioral science discipline.

Influence on Practice

The influence of mid-range theory on practice was not particularly well developed. The practice-theory relationship was described to be analogous to that of the research-theory relationship, in the sense that it was depicted as potentially reciprocal. Just as the practice arena stimulates thinking about researchable questions, it also generates theoretical thinking that is needed to help explain clinical phenomena and anomalies and to help solve problems. Practice problems can serve as the starting point for the theory primacy approach to theory development. Additionally, practice guidelines and standards have been used in a few instances as the basis for mid-range theory development.

Reciprocally, theories clearly have the potential to guide practice. The notion of prescriptive practice theories providing the basis for practice is hardly a new one. However, the influence of middle-range theory on practice is not particularly evident in the literature. At the time of my analysis of the use of theories in practice (Lenz, 1998b), there was rhetoric in the literature advocating it but less evidence that it had occurred. Where described in the literature, the relationship of theory to practice was focused on the grand theories rather than theories of the middle range. When the latter were discussed, they tended to be theories from other disciplines. Moreover, rather than a common core of theories that were drawn upon across practice realms, there understandably seemed to be specialty-specific patterns. A select few of the theories, such as Lazarus and Folkman's (1984) stress and coping theory, were used more generally and were familiar to clinicians in a variety of specialties. Given this exception, the use of most theories was specialty-specific. Practicing clinicians generally believed that their practice was atheoretical until pressed to identify the theoretical ideas that they relied upon. When so pressed, nurses could name one or two mid-range theories.

Trends Summarized

As analyzed in 1997–1998, several trends were apparent: (a) increasing interest in middle range theories and in generating them, (b) inconsistent influence by nurse-developed middle-range theories on nursing research, (c) heavier reliance on mid-range than grand theories as the basis for research but more acknowledged use of grand theories in practice, (d) a lack of evaluation of middle-range theories, including infrequent testing and even less frequent modification, and (e) a persistent pattern of failing explicitly to link one's research and practice to a theoretical foundation. At that point, I expressed guarded optimism that the situation would improve as the discipline began to embrace mid-range theories as the appropriate level for emphasis. So now—nearly 10 years later—what if anything has changed?

Current Patterns

The following discussion focuses on the role of mid-range theory in nursing. Theory generation is examined and the specific theories used in research are identified. Use of theory in practice is then addressed.

Theory Generation

Middle-range theories have been a growing focus in the metatheoretical and theoretical literature of the discipline. General theory texts, once devoted exclusively to metatheory and grand theories, have been modified to include middle-range theories, and new texts have been dedicated exclusively to them. Smith and Liehr's (2003) is an example.

Several new theories have appeared in the literature in recent years. However, the production of new middle-range theories seems to have peaked between 1996 and 1998 and appears to be tapering off but clearly not stopping. Liehr and Smith (1999) noted that the peak in production of mid-range theories in 1997 could have been the result of an issue of *Advances in Nursing Science* (ANS) having been dedicated to the topic. Their review of 10 years of nursing literature as searched in CINAHL revealed 22 theories published between 1988 and 1998. They also noted an increased willingness to label theoretical products as middle-range theories. This, in itself, may help feed the perception that the number of such theories is increasing.

Strategies for Mid-Range Theory Generation

Examples of recently published middle-range theories are listed in Table 4.1 along with the variety of strategies used in their development.

As was the case in the 1997 analysis, a common research-based theory development activity was to develop an explanatory or predictive model based on a summary of the literature. This was depicted as a diagram, tested using path analysis or LISREL, and then the author presented the revised version of the middle-range theory as the product. Examples include Richmond's (1997) model of postinjury disability and Riegel, Dracup, and Glaser's (1998) causal model of cardiac invalidism.

To a greater extent than I observed in my earlier analysis, several of the recent middle-range theories were derivatives of more global nursing theories. For example, Acton (1997) derived a theory of affiliated individuation as a mediator of stress from Erikson, Tomlin and Swain's (1990) modeling and role modeling theory. Jirovec and colleagues (1999) derived a urine control theory from Roy's (Roy & Andrews, 1991) conceptual framework. Olson and Hanchett (1997) derived propositions for an unnamed middle-range theory linking nurse-expressed empathy and patient distress and patient-perceived empathy. The propositions were deduced from Orlando's (1961) nursing model and tested empirically. Algase and colleagues (1996) based their theory of need-driven dementia-compromised behavior on Nightingale's (1969) conceptualization of the environment. August-Brady's (2000) critical analysis of prevention as intervention looked at work derived from the Neuman Systems Model (1995). The studies were described as "flowing from" and "structurally consistent with systems theory" (p. 1304).

Another pattern is that the considerable increase in publications reporting the results of qualitative research has not really been matched by a concomitant increase in mid-range theories developed inductively from qualitative studies. The end products of many qualitative studies have been lists of themes identified from the data, rather than coherent well-articulated theories. There are exceptions, of course. For example, Eakes, Burke, and Hainsworth (1998) developed the middle-range theory of chronic sorrow from 10 qualitative studies concerning various situations.

Concept Analysis and Mid-range Theory

A prevalent pattern, which was also apparent in the earlier analysis, is that considerable theoretical work seems to be occurring at the concept level. The literature contains more and more evidence of concept analyses and concept development activity. Regrettably, relatively little of this work is empirically based, and much of it is preliminary and relatively unsophisticated. The majority of the reports rely on analyses of existing literature using Wilsonian methods, and the results vary widely in their quality and potential contribution (Hupcey, Morse, Lenz, & Tason, 1996).

Table 4.1

Current Mid-Range Theories Identified

Author(s) Date	Content of Mid-range Theory	Source for Generation
Im and Meleis (1999); Meleis, Sawyer, Im, Messias, and Schumacher (2000)	Meleis's theory of experiencing transitions	Developed from the results of five different research studies that have examined transitions using an integrative approach to theory development
Smith and Liehr (1999)	Theory of attentively embracing story	Emerged in the context of the neomodernist and simultaneity paradigms as the authors shared situations in practice and research and linked these encounters to the story literature
Eakes, Burke, and Hainsworth (1998)	Theory of chronic sorrow	Derived through a series of studies and a critical review of existing research
Good (1998)	Theory of acute pain management	Developed from AHCPR guidelines for pain management
Stuifbergen and Rogers (1997); Stuifbergen, Seraphin, and Roberts (2000)	Explanatory model of health promotion in chronic disability	Generated from the literature and through research
Flaskerud and Winslow (1998)	Conceptualization of vulnerable populations	Generated from the literature and through research
Duckett et al. (1998)	Planned behavior-based structural model for breast-feeding	Simultaneous multisample analysis of covariance structures was used to develop the model
Richmond (1997)	Model of postinjury disability	Generated from the literature and through research
Riegel, Dracup, and Glaser (1998)	Causal model of cardiac invalidism	Generated from the literature and through research
Acton (1997)	Theory of affiliated individuation as a mediator of stress	Derived from Erickson, Tomlin, and Swain's (1983) Global Modeling and Role Modeling Theory
Jirovec, Jenkins, Isenberg, and Barardi (1999)	A urine control theory	Derived from Roy's (Roy & Andrews, 1991) conceptual framework
Olson and Hanchett (1997)	An unnamed middle-range theory linking nurse-expressed empathy and patient distress and patient-perceived empathy	Propositions were deduced from Orlando's (1961) nursing model and tested empirically
Algase et al. (1996)	Theory of need-driven dementia–compromised behavior	Based on Nightingale's (1969) conceptualization of the environment
August-Brady (2000)	Theory of prevention as intervention	Based on Neuman's (1995) systems model and more broadly from systems theory

The pervasive concept-level focus that currently seems to be dominating the theoretical literature has pros and cons. On the positive side, conceptual clarity is a necessary underpinning for theory development and also serves as a vital step in measurement. Unfortunately, some concept analyses published in the nursing literature seem to obfuscate rather than to clarify and reflect badly on the entire enterprise. Concept-level work is potentially both interesting and illuminating and can have considerable heuristic value. However, if it never is taken further than an initial analysis, its potential value is severely truncated. With some notable exceptions, concept development activity has not been particularly cumulative within the discipline. Only rarely does theoretical work with a concept reflect continuing refinement and validation. This is the case even though Morse, Hupcey, Mitcham, and Lenz (1996) suggested that concepts can be at many different stages of development, each calling for a different type of empirical study and theoretical communication. With notable exceptions, for example, work by scholars such as Mishel and Morse and their respective colleagues, shows little evidence that concept development has gone on to pave the way for subsequent development of middle-range theories.

Summary of Patterns of Generation

Finally, as was the case in the earlier review, there is little evidence that developers of mid-range theories are continuing to work on them once they are published. Liehr and Smith (1999) observed that the Theory of Unpleasant Symptoms (Lenz, Pugh, Milligan, Gift, & Suppe, 1997; Lenz, Suppe, Gift, Pugh, & Milligan, 1995) was the only one they examined to have undergone "documented, ongoing development in the past decade" (p. 83). Analyses and critiques of existing mid-range theories by persons other than the developers are occasionally published. Cooley's (1999) analysis and evaluation of Corbin and Strauss's (1991) Trajectory Theory of Chronic Illness Management is an example.

Extent of Use of Mid-Range Theories in Research

The most important way that middle-range theories can impact nursing research is to serve as the basis or stimulus for studies. As noted, the mid-1997 analysis of studies published in *Nursing Research* revealed that the majority cited no theoretical basis and of those that did, mid-range theories from the behavioral sciences more commonly provided underpinnings than did nurse-generated theories. Given the emphasis on mid-range theories in the nursing literature during the recent years, it was reasonable to anticipate an increase in their role as the basis for studies during that time. To determine whether there had, in fact, been any change in the theory citation patterns, I repeated the analysis, examining the studies published in *Nursing Research* during the 4-year time period from July 1997 through December 2000. A total of 127 articles were examined. I systematically excluded those from the methodology section of the journal but did include briefs. My findings can be summarized as follows:

1 As was true in the earlier analysis, a majority of the articles cited no theoretical basis for the hypotheses tested or research questions asked.

2 The most prevalent pattern (in 59% of the articles) was to base the current study on a compilation of previous research findings, with no mention of a specific theory or theoretical perspective.

3 In a few instances (9.5% articles), a theoretical explanation was provided as the basis for the research, but no theories were identified or named.

Concerns About Theory-Based Research

In one sense, the failure to base research on theory, or at least to cite the theoretical heritage of the work, was not necessarily surprising. In *Nursing Research* a relatively high percentage of studies have a biobehavioral or physiological emphasis, and reports of such studies often are not explicitly linked to a theory base, but to empirical work. Likewise, reports of the effectiveness of various procedures, such as use of sandbags postangiography and the duration of scrubs, are generally presented without theoretical underpinnings described. However, the pattern was troubling for a couple of reasons.

First, in several of the articles no theoretical credit was given despite the existence of a well-known and documented theory base underpinning the topic. Examples include studies about quality of life, parenting and maternal-infant interaction, self-care, and unpleasant symptoms. The failure to acknowledge the existence of theoretical underpinnings for an area of research leads one to wonder whether the authors were simply unaware of the theoretical heritage for their work, and consequently did not recognize links that actually were there, or were indeed aware of the theoretical underpinnings for the field, but simply failed to acknowledge them because it was deemed unimportant or unnecessary. In either case, the discipline suffers from the failure to make clear the cumulative nature of the science and the links of today's research to extant theory.

Second, a number of articles reporting the development and testing of measurement instruments cited no theory base, nor any explicit conceptualization upon which instrumentation was built. Clear conceptualization is the basis for adequate instrumentation. Failure to explicate the underlying conceptualization of the phenomenon to be measured makes it virtually impossible to assess the construct validity of the tool, to interpret the scores on the instrument, or to judge its degree of fit to the chosen conceptualization of the phenomenon.

It is quite possible that my choice of journals to examine is yielding an artificially low percentage of theoretically based articles because of its particular emphasis on biobehavioral research and page limits. A more comprehensive analysis of the research literature is clearly needed.

Use of Psychosocial Theories

As was the case in 1997, well-known middle-range theories from the psychosocial disciplines influenced nursing studies. This was true in 20% of the reports reviewed. The particular psychosocial theories identified are listed in Table 4.2. Most frequently cited were Lazarus and Folkman's (1984) coping theory and Bandura's (1986) social cognitive and self-efficacy theories. Other theories were as broad as Bass's (1985) leadership model and as specific as Marlatt's (1985) model of relapse prevention. In one or two instances, the authors of current studies reported basing their research on a combination of theories. For example, Richmond (1997) developed and tested a model based on three different

Use of Psychosocial Theories in Nursing Research	
Author(s)/Date	Content of Theory
Lazarus and Folkman (1984)	Coping theory (cited six times)
Bandura (1986)	Social cognitive and self-efficacy theories (cited four times)
Ajzen (1985, 1987)	Planned behavior and reasoned action theories
Aday and Anderson (1974)	Framework for access to health care
Bass (1985)	Leadership model
Cicchetti (1989)	Transactional model of child abuse
Thoits (1986)	Conceptualization of social support
Belsky (1984)	Model of parenting
Rolland (1994)	Family system–illness model
Marlatt (1985)	Model of relapse prevention
Winick (1974)	Drug dependence model
John (1988) and Glaser (1987)	Adult learning theories
Nagi (1991)	Theory of the disabling process
Horowitz (1986)	Theory of posttraumatic stress
Sarason, Shearin, Peirce, and Sarason (1987)	Model of social support perceptions

models or theories of variables influencing postinjury disability. These included Nagi's (1991) theory of the disabling process, Horowitz's (1986) theory of posttraumatic stress, and Sarason, Shearin, Peirce and Sarason's (1987) model of social support perceptions. An observation worthy of note is that all of these theories are at least 15 years old.

Some investigators credited the basis of their studies to broadly defined theoretical perspectives that were not tied explicitly to a given theorist or theory. These included the "public health model," used as the basis for an early intervention program, "epidemiology," "classic psychosomatic hypotheses," and "models of self concept," only one of which was actually cited. When this broadly sketched approach is used, it is difficult to ascertain exactly what is meant, let alone critically evaluate the appropriateness of the theory or interpret the results in light of the theory base.

Mid-Range Nursing Theories and Research

Nursing theories provided the basis for only 9.5% of the studies and all but one were based on theories of the middle range. They included Corbin and Strauss's (1992) illness trajectory model, Pender's (1996) health promotion model, Piper's fatigue model (Piper, Lindsey, & Dodd, 1987), Brooten and colleagues' (1988) quality-cost framework, Pollock's (1986) stress-adaptation model, Smith's (1999) caregiving effectiveness model, Benner's (2001) skill acquisition model, Swanson's (1991) caring theory, Nyamathi's (1989) comprehensive health seeking and coping paradigm, and Hall and Buckwalter's (1987) conceptual model for the care of patients with Alzheimer's disease.

It may be noted that one book on the analysis and synthesis of research based on one grand theory was published in 1999 (BBARNS). The analysis includes 163 studies published between 1970 and 1994. Of the research evaluation, 116 studies met the criteria of links to the grand theory and scientific soundness and were used to test the 12 generic propositions of the model. The findings of each study were described as supporting or not supporting ancillary (that is, middle-range) and practice-level propositions.

Conceptualizations or concept analyses, rather than fully developed theories were also cited. For example, authors referred to Ketefian's (1981) conceptualization of moral reasoning and Flaskerud and Winslow's (1998) conceptualization of vulnerability. One of the interesting developments has been the use of nursing classifications as the theoretical basis for research. The NANDA classification was cited as the theoretical basis for a study carried out to validate diagnoses; similarly the NANDA-NIC-NOC connection has been referred to in some intervention and outcome studies. Practice guidelines were also used as the theoretical basis for a middle-range theory that informed a study of pain management (Good, 1998)

Patterns Summarized

Some patterns worthy of note are the following: (a) the nursing theories tended to be newer than the psychosocial theories, (b) at least three were identified as influential in the previous (1997) analysis, (c) most were by relatively well-known, often-cited scholars who over the years have made multiple contributions to the literature and have mentored many doctoral students, and (d) there was a limited tendency to combine nurse-generated theories with those generated by other disciplines. These patterns are consistent with the results of the earlier analysis. One observation is that some of the most frequently cited theories identified previously, for example, Mishel's (1988) middle-range theory of uncertainty in illness, were cited much less frequently as the basis for research published in *Nursing Research*. The role of these middle-range theories in influencing research published elsewhere was not ascertained.

Consistent with the previous analysis, self-citation was a common pattern. In one article, the author cited her own theory as the basis for the current study (a common practice in all disciplines), but had a total of 12 self-citations in the same article. Another article included 8 self-citations in addition to the theory.

One role of theory is as the end product of research endeavors. There was evidence that theory development is being carried out. The most commonly depicted end product was an explanatory or predictive model that could be represented by a diagram. In some instances, the research being reported had tested a model generated from the literature, and the model was then revised. Examples included Richmond's (1997) model of postinjury disability and Riegel, Dracup, and Glaser's (1998) causal model of cardiac invalidism. Other theoretical products that could be labeled mid-range theories included Stuifbergen's (Stuifbergen & Rogers, 1997; Stuifbergen, Seraphin, & Roberts, 2000) explanatory model of health promotion in chronic disability, Flaskerud and Winslow's (1998) conceptualization of vulnerable populations, and Duckett and colleagues' (1998) planned behavior-based structural model for breast-feeding. The Stuifbergen model was applied in more than one study by the author, but there was no evidence that the others—admittedly quite recent—have yet influenced the published literature of the field.

It was disappointing that there were so few theories that were generated from qualitative research. Surely that is one of the research strategy's most promising potentials. Although themes are typically identified, there is a general failure to try to weave the themes into a theory.

Impact of Mid-Range Theories on Nursing Practice

There was little evidence in the literature that theory-based practice has become any more viable a notion recently than was the case in the past. Although articles reporting the application of grand theory in practice continue to be published, mid-range theories are rarely cited in the general literature and in any specialty literature other than psychiatric and maternal-child nursing. An occasional intervention study claims to be theory based, but often the specific theories are not named.

On the other hand, a very real change in the recent years has been a tremendous upswing in references to evidence-based practice. The phrase has become a buzzword, it seems. There is clearly nothing wrong with evidence. However, it is of some concern that the evidence that is cumulating is not being systematically examined for its commonalities and summarized by empirical generalizations, let alone studied from the perspective of its theoretical implications. Theory is, after all, an effective and efficient way to summarize and integrate results of multiple studies and to move the findings to a more abstract level that can be applied across clinical situations. Theory can help with explaining what is happening, with designing effective interventions, and with predicting what will occur. It can serve as a heuristic reminder of the various aspects of a clinical phenomenon that need to be taken into account. Particularly middle-range theory, if appropriately generated and tested, can serve as a very viable resource for the practicing nurse, yet, it seems to be forgotten in the flurry to base practice on evidence.

It is curious to me that when expert nurses practice, they base their actions on evidence that they have gleaned over a variety of experiences, both direct and indirect. They use analogous thinking to extrapolate from one situation to another and make their clinical judgments accordingly. On the other hand, students who are contemplating the study of a particular phenomenon will often argue that they must, in essence, reinvent the wheel, because no one has studied that very specific clinical population or situation previously. They seem unwilling to generalize from what is already known about the phenomenon in similar populations. In other words, they seem unwilling to carry out theoretical thinking. What's the problem? Lack of practice is likely one aspect. Today's nursing education in many instances is very much oriented to technical skills, and graduate education for advanced nursing practice is guided considerably by the medical model. There is precious little time to think about theorizing or to entertain alternative world views.

Implications and Recommendations

What is the bottom line regarding the impact of mid-range theory on nursing research and practice? Basically, the impact seems to be relatively limited. Disappointingly little progress was evident in the 5 years since the last analysis. The majority of research reports continue to neglect admitting that theory had a role. Where acknowledged, there is continued heavy reliance on somewhat outdated psychosocial theories and relatively less on nursing theories. Where nursing theories are guiding research, they tend to be middle range, rather than grand in scope, and also tend to be the works of productive scholars whose reputation is well established in the discipline. Nevertheless, the majority of research reports do not report that the research was grounded in any theory base at all.

Likewise, the practice world seems to be relying very heavily on evidence, but little attention is being given to the relationships of that evidence to theory. The benefit of mid-range theories is their proximity to and congruence with evidence generated in the practice situation. Unfortunately, they are not being used with great frequency, nor is attention being paid to developing them from the evidence that is currently being accrued to direct practice. The considerable promise held out by the growing attention to mid-range theory by the metatheorists has not been realized as yet.

How can the issues identified be improved? The following recommendations are made to improve the state of the art of the use of mid-range theory and help to realize the potential envisioned.

1 Undergraduate and master's education might be revised to incorporate more mid-range theory. Just as priority is now being placed on incorporating research findings—that is, evidence—into teaching, middle-range theories could become just as central at all levels of the curriculum.

2 Similarly, doctoral programs can be revised to incorporate more theory-building experiences. At this point, every doctoral program addresses middle-range theory to some extent; virtually all include opportunities to analyze and evaluate theories; and most explicitly incorporate theories in required coursework. Fewer programs address theory-building strategies and include assignments that require the generation of theory.

3 In compiling evidence about given phenomena, nurses can be encouraged not to limit evidence to discrete empirical findings but to begin to generate empirical generalizations that summarize evidence and then to view those generalizations within the context of existing or evolving theory.

4 In all areas of nursing, we can encourage analogical thinking. Do not allow students or investigators to get away with saying that they want to do an exploratory study when there is already much known about a phenomenon and relevant theory exists. Insist that they acknowledge the existence of a theoretical basis for their work when it, in fact, is there.

5 We can insist that theory building be part of the empirical research enterprise. End products of a program of qualitative research should be theories, not just themes. End products of model testing studies should be fully described and elaborated models or theories, not just revised diagrams that are too confusing to understand and too dry to read. This requires active collaboration between theorists and researchers.

6 An important strategy is to encourage clinicians to think theoretically. In addition, we can also encourage theory developers to think clinically. For example, encourage them to write in clear and understandable language, and to publish in journals that clinicians read. The clinical scholar role could be instrumental in enhancing the links between mid-range theory and practice.

In summary, we need to continue to examine and promote the use of middle-range theories in research and practice. If the promise of middle-range theories is to be realized, there needs to be a lot more explicit attention to how such theories can be and are being used to good advantage.

REFERENCES

Acton, G. J. (1997). Affiliated-individuation as a mediator of stress and burden in care-givers of adults with dementia. *Journal of Holistic Nursing, 15*, 336–357.

Aday, L. A., & Anderson, R. M. (1974). A framework for the study of access to medical care. *Health Services Research, 9*, 208–220.

Ajzen, I. (1985). From intentions to actions: A theory of planned behavior. In J. Kuhl & J. Beckman (Eds.), *Action control: From cognition to behavior* (pp. 11–59). Berlin: Springer-Verlag.

Ajzen, I. (1987). Attitudes, traits and actions: Dispositional prediction of behavior in personality and social psychology. *Advances in Experimental Psychology, 20*, 1–63.

Algase, K. L., Beck, C., Kolanowski, A., Whall, A., Berent, S., Richards, K., & Beattie, E. (1996). Need-driven dementia-compromised behavior: An alternative view of disruptive behavior. *American Journal of Alzheimer's Disease, 11*(6), 10-19.

August-Brady, M. (2000). Prevention as intervention. *Journal of Advanced Nursing, 31*, 1304–1308.

Auvil-Novak, S. E. (1997). A middle-range theory of chronotherapeutic intervention for post-surgical pain. *Nursing Research, 46*, 66–71.

Bandura, A. (1986). *Social foundations of thought and action: A social cognitive theory.* Englewood Cliffs, NJ: Prentice-Hall.

Bass, B. M. (1985). *Leadership and performance beyond expectations.* New York: Free Press.

BBARNS. (1999). *Roy Adaptation Model-based research: 25 years of contributions to nursing science.* Indianapolis, IN: Center Nursing Press.

Belsky, J. (1984). The determinants of parenting: A process model. *Child Development, 55*, 83–96.

Benner, P. E. (2001). *From novice to expert: Excellence and power in clinical nursing practice.* Upper Saddle River, NJ: Prentice-Hall Health.

Brooten, D., Brown, L. P., Munro, B., York, R., Rohen, S., Roncoli, M., & Hollingsworth, A. (1988). Early discharge and specialist transitional care. *Image: Journal of Nursing Scholarship, 20*, 64–68.

Cicchetti, D. (1989). How research on child maltreatment has informed the study of child development: Perspectives from developmental psychopathology. In D. Cicchetti & V. Carlson (Eds.), *Child maltreatment: Theory and research on the causes and consequences of child abuse and neglect* (pp. 337–431). New York: Cambridge University Press.

Cooley, M. (1999). Analysis and evaluation of the trajectory theory of chronic illness management. *Scholarly Inquiry for Nursing Practice, 13*, 75–109.

Corbin, J. M., & Strauss, A. (1991). A nursing model for chronic illness management based upon the trajectory framework. *Scholarly Inquiry for Nursing Practice, 4*, 155–174.

Duckett, L., Henly, S., Avery, M., Potter, S., Hills-Bonczyk, S., Hulden, R., & Savik, K. (1998). A theory of planned behavior-based structural model for breast feeding. *Nursing Research, 47*, 325–336.

Eakes, G. G., Burke, M. L., & Hainsworth, M. A. (1998). Middle-range theory of chronic sorrow. *Image: Journal of Nursing Scholarship, 30*, 179–184.

Erickson, H. C., Tomlin, E. M., & Swain, M. A. P. (1983). *Modeling and role modeling: A theory and paradigm for nursing.* Englewood Cliffs, NJ: Prentice-Hall.

Flaskerud, J. H., & Winslow, B. J. (1998). Conceptualizing vulnerable populations health-related research. *Nursing Research, 47*, 69–78.

Glaser, R. (1987). Thoughts on expertise. In C. Schooler & K. W. Schaie (Eds.), *Cognitive functioning and social structure over the life course* (pp. 81–93). Norwood, NJ: Ablex Publishing.

Good, M. (1998). A middle range theory of acute pain management: Use in research. *Nursing Outlook, 46*, 120–124.

Hall, G. R., & Buckwalter, K. C. (1987). Progressively lowered stress threshold: A conceptual model for care of adults with Alzheimer's disease. *Archives of Psychiatric Nursing, 1*, 399–406.

Horowitz, J. J. (1986). *Stress response syndrome* (2nd ed.). Northvale, NJ: Jason Aronson, Inc.

Hupcey, J., Morse, J. M., Lenz, E. R., & Tason, M. C. (1996). Wilsonian methods of concept analysis: A critique. *Scholarly Inquiry for Nursing Practice, 10*, 185–210.

Im, E., & Meleis, A. I. (1999). Situation-specific theories: Philosophical roots, properties, and approaches. *Advances in Nursing Science, 22*(2), 11–24.

Jirovec, M. M., Jenkins, J., Isenberg, M., & Barardi, J. (1999). Urine control theory derived from Roy's conceptual framework. *Nursing Science Quarterly, 12*, 251–255.

John, M. (1988). *Geragogy: A theory for teaching the elderly.* New York: Hearth Press.

Ketefian, S. (1981). Moral reasoning and moral behavior among selected groups of practicing nurses. *Nursing Research, 30*, 171–176.

Kim, H. S. (1996). Reflections on building a cumulative knowledge base for nursing: From fragmentation to congruence. Invited papers of the 4th and 5th symposia of the Knowledge Development Series. In *Building a cumulative knowledge base for nursing from fragmentation to congruence of philosophy, theory, methods of inquiry and practice.* (pp. 63–67). Kingston, RI: University of Rhode Island College of Nursing.

Lazarus, R., & Folkman, S. (1984). *Appraisal and coping.* New York: Springer.

Lenz, E. R. (1998a). The role of middle-range theory for nursing research and practice: Part 1. Nursing Research. *Nursing Leadership Forum, 3*(2), 62–66.

Lenz, E. R. (1998b). The role of middle-range theory for nursing research and practice: Part 2, Nursing Practice. *Nursing Leadership Forum, 3*(1), 24–33.

Lenz, E. R., Pugh, L. C., Milligan, R. A., Gift, A. G., & Suppe, F. (1997). The middle range theory of unpleasant symptoms: An update. *Advances in Nursing Science, 19*, 14–27.

Lenz, E. R., Suppe, F., Gift, A. G., Pugh, L. C., & Milligan, R. A. (1995). Collaborative development of middle-range nursing theories: Toward a theory of unpleasant symptoms. *Advances in Nursing Science, 17*, 1–13.

Liehr, P., & Smith, M. J. (1999). Middle range theory: Spinning research and practice to create knowledge for the new millennium. *Advances in Nursing Science, 21*, 81–91.

Marlatt, G. A. (1985). Relapse prevention: Theoretical rationale and overview of the model. In G. A. Marlatt & J. R. Gordon (Eds.), *Relapse prevention: Maintenance strategies in the treatment of addictive behaviors* (pp. 103–170). New York: Guilford Press.

Meleis, A. I., Sawyer, L. M., Im, E., Messias, D. K. H., & Schumacher, K. (2000). Experiencing transitions: An emerging middle range theory. *Advances in Nursing Science, 23*(1), 12–28.

Merton, R. K. (1968). *Social theory and social structure* (Enlarged ed.). New York: Free Press.

Mishel, M. H. (1988). Uncertainty in illness. *Image: Journal of Nursing Scholarship, 20*(4), 225–232.

Mishel, M. H. (1990). Reconceptualization of the uncertainty in illness theory. *Image: Journal of Nursing Scholarship, 22*(4), 256–262.

Morse, J. M., Hupcey, J., Mitcham, C., & Lenz, E. R. (1996). Concept analysis in nursing research: A critical appraisal. *Scholarly Inquiry for Nursing Practice, 10*(3), 253–277.

Nagi, S. Z. (1991). Disability concepts revisited: Implications for prevention. In A. M. Pope & A. R. Turlow (Eds.), *Disability in America: Toward a national agenda for prevention* (pp. 309–327). Washington, DC: National Academy Press.

Neuman, B. (1995). *The Neuman Systems Model* (3rd ed.). Norwalk, CT: Appleton & Lange.

Nightingale, F. (1969). *Notes on nursing: What it is and what it is not.* New York: Dover Publications. (Original work published 1859)

Nyamathi, A. (1989). Comprehensive health seeking and coping paradigm. *Journal of Advanced Nursing, 14*, 281–290.

Olson, J., & Hanchett, E. (1997). Nurse-expressed empathy, patient outcomes, and development of a middle range theory. *Image: Journal of Nursing Scholarship, 29*, 71–76.

Orlando, I. J. (1961). *The dynamic nurse-patient relationship.* New York: G. P. Putnam's Sons.

Pender, N. J. (1996). *Health promotion in nursing practice* (3rd ed.). Stamford, CT: Appleton & Lange.

Piper, B., Lindsey, A. M., & Dodd, M. (1987). Fatigue mechanisms in cancer patients: Developing nursing theory. *Oncology Nursing Forum, 14*(6), 17–23.

Pollock, S. E. (1986). Human response to chronic illness: Physiological and psychological adaptation. *Nursing Research, 35*, 90–95.

Polk, L. L. (1997). Toward a middle range theory of resilience. *Advances in Nursing Science, 19*(3), 1–13.

Richmond, T. S. (1997). An explanatory model of variables influencing post-injury disability. *Nursing Research, 46*, 262–267.

Riegel, B. J., Dracup, K. A., & Glaser, D. (1998). A longitudinal causal model of cardiac invalidism following myocardial infarction. *Nursing Research, 47*, 285–292.

Rolland, J. (1994). *Families, illness and disability: An integrative treatment model.* New York: Basic Books.

Roy, Sr. C., & Andrews, H. (1991). *The Roy Adaptation Model: The definitive statement.* Norwalk, CT: Appleton & Lange.

Sarason, B. R., Shearin, E. N., Peirce, G. R., & Sarason, I. G. (1987). Interrelations of social support measures: Theoretical and practical implications. *Journal of Personality and Social Psychology, 52*, 813–832.

Smith, C. E. (1999). Caregiving effectiveness in families managing complex technology at home: Replication of a model. *Nursing Research, 48*(3), 120–128.

Smith, M. J., & Liehr, P. (1999). Attentively embracing story: A middle-range theory with practice and research implications. *Scholarly Inquiry for Nursing Practice, 13*, 187–204.

Smith, M. J., & Liehr, P. (2003). *Middle range theory for nursing.* New York: Springer.

Stuifbergen, A. K., & Rogers, S. (1997). Health promotion: An essential component of rehabilitation for persons with chronic disabling conditions. *Advances in Nursing Science, 19*(4), 1–20.

Stuifbergen, A. K., Seraphin, A., & Roberts, G. (2000). An explanatory model of health promotion and quality of life in chronic disabling conditions. *Nursing Research, 49*, 122–129.

Suppe, F. (1992). Paradigms, socialization and nursing science. *Proceedings of the 1992 annual forum on doctoral education in nursing.* Baltimore: University of Maryland School of Nursing.

Suppe, F. (1996). Middle-range theory: Role in nursing theory and knowledge development. In L. M. Allen-Holmes, H. S. Lee, & M. T. Quinn (Eds.), *Proceedings of the sixth Rosemary Ellis scholars retreat. Nursing science: Implications for the 21st century* (pp. 38–77). Cleveland, OH: Frances Payne Bolton School of Nursing.

Swanson, K. (1991). Empirical development of a middle-range theory of caring. *Nursing Research, 40*, 61–66.

Thoits, P. A. (1986). Social support as coping assistance. *Journal of Consulting and Clinical Psychology, 54*, 416–423.

Winick, C. (1974). A sociological theory of the genesis of drug dependence. In C. Winick (Ed.), *Sociological aspects of drug dependence* (pp. 3–13). Cleveland, OH: CRC Press.

Linking the Nature of the Person With the Nature of Nursing Through Nursing Theory and Practice and Nursing Language in Brazil

Marga Simon Coler
Maria Miriam Lima da Nóbrega
Telma Ribeiro Garcia
Matthew Coler-Thayer

T he International Conference on Emerging Nursing Knowledge 2000 was a culminating event highlighting the 20th century as an era that marked rich growth in nursing knowledge development linked to an ontological and epistemological explication of nursing. This chapter offers a perspective on the Nursing Knowledge Consensus Conference Position Paper (see chapter 1) from the perspective of Brazilian nurses. A particular focus of this discussion is on nursing language in general and especially in Brazil. Our approach is to use an international perspective in linking the nature of person with the nature of nursing through nursing theory, practice, and nursing language.

The Brazilian Analysis

Beginning with concept analysis of the key words appearing in the consensus statement, we recognized that an analysis of the linguistics of these words was needed to reach common understanding. By reading and rereading the consensus statement one is able to comprehend more fully the four components outlined in the statement. When these key concepts were translated into Portuguese, we discovered a rich, all-encompassing array of words. However, this array, for our taste, was a bit complex for international application.

Initial Review of Theoretical and Philosophical Bases

In examining the document to unravel its complexity, we recognized the variety of schools of philosophical thought evident throughout. The well-rounded philosophical document reflected much thinking on the part of the developers. A Cartesian dualistic approach emerged when we read about the inherent goodness of people. The work incorporated spirituality when it labeled the soul as an existential reality. The position was strong in the vein of existentialism, which was evidenced by reference to Sartre's claim of authenticity. Existentialism was further represented by the phrase, the "essence of Nursing lies in modes of being." Heidegger's view of the perspective of being-with-others is inherent in the global vision guiding the 2000 international conference and is substantiated by the phrase that, "the nurse is open to another person's reality."

There was also a potent vein of systems theory woven into the fabric of the consensus statement. Elements articulated the open systems of person, environment, and nursing acting in symbiotic coexistence. Such philosophy leads into the arena of globalism and the prospect of integrating a diversity of nursing visions. This goal can be increasingly seen as a meeting of multiple perspectives in the science and art we call nursing. As was affirmed by Capra in 1996, systems theory perceives reality as a network of relations and descriptions of reality as a network of interconnectedness of conceptions and models, all of equal importance.

Systems theory teaches us that what is living is in a continual state of permanent reorganization; every moment is a new moment, and every state, a new state. Uncertainty, a product of disorder, enriches life and living. It can contribute to transformation and innovation. Uncertainty, of course, is occurring presently in nursing, including among the participants of the 2000 conference. Louis Pasteur, the noted French scientist, observed that science advances from provisional responses to a series of questions that are increasingly subtle and profound in the essence of natural phenomena (Capra, 1996).

The consensus statement documents the effort to synthesize many perspectives that can be identified in the development of knowledge in nursing. Although development of the consensus statement was an endeavor to thoroughly examine the essence of the nursing phenomena (Kim, 1997), it must be considered a provisional response to ontological and epistemological questions of nursing.

Translation Process

The task of translating the consensus statement required the use of dictionaries, thesauri, and linguistic tools. As is frequently the case with many professions, our ongoing work lacked experts in linguists and philosophy. The consensus statement was endorsed by colleagues in the Northern Hemisphere, and we were seeking to understand how it would work in the Southern Hemisphere system of nursing. Brazilian nursing is a system that has translated and adopted the Classifications of the North American Nursing Diagnosis Association (NANDA) and the International Classification of Nursing Practice (ICNP). As consumers, we are using this product to test its relevance and value within in the culture of Brazilian nursing.

Linguistic Analysis

The translation of the consensus statement was informed by Brazilian colleagues who labored over the English version. Statements were translated into simple declarative sentences with a space for the respondent to comment. We were careful in the translation to replicate the language as much as possible and to represent the same philosophy regarding the ontology of the person, the ontology of nursing, nursing theory, and the linkage of the three.

Interpretation and communication related to the essence expressed in the statement required, in some cases, a semantic revision to compensate for the gap between what we called the ivory tower and the world of direct care. In the process, we have interpreted esoteric vocabulary that, on face translation, could have been misinterpreted. In short, we began the process of linguistic analysis. This type of analysis is attributed to the Semantic Line of Saussure by Lopes (1979). Basically, according to Saussurian thinking, a linguistic element is a pure value. Its significance lies in its discernible syntax from other elements in a sentence (parole) and, in its discernible paradigms, associative, syntactic, and structural relationships.

Associative relationships are those words that appear in a class. For example, the umbrella, *education*, is a major category for associates such as school, learning, and teaching. All of these words have the similar semantic base—education. Another example of associative relations is that which would link a word with its synonym (Miller, 1998). Therefore, a synonym for the word *consensus* would yield a response of *general agreement* in the majority of persons who would be asked to associate the former with a word that has the same meaning. An antonym association might be *disagreement*. Figure 5.1 demonstrates such association in the process of translation.

Paradigmatic Analysis

A paradigm is a class of elements that can be inserted in the same point in the same context. These elements are substitutable, commutative, or exchangeable. Paradigmatic relations are patterns or prototypes. Paradigmatic relationships are also associative (Lopes, 1979). This is demonstrated by the first sentence under Scientific Principles and Values in the section on the ontology of the person. This sentence characterizes the person by the words *wholeness, complexity, consciousness*. The descriptors translated into Portuguese included terms such as: *totalidade, complexidade, consciência*. However, the word, *consciousness*, might also have been translated into *percepção*, which may be "back" translated in English

EDUCATION is a major category for *associates* such as school, learning, and teaching. All of these words have the *similar semantic base, EDUCATION*.

➢ Words or word phrases that link a word with its synonym

   English: Consensus   (General Agreement)

   Portuguese: Consenso   (Concordância, Acordo)

➢ Antonyms, too, are associations

   English: Consensus   (Disagreement)

   Portuguese: Consenso   (Discordância; Desacordo)

Associative interpretations/relationships of words that appear in a class as shown when translating.

as *perception, insight, feeling*, and so forth, or *sentimento*, which would "back" translate into *sentiment, emotion, perception*, and even *sorrow*. All of these words are associative prototypes of consciousness. Not only does the translation depend on common usage, which may differ from esoteric nursing vocabulary, but also on the state of mind of the translator and recipient of the message at a given point in time (see Figure 5.2).

Paradigmatic Exemplar

In describing a paradigmatic sense, we shall present one other example that creates problems for linking the consensus statement and the global perspective. This appears in the statement under the subheading Scientific Principles and Values of the Ontology of Nursing. Here, we find a phrase stating, "The nurse uses both philosophic and scientific

PATTERNS or PROTOTYPES (not synonyms, but they share a commutative relationship (for example, husband/wife)

➢ Wholeness, Complexity, Consciousness   PERSON

➢ Totalidade, Complexidade, Consciência   PESSOA

or

➢ Philosophical, Scientific Knowledge   EMPOWER

➢ Conhecimento, poder

   AUTODETERMINAÇÃO

   EMPOWERMENT   ("entre nos brasileiros é veiculada")

   AUTODETERMINAÇÃO   ("não compreendi")

Paradigmatic interpretations/relationships between words when translating (may also be associative).

knowledge to empower others." We could not find the word *empower* in our Brazilian dictionaries. After much discussion, we labeled, *empower* as a neologism and translated it into what we believed to be relevant Portuguese as *empoderar*. Respondents to our questionnaire had no sense of the word and answered with question marks or asked what the word meant. A suggestion was offered as a possible substitute by a respondent well versed in English. The suggestion was, *autodeterminação,* or *self-determination.* One doctoral student was apparently familiar with the word.

Syntactic Relationships

To look at syntactic relationships is to study the internal structure of sentences, the relationships of words to one another, and to phrases (Salzmann, 1998). In particular, syntax studies the principles and processes for construction of sentences in a particular language. The goal of syntactic investigation is "the construction of a grammar that can be used as a devise of some sort for producing the sentences of the language under analysis" (Chomsky, 1965, p. 11). In the case of this effort, we tried to connect words to form phrases that made sense in Portuguese. For example, such words as in the phrase, *A human being is evolving, in process, fluid, and changing* appeared in our instrument as, *Está em evolução em processo, fluindo, mudando.* Only months after translating the phrase into succinct Portuguese, and following validation with Brazilian coauthors, it became evident that a change in grammatical structure occurred in the translation process. *Está em evolução* could have been perceived as *She/he/it is in evolution.* Because the human being was implied, the written responses focused on the changes as the work of nursing at the beginning of the process, as subjects in the sentence. To accomplish this focus, the authors translated sentences in segments as is illustrated in Figure 5.3.

ONTOLOGY OF THE PERSON

Understanding the human person

as individuals, families, communities, and groups,

is the focal point

of knowledge development

in nursing

ONTOLOGIA DA PESSOA

A compreensão da pessoa humana

(indivíduos, famílias comunidades e grupos)

é o ponto focal

do desenvolvimento do conhecimento

em enfermagem

Syntactic interpretations/relationships shown when translating units of vocabulary.

Structural Relationships

In structural relationships, one analyzes the fit of a word within a phrase or sentence. Structure also demonstrates relationships between words, which can vary from one language to another (e.g., the placement of nouns in relationship to verbs). Another example is the use of word gender (Salzmann, 1998). This relationship fits the illustration in Figure 5.3, demonstrating the connectedness between syntax and structure. Once again, our continuous search in the literature of linguistics shows strong relationships among syntactic, structural, paradigmatic, and associative components to the point where a recent purchase of ours was the work by Chomsky, *Syntactic Structures* (1976).

Aside from collaborative discussions, semantic references provided direction for the difficult words that defied our debates. Along this vein was the use of a computerized linguistics program (*WordNet*), which was discovered via an article in the *American Scientist* (Hayes, 1999). A creation of Miller and colleagues at the Cognitive Science Laboratory at Princeton University, it is a user-friendly linguistic program that helped lighten the linguistic jargon of Saussure. The emphasis in *WordNet* is on relationships between words rather than on the pure words. Therefore, the team could move from an analysis of a pure word in translation, to how the word related to others. *WordNet* introduced the concept of synonymy and synsets where words of a similar meaning were grouped together. It is a sort of thesaurus, which is a must in the art of translation. Hayes (1999) described synonymy as the glue of *WordNet*. Synonyms can replace each other in a sentence and might be feasible for use in the translation of a philosophical document where certain words are untranslatable symbols that, in English, for example, might represent a given nurse theorist's perspective in the field of knowledge. What we questioned is whether or not a synonym in another language might destroy the essence of the original thought of the theorist. What has occurred historically, however, gave us support in that Heidegger wrote in German and Sartre in French. For decades scholars have studied the translated philosophies and even incorporated these works into the philosophy of nursing and thus showed a trust in the translated word. What is critical to remember, however, is that one day the word may be changed with input from those

---

- **Attributed to the semantic line of Saussure.**

  ...a linguistic element is a pure value. Its significance lies in its discernible syntax from other elements in a parole and in its discernible paradigm or associative relationship

- **Analyzes the fit of a word within a phrase or sentence.**

- **Relationships between words (can vary from one language to another).**

  For example, where nouns are placed in relationship to verbs; the use of word gender.

Structural interpretations/relationships between words.

using the document in another language. This discussion of structural relationships is summarized in Figure 5.4.

Summary of Linguistic Analysis

In a paper presented at the 14th Conference of the North American Nursing Diagnosis Association (NANDA), Sister Callista Roy stated that "what a unified nursing language requires [is]: semantic typing for the concepts, identifying semantic relations, mapping of terms from different vocabularies, relating vocabularies and identifying synonyms" (Roy, 2000, n.p.). Dochterman and Jones (Chapter 15) used the term *harmonization* as a process, which assures that a unified model results from collaboration, when they wrote on unifying the languages of NANDA, NIC, and NOC. This is congruent with our thinking and is what we have done and continue to do as we refine our study to contribute to the formulation of a new global consensus statement.

In this spirit, we began with a semantic analysis of the concepts presented in the consensus statement. Our translation was listed under their major headings: The Ontology of the Person, The Ontology of Nursing, Nursing Theory, and Linking the Nature of Person, the Nature of Nursing, and Nursing Theory to Nursing Practice.

Survey of Brazilian Nurses

A questionnaire consisting of the translated lists preceded by instructions was given to a selected group of respondents. Respondents were asked to indicate affirmatively or negatively if the words or phrases in the translated format were applicable to Brazilian nursing practice and to insert comments next to the item if he or she felt that comments were indicated. There was also a section for additional comments at the end of each major category.

Method

The questionnaires were sent via e-mail as well as dispersed manually to a sample of academicians, graduate students, and nurses in the service arena. Twenty-four responses were received from 33 questionnaires distributed. The investigators assigned a number to each respondent and responses were color-coded by respondent category and then entered into the instrument.

In discussing our findings, we need to point to our small sample size ($n = 24$) and that only two of the respondents are from the service arena. Both of the nurses in practice stated in a letter that the vocabulary was incomprehensible; therefore, they did not address any of the items on the questionnaire. Had there been a higher response rate of nurses in practice, the investigators feel that the findings from the two clinicians would have been amplified. It is probable that the majority of responses would have been similar or would have recorded negative responses or comments. The closest we came to comments from nurses in the service arena was the stratum of new master's degree students who were within 2 weeks of beginning their first semester. Many had been direct care providers, but were nurses who had selected to begin graduate studies.

Findings

Our data indicated that the affirmative responses were far greater in all of the strata than the negative responses. The raw numbers of affirmative and negative responses are presented in Table 5.1 for Ontology of the Person and Ontology of Nursing.

The written comments about the statements concerning the ontology of the person included the notion that these concepts permeate the theoretical formation of Brazilian nurses but that they do not always permeate practice. They are principles inherent in the human being, but in reality their effectiveness in the lives of persons is dependent on such factors as education, knowledge, socioeconomic conditions, and so forth. Further, one respondent noted that relative to the ontology of nursing, the first block of assertions were fundamental in humanistic theories. However, it merits questioning if they were supported in the biological realm. Another particular observation was that nursing, even though in growth and transformation, is still a class of little social mobilization, especially in the battle for better working conditions, salaries, and recognition. Further, nursing is a discipline that tries to impose itself in the health sector in Brazil but seems to have lost areas already conquered—one of these being the hospital. Finally, a respondent summarized that although all of the principles and values are present in the schools of nursing and in the literature, their realization in practice often suffered because of restrictions of the economy and policy.

The responses of the sample to the consensus statement related to Nursing Theory and the Links Between Theory and Practice are presented in Table 5.2.

Some general comments by the respondents regarding this section were that the theories are not well known by the Brazilian nurses who lack graduate education. However, they are important for the growth of the profession and are in continuous evolution. One respondent noted that theory demands reflection and change. Another commented that various topics are ideal and not real, but they ought to be maintained. We have to have dreams to build the tomorrows. It was also noted that Brazilian nurses use theories in practice via the nursing process. However, they do not know the essential content of theories.

Table 5.1	Responses to Items From Consensus Statement Related to Ontology of the Person and Ontology of Nursing			
	Ontology of Person (13 items)		Ontology of Nursing (38 items)	
Respondent Category	Affirmative Responses	Negative Responses	Affirmative Responses	Negative Responses
Doctorally Prepared $n = 9$	103	4	103	4
Other University Faculty $n = 2$	27	0	27	0
Terminating MS Students $n = 5$	24	13	24	13
Beginning MS Students $n = 3$	30	8	30	8
Nurses in Practice Arena $n = 2$	NR[a]	NR[a]		

[a] Response to inapplicability of Consensus Paper was by letter.

Table 5.2	Responses to Sample From Consensus Statement Related to Nursing Theory and the Links Between Theory and Practice				
		Nursing Theory (20 items)		Linking the Nature of the Person, the Nature of Nursing, and Nursing Theory to Nursing Practice (23 items)	
Respondent Category		Affirmative Responses	Negative Responses	Affirmative Responses	Negative Responses
Doctorally Prepared $n = 9$		163	1	151	9
Other University Faculty $n = 2$		28	0	45	0
Terminating MS Students $n = 5$		93	5	67	55
Beginning MS Students $n = 3$		39	3	64	4
Nurses in Practice Arena $n = 2$		NR[a]	NR[a]	NR[a]	NR[a]

[a] Response to inapplicability of Consensus Paper was by letter.

In examining the responses related to Nursing Theory, the investigators concluded that the principles should, but do not apply to the Brazilian reality, except in research. Nursing theory is taught at the graduate level only, therefore there is little application of theory in practice. Concerning the last section, Linking the Nature of Person, the Nature of Nursing, and Nursing Theory to Nursing Practice, a similar observation is that there is little application of theory to practice. In the data we noted that there were contradictions between what should be and what is. For example, the principle states that "the person is characterized by wholeness, complexity, and consciousness." In reality, the person is not seen holistically, but in parts. The principles and values should be applicable, but are not part of the reality of the nurse, nor the clients.

The team also offers some comments regarding specific terminology. We suggest the use of the term *reciprocity* in place of the word *mutuality*. Second, we recommend that the term *self-determination* replace *empowerment*, and that the term *intimidation* be deleted.

A final conclusion is that there is a wide gap between the ideals expressed in the consensus statement and reality, which should be the rights of nurses and of those they serve. However, in Brazil the gap between the ideal and the real is a giant chasm.

Summary

To summarize, in general we noted that because of the philosophical nature of the consensus statement, the language is only available to a select few of those working in academia. Therefore, we conclude that the principles need language modifications to be understood by all nurses. Second, for respondents who agreed with the applicability of the consensus statement, affirmative responses were much more frequent than were negative ones. Further, we conclude that Brazilian nursing exists in a health system that fragments the person. The model reflected in the consensus statement is used in teaching, but the workplace does not accept the vision.

In addition, for each section of the consensus statement, we offer specific observations. In considering the ontology of the person, comments indicated that the principle is correct, but its realization is not always possible. Public policy and social practices, furthermore, are constraints to the realization of the principles. Relative to the ontology of nursing, adverse working conditions, including salary, are major constraints.

The model of care in practice is illness-oriented, rather than focused on the whole person. For nurses in Brazil, the environment and the working conditions discourage the application of such idealistic principles. Finally, *empowerment* is not a part of the vocabulary of Brazilian nursing.

Discussion

As was implied by Roy in the NANDA presentation, the passage of time (even from 1998, when the consensus statement was drafted, until the year 2000, when it was in the first step of analysis in Brazil) will produce new ways of thinking and interpretation. Both time and culture will influence semantic interpretation in this new century. NANDA classification is moving closer to that of the ICNP. In nursing we are evolving to an era of classifying our nursing phenomena according to domains and classes. Nursing diagnoses, interventions, and outcomes are being stated in terms of multidimensionality. Such thinking will automatically influence the interpretation of nursing knowledge, which in the consensus statement focused on holism.

Our concentration in 1998 was on the individual person. Today, in the world, but especially in Brazil with its Unified Health System, we are moving our focus to social components. Our interpretation of knowledge, therefore, will become increasingly socially oriented. Once again, the major nursing classification systems, products of post-1998 thinking, increasingly emphasize the impact of environmental and other social conditions. This type of ongoing evolution, a flow of energy between open systems, necessarily has a cultural impact on the interpretation of semantic components.

The findings of our small Brazilian sample, in the year 2000, indicated that the consensus statement needs linguistic revision in order to communicate the meaning of words that are not only English but also esoterically philosophical. The translations we have made have been of the linguistic symbols and of their associations in Brazilian Portuguese through the application of semantics. We have replaced words that were apparently understood only by students and professors in academia with synonyms.

Because we, the authors, are "ivory tower folks," our colleagues in the service area were more difficult to contact. Because e-mail is generally not accessible to them, data collection to obtain a broader perspective means using alternative methods of contact. We made several attempts. One was through colleagues who had students in the clinical area and had access to nurses working there. This approach also did not work out because using busy academicians as the link of communication is sometimes a weak approach. Another attempt was to try to convene a specialty group offering a workshop on nursing knowledge and then distributing the questionnaire. Two attempts in communicating with a key person in that group also failed, and then, between a 2-month strike, meetings away, and vacation, the months flew by, and time did not permit further follow-up. Our next step will be to survey more assertively those colleagues working in the service arena. This will be the next stage of our work, after the global components have been added and the present consensus statement has been revised to meet the needs of more nurses.

Conclusion

The input we have received from Brazilian nurses has served to identify words and grammar that will need further exploration in our continuing effort to give input to a global vision of nursing knowledge. Our presence among colleagues at the International Knowledge Conference 2000 and our research have served to stimulate us to continue activism in procreating a global vision of nursing knowledge. We look forward to our next phase of research and dissemination of Brazilian findings.

Background of author Marga Simon Coler

As the lead author and conference presenter of this joint work, I consider myself not a philosopher but a scientist whose philosophy is based on pragmatism with a vein of existentialism. Because I am involved in semantic interpretations, I have a professional and personal need for succinctness and pragmatism. My major research focus involves semantic analyses of the classification systems of the North American Nursing Diagnosis Association (NANDA) and the International Classification of Nursing Practice (ICNP) of the International Council of Nurses. I specialize in translation, an area that predicates my pursuit for linguistic clarity. As we explore our cultural and ethnic origin, we find also that which Chomsky termed "universal grammar," the innate ability of grammatical acquisition.

As miracles would happen, I received an invitation to represent Brazil in an attempt to expand the dialogue regarding the consensus statement to a global arena. My initial thought was to decline the invitation because I wondered how I, an American, a Professor Emeritus from the University of Connecticut School of Nursing, could authentically represent Brazilian nursing. I dwelt on the subject for some time, linking it to my personal philosophy. Using ethics and logic, I was able to justify the invitation on the following grounds. First, I have worked with Brazilian colleagues off and on since 1976, when as an Educational Consultant of Project HOPE, I worked with colleagues in Academia at the Federal University of Pernambuco in an attempt to launch a master's program in nursing. My 2 years of groundwork led to an enriching personal and professional experience regarding Brazilian nursing. Then, in 1985, when I was a member of the University of Connecticut faculty, I discovered Partners of the Americas. Through this program the State of Connecticut had as a sister state Paríba, Brazil, a neighboring State of Pernambuco. Upon that discovery, I wrote a proposal, which was endorsed by Partners. I conducted a mini-research project to study transcultural application of Nursing Diagnoses (Coler & Hafner, 1991). During my 2 weeks in that country, I linked with the psychiatric nursing faculty of the Federal University of Paraíba. I taught them about nursing diagnosis and began collaborative research projects to help them utilize nursing diagnoses. The new link led to several visits of faculty from that university to the

University of Connecticut and to their participation in NANDA conferences, presenting posters and papers regarding the research projects we had engaged in. The diagnostic word spread throughout Brazil via a small manual that four of us prepared and published (Farias, Nóbrega, Perez, & Coler, 1990).

This was followed by another year of a residency in Paraíba as a Fulbright Fellow, validating NANDA nursing diagnoses. During this time, as a collaborative venture between the U.S. Embassy, the administering agency of my Fulbright, and several universities in Brazil, I was able to teach other nurses about nursing diagnoses and had contact with Brazilian colleagues throughout the country. Later I spent another year in Brazil during my sabbatical at the University of Connecticut, doing more research on the language of nursing. Presently, I am in the fourth year of my role as a Visiting Professor at the Federal University of Paraíba, continuing my work in the translation of nursing classification systems, always using the tools of linguistic analyses.

Still, all of my formal education was obtained at North American Universities, and there are thoughts, feelings, and behaviors that will always be stamped as North American. However, because I have participated in research with Brazilian colleagues and because I have shaped the thinking of many postgraduate students and practicing nurses, I feel that I can represent the country.

This paper was coauthored by an American citizen/Brazilian resident, two Brazilian colleagues—fellow academicians—with whom I have worked and debated over the years, and a philosopher. I was on the doctoral committee of both nurses, and one was my first master's degree advisee in Brazil. Both are also involved in semantics as applied to the two aforementioned classification systems.

REFERENCES

Capra, F. (1996). A teia da vida: Uma nova compreensão científica dos sistemas vivos. [The theme of life: A new scientific understanding of the systems of life] São Paulo, Brazil: Cultrix.

Chomsky, N. (1965). *Syntactic structures*. The Hague, The Netherlands: Mouton.

Coler, M., & Hafner, L. (1991). An intercultural assessment of the number and intensity of crisis precipitating factors in three cultures: USA, Brazil and Taiwan. *International Journal of Nursing Studies, 28*, 223–235.

Farias, J., Nóbrega, M. M., Perez, V., & Coler, M. S. (1990). *Diagnóstico de enfermagem, uma aboradagem conceitual e pratica*. João Pessoa, Paraíba, Brazil: Santa Marta.

Hayes, B. (1999). The web of words. *American Scientist, 87*, 108–112.

Kim, H. S. (1997). Terminology in structuring and developing nursing knowledge. In I. M. King & J. Fawcett (Eds.), *The language of nursing theory and metatheory*. (pp. 27–36). Indianapolis, IN: Center Nursing Press/Sigma Theta Tau, International.

Lopes, E. (1979). *Fundamentos da lingística contemporânea. [Fundamentals of Contemporary Logistics]*. São Paulo, Brazil: Cultrix.

Miller, G. (1998). Nouns in WordNet. In C. Fellbaum (Ed.), *WordNet*. Cambridge, MA:
    The MIT Press.
Roy, C. (2000). *Theoretical implications of standardized nursing languages and electronic
    databases.* Paper presented at the 14th Conference of the North American Nursing
    Diagnosis Association, Orlando, FL.
Salzmann, Z. (1998). *Language, culture & society*. Boulder, CO: Westview Press.

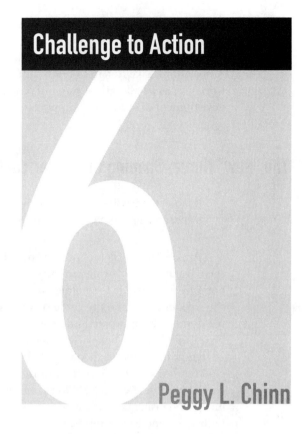

Challenge to Action

Peggy L. Chinn

his chapter presents a challenge to action based in part on my participation in the Nursing Knowledge Conferences. What I witnessed over the years those conferences were held was the very best of nursing, applied in a formal, professional group. The organizers seemed to trust the process, knowing that everything will come together in its own time; trusting, if you will, the inherent wholeness of all things, including conferences. Thus, we can be involved in a process in which we contribute to the exciting journey of international dialogue. I want to draw attention to the situations in which we, as nurses, find ourselves, and how being situated in time and place shapes and shifts our views of nursing, nursing knowledge, and our relationships with the world. I hope to challenge all of us to keep the dialogues open, to learn from the example of the conferences' evolving process as we truly listen to one another, hear with all of our sensibilities, and respond by reaching across boundaries to move toward new awarenesses. I submit that this is not simply an exercise to tickle our brains and challenge our propensities for parochialism. Instead, what we engage in has the potential to expand our minds, our hearts, and our very being, opening windows of opportunity for nurses worldwide to address global health problems.

I will address three major challenges. First, I will discuss where we are situated in history, examining the questions: Are we becoming the same old nurse with a few modern improvements? What exactly is the problem here—is it embedded in the word "old"? Or "same"? Or "modern"? Second, I will examine where we are situated socially and spatially. Specifically, I will ask a number of questions concerning our identity, our ontology. Metaphorically, I will examine the question: What is the difference between nursing a drink and doctoring a drink? Finally, I will propose a fifth dimension to the four essential features of contemporary nursing practice as set forth by the American Nurses Association. Like Senge's (1990) "fifth discipline" (learning), the fifth dimension that I propose as a hallmark of nursing practice is so obvious that it is almost invisible—the development of systems of support to promote health and to improve the quality of life.

The "New" Nurse: Shaping Our Historical Destinies

It is necessary that we should always be expecting that a new knowledge will arise, transcending another that, in being new, would become old. (Freire, 1998, p. 32)

Anna Howard Shaw, who was noted at her death in 1919 as the "strongest force for the advancement of women that the age has known" (Faderman, 1999, p. 40), fought not only for suffrage for women in the United States but also for the right to education, the freedom to enter any trade or profession, and all manner of radical (for the time) freedoms to bring women into contact with the larger life of the world, becoming more broad minded and better developed. Anna Howard Shaw was the lone woman in the 1876 graduate class in theology at Boston University. She served as a minister on Cape Cod for 7 years, then returned to Boston University to earn a medical degree in 1886. In a speech in the early 1890s, in order to allay fears that women were becoming too manly and losing their femininity, Shaw noted: "The new woman is the same old woman, with a few modern improvements" (Faderman, 1999, p. 46)—the quote that inspired this section of this chapter.

Without going further into the history of women in general, suffice it to say that nursing worldwide has developed and grown hand-in-hand with the larger struggles for women's rightful identity and freedoms. In many countries, women have suffered for decades through struggles, and now others benefit immensely from the investment of those who went before. In some parts of the world, women and nurses still face immense challenges and limitations, often related to the fears noted by Shaw concerning women and gender. It is important to note that the association of nurses with gender is not universally female. In Gaza, for example, practically all nurses are men, for women are not accepted as workers in public life. What does appear to me to hold constant across situations is the powerful force that gender identity plays in shaping our historical destiny. Gender identities and challenges are embedded in nursing ideology, practice, mythology, and, indeed, our ontology.

If we translate Shaw's quote to read "The new nurse is the same old nurse, with a few modern improvements," we raise a number of questions and challenges concerning our temporally located historical situation. The good news is that in this quote nurses can recognize the opportunity to shape historical destiny, to take full ownership of who they are, situated in a historical context where there is meaning to the notions of what is old and what is new, what is modern, what is premodern, and postmodern.

If the new nurse is the same old nurse, then is there really anything new? What are the modern improvements? As I raised the question earlier, is the problem embedded in the word "old" or "new" or "same" or "modern"? I am sure that within nursing there are many interesting perspectives on these questions. Here are a few possibilities. As Jean Watson has so beautifully set forth in her book, *Postmodern Nursing and Beyond*, we live in a time of deep archetypal awakenings, when the old becomes new, and the changes leave us feeling like we are in the center of a whirlwind. As Watson says,

> These changes . . . move between text and hypertext to hidden text, jumping from 'word processing' to 'thought processing,' leaping from text to subtext to intertext; from actual to virtual, no longer aware of differences, no longer dealing with logical, linear thought or data. Such quantum leaps in human experience require that we reconsider our very concept of being. (Watson, 1999, p. xiv)

As Watson described, the "old" for nursing includes our association with the sacred feminine archetype—and in this deep transformative archetype, all things can be made new and become whole. Most nurses, regardless of cultures of origin, have not been so privileged as to grow up believing in the fundamental worth and value of that which is female, that which comes from women's experience, from women's perspectives on the world. Quite the contrary. As Watson points out, nursing has been marginalized, blamed, and ignored, and dismissed as part of the problem in health care, rather than being recognized for the marvelous potential that it has to bring about the most fundamental solutions in health care. My fear is that as more and more sectors of societies worldwide begin to recognize nursing's potential, nurses will continue to deny what they know, and who they are, and will not be ready for the challenge. My hope is that sufficient numbers of us are awakening to nursing's real potential and are willing to take brave steps to accept the challenge.

Indeed, in my view, at this point in history, the fundamental problem with the image of the "new nurse" is embedded in what we think of as "modern improvements" rather than in our association with that which is female (although this is still a challenge for us). In the United States, most of our undergraduate programs now only pay lip service to the fundamental knowledge of the discipline, spending instead hour upon hour giving lectures that are barely discernible from that given across the street in the medical school. We have almost completely dismantled master's education as that which advances the application of nursing knowledge in practice, so that now, most of the United States master's programs are serving a master (literally and figuratively) driven by a medical model of curriculum, pedagogy, and practice. Many of the master's programs in this country have deleted content related to nursing theory and research from the curriculum. Instead, we qualify students to take specialty certification exams, the contents of which are almost exclusively medical knowledge. The qualifying process involves counting up hours spent in specific settings, doing certain kinds of (mostly) nonnursing tasks that can be quantified, largely ignoring the cultivation of the being of the nurse, the creative impulses that spring from deep insights into the nature of human experience. I heartily endorse nurses learning what it takes to address people's fundamental primary health care concerns, regardless of disciplinary origin. However, we too often do so at the expense of the knowledge that forms the foundation of our own discipline, and we thereby sacrifice the quality of nursing care that we provide.

Amazingly, nurses who trudge through these intensive "memorize and do" programs somehow still emerge with a vision of what nursing has been and what it could be. They continue to yearn for something more, for something meaningful, for a return to the old and sacred roots of human caring and connection. But wanting something and having it are two different things. Graduates of many master's programs in the United States do not have the insights that come with a deep grasp of the knowledge of the discipline of nursing. In my experience, nurses in this country who enter nursing doctoral programs discover there for the first time nursing's rich heritage, both politically and theoretically. As the insights begin to flash, they experience deep recognitions of what they knew before, but could not acknowledge, of forebearers who already have walked paths they have longed to walk, and of nursing perspectives that are so sensible and inspiring, and yet so hidden.

What goes on in the United States is certainly not the norm for other countries, and few, if any, other countries have formalized an advanced practice role for nurses in the way that we have. The textbooks that are published in the United States, however, are tailored for our unique approaches and role identities and remain in use by nursing programs worldwide. In a soon-to-be completed analysis of American nursing textbooks published in this country, Lynn Giddings of New Zealand has found an alarming absence of concepts of health and increasingly eroding perspectives that come from nursing's traditional values of promoting health and well-being. In effect, through the mechanism of textbooks published in this country, we perpetuate the American ideological colonization of other countries, much to our peril worldwide.

The Crossroads

So where do we stand vis-à-vis that which is "modern"? Are we ready to deconstruct the modern and reconstruct a genuinely new and transformative reality that brings into clear focus how we shape our historical destiny? Is it possible to consciously bring forward that which we value in the old, work with the realities of our present time in history, and create a vision for the future? I believe that not only is this possible, it is imperative, and it is inevitable. The communities served by nurses are speaking very clearly about the kinds of health care they prefer. As humans we have stretched the limits of what this glorious planet can accommodate. These limits call for an old and new concern. How we as humans treat the earth can influence how we will inhabit the earth without killing one another off. How we balance our needs for human meaning, existence, and nurturing with the marvelous potentials created by science and technology are challenges we must consider. Nursing, by returning to our traditional roots of caring, protecting, and nurturing, can embrace our historical moment in dramatic ways.

> Caring is both old and new. As something old it is tradition, literally something that has been handed on in the oral tradition of women (and enlightened men) as folklore through time: the timeless. As something new, it is thinking in ways that mix the tradition and past wisdoms with a new awakening of caring knowledge and moral ideals and practices to counter the social crises of the modern era . . . We seek the point of intersection between the time and the timeless, the heaven and the earth, the masculine and the feminine spirit of our ground of being. (Watson, 1999, p. 87)

Standing at this threshold, we have an opportunity to turn the course of history. Dramatic changes are needed to create a preferred future. There are many nurses who have not forgotten our heritage, and nursing has ever-stronger doctoral programs worldwide preparing nurse scholars in the very best sense of the term. Nursing has the opportunity to move into a postmodern period, claiming both the old and the new. As a discipline, nursing can claim the important skills, including the medical skills that came with modernity. We can recognize their limits and move beyond into a world where we value that which stands at the heart and center of that which nursing values. As a community, nurses may disagree on certain points concerning that which is at the heart. But there are far more points of agreement than disagreement, and, as a discipline, we can integrate our differences within the whole, forming a vision that comes from our solidarity—a vision of health for all peoples of the world, spoken in many voices, carrying many tunes, and using many languages.

To Be a Nurse: Creating Our Identities From the Margins

So who is nursing to be? Part of the response that we give to this question depends on how nurses are situated in the world relative to our cultures, to those we serve, and to institutions and governments. For the most part, nurses stand at the margins, not at the center of these groups. Although our marginal position disadvantages nurses in the mainstream (read: male-stream) power structures, it also advantages the discipline in important ways. It positions nursing to seize the opportunity to work around and through structures that have yielded great power in the course of history. From the position of a discipline at the margins, nurses can move in and around boundaries with some degree of ease, for we are familiar with the territory on all sides of the margins.

From a position on the margins nurses are well qualified to consider the question: What is the difference between nursing a drink and doctoring a drink? To nurse a drink is to make it last throughout the entire evening, savoring the occasional sip, integrating the act of drinking with the conversation, the movement, and the social interactions of the occasion. Doctoring a drink is another matter entirely. To doctor a drink means to fix it up with something—sometimes even something quite dangerous and sometimes unbeknownst to the drinker. Despite this ominous possibility nurtured in the best and worst of literary and performance arts, surely none of us would argue with the desirability of fixing a drink to make it more palatable, more interesting, or to correct an error in the recipe. Likewise, I believe that people all welcome that which can "fix" our sick and tired bodies when we need "fixing." However, I am not so sure that we recognize and value the skills that it takes to nurse—to nurture and take care of a person, integrating all we know about the situation that the person is in. Most important, I am not sure that we know how to embrace both possibilities—nursing and doctoring. Do we not need the best of both? Should not doctoring be done with careful attention and nurturing of the person? Should not nursing be done with attention and intention to move toward wholeness, toward healing?

Recently colleagues from the Netherlands raised the issue of doctoring, wondering if folks who "doctor" are interested in the kinds of questions we are raising relative to nursing. They make the important point that many of the issues nurses are addressing are common to other disciplines, including medicine. This is exactly what nursing's position at the margins allows us to see. In my view, those who practice medicine are well served by considering how they "doctor." Many physicians are indeed involved in doing so. Widespread dissatisfactions with medical care, at least in the United States, seem to stem from medicine's long-standing neglect of who they are, what masters they serve, and from what assumptions do they base their practice. Indeed, as Watson and others have noted, medicine is changing, and much of the change is influenced by the same kinds of transformative shifts that influence us in nursing, shifts that are taking place in our postmodern time. Watson notes that

> medicine is shifting from an exclusive emphasis on diagnosis to a concern with meaning and the subjective aspects of what the experience is for the person (ironically, the domain of nursing in its previous definition with its emphasis on human response to actual or potential health problems). Could it be that as nursing once again takes on some discarded appendages of medicine, such as the technical diagnosis language, it becomes the medical technician, while medicine expands its boundary into complex caring—healing practices? (Watson, 1999, p. 42)

This statement illustrates the vital nature of the matters that have concerned those involved in knowledge development. The social and institutional contexts in which many nurses practice already reduce nurses and nursing to medical technicians and assistants. This is ironic because nurses have fought so diligently over so many decades to overcome the "handmaiden" image of nursing. Yet some of the very pathways that we collectively have taken to overcome that image have led us straight down the narrow path of technician and assistant. Nurses function at a very different level than that of the old handmaiden— they do not simply hand over the scalpel or make ready the charts and the sterile field for the doctor. Rather, nurses today make diagnostic distinctions, interpret technically sophisticated electronic monitors and laboratory results, and prescribe medications. Still nurses must ask, what master do we serve? And more fundamentally, who are we, and who have we become when our practice is reduced to this?

I do not advocate defining who we are in the interest of defining our discipline as unique, for fundamentally all disciplines whose purpose is to serve others share many values and characteristics in common. Rather, I liken the project of determining who we are to the human lifelong quest for self-understanding and self-knowing. This quest is as necessary as breathing. Unless we know who we are as nurses, what we believe, who we serve, and what we value, nursing becomes the instrument of other interests, of other powers, and indeed nursing barely exists, if it exists at all. Nursing's ability to articulate the discipline within the context of society and other related disciplines is essential for the health and well-being of nursing and is essential to our ability to serve others. Knowing who we are as nurses makes it possible for us to not only identify the outcomes of our practice, but also to address the more complex issues underlying decisions about the desired outcomes that we seek. When nurses are confident about their identity, nurses can embrace all the ways that we are like others and celebrate what we share in common. What we share becomes a source of great joy, rather than a threat. Personally, I long for the day when I can enter a building that houses the caring/healing, nursing/medical arts, knowing that I will encounter another person who listens, who accepts, and who responds to me as a person. In that building, there will be more nursing, not less; more caring, not less; more healing of whole persons and their experiences, not less. *Perhaps* more nurses. *Perhaps* more doctors. But all will be practicing the exquisite art of healing and caring. Indeed, nursing's being will be present, palpable, and real, regardless of whether we encounter a physician, a receptionist, a pharmacist, or—a nurse.

The Fifth Dimension: Supporting Health and Quality of Life

The final area in this challenge to action is to consider adding a fifth dimension to the four essential features of contemporary nursing practice set forth by the American Nurses Association (ANA; 1995, p. 6). A few years ago I began taking about this issue. Like Senge's (1990) fifth discipline (learning), the fifth dimension that I proposed as a hallmark of nursing practice is so obvious, yet it was entirely absent in that edition of ANA definition of nursing and is still hardly visible in the current edition (ANA, 2003, p. 5). The addition I was proposing is "the development of systems of support to promote health and quality of life for all." This is a very old but fundamental tenet of nursing. However, because it is completely absent in the ANA social policy statement of 1995 that defines nursing, apparently it was also very new at that time and still not a strong tenant by 2003. The ANA features are highlighted here because they reference characteristics of nursing that point to practice and provide a widely available stance from which to critique and examine our identity and social purposes. The four features that the ANA named at that time are consistent with, but bot inclusive of, the consensus statement derived at the 1998 knowledge conference and featured in chapter 1 of this book. The essential features as stated by ANA at that time were:

1 Attention to the full range of human experiences and responses to health and illness without restriction to a problem-focused orientation.
2 Integration of objective data with knowledge gained to form an understanding of the patient's or group's subjective experience.
3 Application of scientific knowledge to the processes of diagnosis and treatment.
4 Provision of a caring relationship that facilitates health and healing. (American Nurses Association, 1995, p. 6).

It is interesting and enlightening to consider the ANA features in light of the scientific principles and values associated with the ontology of nursing in the consensus statement. In brief, these four principles are:

1 The essence of nursing lies in modes of being, including the nurse's true presence of his or her whole self.
2 The nurses use of the mode of being with and being for, in the process of human-to-human engagement.
3 Nursing by its nature brings intentionality to the therapeutic process.
4 In addition to being for the other, the nurse acts for the other.

The document also emphasized cultural competence as a core element of nursing. Caring by the nurse is transcultural. To be transcultural is more than a value, it is a demand for action. As a discipline with a social mandate, nurses take responsibility for social transformation. Political activism is one form of valuing and acting within the discipline.

When the features described by the ANA were updated in 2003 the additions related to advancement of knowledge and to influence on social and public policy to promote justice. Still the focus on development of systems of support to promote health and quality of life for all is hardly strengthened.

The features described by the ANA and consensus statements serve different purposes, but taken together they portray a picture of nursing as well situated to fully embrace our traditional function of developing systems of support to promote health and improve the quality of life. This essential feature of nursing implies political engagement. Conscious engagement with the world is fundamental in order to transform the world. Praxis is thoughtful reflection and action that occur in synchrony, directed toward deliberative transformation of the world (Chinn, 2001, p. 7). Praxis is values made visible in the world through action. It requires a clear sense of the values on which one wishes to build actions, a vision of the transformations one seeks in the world, and conscious engagement with the world.

Engagement with the world of health care in praxis requires a special kind of consciousness. Freire (1998) describes it in this way:

> *Consciousness of,* an intentionality of consciousness does not end with rationality. Consciousness about the world, which implies consciousness about myself in the world, with it and with others, which also implies our ability to realize the world, to understand it, is not limited to a rationalistic experience. This consciousness is a totality—reason, feelings, emotions, desires; my body, conscious of the world and myself, seizes the world toward which it has an intention. (p. 94)

It is this type of consciousness that makes possible the kind of engagement I believe to be at the heart of nursing. It is an engagement that makes it possible for us to work as partners with communities to envision their desired outcomes for health and quality of life. It is an engagement that gives rise to nurses' political voices in the world. Once one is consciously engaged with the world, one's interactions with others in the world take on a quality that can be called caring/healing, and one can no longer sit on the sidelines. Rather, one engages with the world, energized by a passion to contribute to the world in a meaningful way. In the *Nursing Manifesto: A Call to Conscience and Action* (2000), we described what I think can emerge from nurses' conscious engagement with the world:

> We call forth in all nurses the possibilities inherent in discovering one's own truth and living fully as a person and nurse from this truth. We call forth a willingness to reach for making a critical difference toward betterment of humankind. We call forth the power to act forcefully out of conscience to shape a future that is consistent with our values. We call forth the reawakening of our personal and professional sovereignty to determine our own destinies and to act individually and collectively to transcend the forces that would constrain us. We call forth the passion of practicing nursing from this state of sovereignty and rightfully claim governance of our discipline. We call forth a repudiation of patterns that we create, or that are imposed upon us, that inhibit the full expression of our beings as nurses and persons. We call forth the opening of our hearts to reveal the prospects for action that carry us beyond the negative forces of passivity, contempt, frustration, cynicism, and despair; forces that keep us from living our wholeness and creating a world of peace and healing (A Nursing Manifesto, p. 90).

Conclusion

Last, I turn to a work by David (2000), who provides a passionate analysis of nursing's gender politics. She calls for nurses to develop strategies out of the margins to change our own consciousness as the first step in demanding changes from others in the health care system. David states

> What is needed is a shift from silent, divisive sufferers to collective, proactive risk takers engaging in what Hooks [bell hooks, *Talking Back.* Boston, South End Press, 1989] refers to as "talking back." Talking back is a movement from silence to speech, a primary act of resistance that confronts the dehumanizing politics of domination that renders nurses voiceless and nameless. Talking back is a courageous, defiant act . . . Moving from silence to speech has potential to transform nurses as they attempt to name and understand the representations and practices that define and marginalize the social identity of nurse. (David, 2000, p. 90)

Over the next several decades, I do not want to hear the song "Where have all the nurses gone." Instead, I want to hear voices of nurses raised in harmony to speak out on behalf of health and quality of life. Voices that sing gentle lullabies to calm troubled spirits. Voices that scream in opposition to violence and injustice. Voices that speak with utter confidence to defy those who would restrict the fundamental rights of people for health and happiness. Voices that challenge social and political structures that assure benefits for some and disadvantage for others. Voices that speak in eloquent poetry of visions for the future. And voices that convey generosity of spirit, understanding, respect, and love for our sisters and brothers in nursing around the world, as we all grow and develop in our own places and times. As we proceed with the challenge to action, it is my hope that all nurses everywhere will engage in the kinds of discourses that nurture our collective voices around the world.

REFERENCES

American Nurses Association. (1995). *Nursing's social policy statement*. Washington, DC: American Nurses Publishing.

Chinn, P. L. (2001). *Peace & power: Building communities for the future* (5th ed.). Sudbury, MA: Jones & Bartlett.

David, B. A. (2000). Nursing's gender politics: Reformulating the footnotes. *ANS. Advances in Nursing Science, 23*(1), 83–93.

Faderman, L. (1999). *To believe in women: What lesbians have done for America: A history*. Boston: Houghton Mifflin.

Freire, P. (1998). *Pedagogy of the heart*. New York: Continuum.

A nursing manifesto: A call to conscience and action. (2000, July 30). Retrieved June 30, 2006 from www.nursemanifest.com.

Senge, P. M. (1990). *The fifth discipline: The art and practice of the learning organization*. New York: Doubleday.

Watson, J. (1999). *Postmodern nursing and beyond*. New York: Churchill Livingstone.

Part

Philosophical Basis for Knowledge

Introduction

Exploring the philosophical underpinnings of knowledge development in nursing from three different perspectives will offer the reader the opportunity to analyze, critique, and synthesize commonalities and acknowledging uniqueness of each perspective. This approach can guide movement toward philosophical unity and recognition of the beliefs and values that underlie nursing knowledge development overall.

The *problem solving perspective* is a recognized way to discover and uncover science. Nurses were first introduced to this perspective early in their careers. The nursing process is an essential component of nursing practice and is grounded in a problem-solving approach to patient care and reflected as foundational in the standards of professional practice (American Nurses Association, 2003). Currently, this process is more commonly referred to as clinical reasoning. The goal, however, remains the same—namely, assessment, problem identification, outcomes planning, and isolation of specific interventions useful in achieving a desired goal. Observation, monitoring, and the use of subjective and objective (measurable) data are integral to evaluating the improvement and resolution of a problem.

Within this discussion, Beth Rodgers (in chapter 7) explores the genesis of knowledge development from a *problem-solving perspective*. The author reflects on how philosophers, including Aristotle and Laudan, have used this approach to uncover new knowledge, isolate problems, and discover new answers. She challenges nurses, using a problem-solving perspective, with a critical question, "What are the problems that nursing as a discipline solves?" The answer to this question is an important one. First, the naming of the problem gives nurses a focus and guides the development of nursing's phenomena of concern. Second, problem identification can be useful in defining and shaping the content of practice and nursing curricula. Finally, the problem-solving perspective offers direction for scholarly inquiry and research and contributes to the developing knowledge of the discipline.

Knowledge as process has a significant heritage in nursing. Nurses can easily identify the times they have participated in dialogue with individuals and groups. Usually, it was these experiences that helped to establish relationships and enabled nurses to know patients (families and communities) and their experiences. The narrative (Benner, 1996) has been an effective strategy used by many nurses to reflect patients' perceptions of their journeys toward uncovering meaning, promoting health, relieving suffering, or enabling a peaceful death. This engagement between the nurse and patient exemplifies the philosophical perspective of *knowledge development as a process.*

Margaret Newman and Dorothy Jones' presentation in chapter 8 offers one theoretical perspective that celebrates the use of the dialogue as a process within the nurse–patient partnership. The intentional presence of the nurse within a nurturing environment of care helps create a safe space for personal discovery, pattern recognition, reflection, insight, and choice. Knowledge gained by using a process perspective, particularly as described by Newman, provides an integrated, wholistic understanding of the person. The process illuminates patients' (groups') experiences and can inform care by directing the development of new approaches to health, change, and personal transformation.

Knowledge development within the *poststructuralist feminist perspective* has emerged significantly in recent years. It offers another process-oriented perspective on knowledge development, useful in nursing as a way of viewing the human condition. In chapter 9, Janice Thompson suggests that the attraction to this perspective is its exploration of the use of power, particularly within communities; political implications of power, especially within oppressed groups; and the value of coalition building to advance political and personal agendas and foster emancipation from opression. The author suggests that nurses are in a position to use the knowledge gained from this perspective, both social and political, in order to find a voice and move the discipline from silence to one that informs social consciousness, offers strategies to resolve conflicts, and promotes the greater good and health as a right of all.

Sr. Callista Roy, in chapter 10, continues to advance the philosophical base for nursing knowledge development in a way that embodies both of the perspectives discussed. Using a personal journey in search of truth and the philosophical assumption of veritivity, Roy suggests that nurses are in a position to inform global change, promote equity, and foster human rights and dignity for all. She identifies strategies for achieving this goal, by further development of the ontological and epistemological perspective of *knowledge as a universal cosmic imperative*. Within this perspective, concepts related to unity, purposefulness, promise, imperative as action, and nursing practice are expanded. Roy charges nurses to answer a call to action to create a global health delivery system that promises all citizens a place to live, grow, and discover the potential of what it means to be human.

The discussion of the philosophical basis of knowledge development concludes with Dorothy Jones's synthesis in chapter 11. She integrates the philosophical perspectives of Rodgers, Newman, and Thompson in relation to five specific elements—namely, person, nursing, language, interventions/actions, and outcomes. The reader is given an opportunity to reflect on the interrelationships, as well as the value of each perspective. We can in this way uncover areas of philosophical unity, and identify differences associated with knowledge development from each point of view.

References

American Nurses Association. (2003). *Nursing's social policy statement*. Silver Spring: MD: ANA.

Benner, P. (1996). *Caregiving: Readings in knowledge, practice, ethics, and politics*. Philadelphia: University of Pennsylvania Press.

Knowledge as Problem Solving

Beth L. Rodgers

ursing scholars have spent about 3 decades discussing various philosophical aspects of our discipline. In our striving to meet what we perceived to be a need to demonstrate a specific identity as a discipline, we have explored with vigor such topics as the nature of science, the nature of truth, the development and verification of theory, and how all of these pieces fit together to constitute nursing as a legitimate, unique, and ideally, a scientific discipline. As a discipline, we have not resolved these issues completely. In fact, we will never consider them totally resolved because doing so might cause us to become complacent, and such complacency would make nurses less likely to seek new and possibly better ways of conceptualizing who we are and what we know.

This initial period of nursing's philosophical development can be likened to the adolescent phase of human development. Similarly, the discipline has emerged from this period with a reasonable sense of who we are, even though we might not be satisfied totally with our ability to fully articulate its dimensions. Given nursing's association with the complex and ever-changing realm of health care, there is a continual need to deal with questions regarding the nature of nursing and its purpose. This approval will ensure that the discipline remains contextually focused and relevant. To date many of the answers we have adopted to respond to fundamental questions have moved us little beyond the level of dogma and tradition (Rodgers, 1991). It will benefit our progressive growth to continue to examine our nature, while looking to increase our own understanding of nursing as a discipline. The goal of these efforts can help ensure a positive and productive direction for our growth in knowledge and its relevance to the challenges of health care.

Passing through this adolescent phase, nursing is in a position of openness to new ideas, new questions, and new ways to frame what it is that we do and especially to describe the content of nursing knowledge. One of the contemporary challenges nursing faces is exploring what we do, not on an instrumental basis, but as scholars and scientists, as seekers and developers of knowledge. How can we, or should we, invest our scientific and creative energies as we work to develop the knowledge base for our discipline?

Approaches to Explore Nursing Science

Throughout the literature on epistemology and especially the philosophy of science, we can find many potential answers to the question of how to develop knowledge for nursing. Some authors suggest devoting energy to the development of formal theories (Ayer, 1959; Carnap, 1956; Hemple, 1966). Others support the acquisition of truth or, at least, less falsehood (Popper, 1963/1976, 1972/1979). There are authors who support the articulation and expansion of paradigms (Kuhn, 1962, 1970) or research given traditions (Laudan, 1977). Toulmin's (1972) work suggests knowledge development by expanding and clarifying our conceptual repertoire. Other approaches emphasize emancipation and uncovering the power and authority structures that pervade human interactions (Gadamer, 1975, 1976; Habermas, 1968; Horkheimer & Adorno, 1972) to the goal of achieving hermeneutic enlightenment.

Recently, the call has been added to examine subjective lives through the analysis of narratives and discourse, particularly to uncover the power structures that are pervasive in the worlds of women and persons marginalized from the mainstream of society (Bowers & Moore, 1997; Harden, 2000; Harding, 1991). All of these and other goals have been argued by philosophers and nurse scholars to be the proper objective of our knowledge development efforts. Each has its strengths and limitations and some characteristics of both prescriptive and descriptive credibility.

It is possible to adopt one of these positions to provide direction for further knowledge development. Such dialogue about what nursing should be doing has appeared consistently in our literature. Currently, it seems that as a discipline we are most inclined to accept one of two positions. Some encourage pluralism of ideas about knowledge development processes, in the belief that all contribute different yet important elements to knowledge. Others choose to develop their own philosophies and methods in an attempt to capture the best of each of these ideas. We see this in research sometimes through the merging of a variety of disparate methods.

These options raise questions about philosophical incongruencies among these viewpoints. Each essentially has a unique perspective and speaks a different language. It is not possible merely to select the elements of each perspective that appeals to us, blend them together, and expect to have a consistent and defensible whole. There is another possibility, however, that has not been addressed in detail. There is the possibility that a common epistemological thread underlies these different philosophical approaches.

Although the specific methodologies used to study these viewpoints may be quite different, the scholarly efforts that exist within these various traditions might all be viewed as efforts toward solving problems important in our discipline.

Problem Solving as the Product of Knowledge Development

On a superficial level, it is tempting simply to accept the view that the development of knowledge is a problem-solving process and then just get on with it. What better outcome could we expect from our knowledge base than to make progress in solving some of our disciplinary and clinical practice problems? But, we are dealing with philosophical issues and perspectives, and as any student of philosophy knows, things are never that simple.

Initially, nursing needs to look more in-depth at what it means to view knowledge as problem solving. This task is made more difficult by the fact that philosophers and historians of science have paid little direct attention to this aspect of knowledge development. We can approach the task by looking at the prevailing ideologies in modern philosophy as a basis for comparison, especially at the recently dominant position of *Logical Positivism*. Logical Positivism and related writings compelled us to look at the *products* of knowledge development activity rather than at the processes involved. The appropriate product of such activity for some time has been considered to be theory, particularly formal or propositional theory. Knowledge development activity, which we can refer to as science, was considered to have progressed as new theories were developed and as newer theories were regarded as *better* than the earlier theories. Better in this context meant that the new theory was supported by more facts and withstood more precise testing; in other words, it was more *true* than previous theories.

This emphasis on theoretical products to demonstrate advancement of knowledge is quite troublesome. It treats theories as if they can be compared, that they can be looked at side by side. From this comparison then, we could determine whether one should take the place of the other in the name of advancing the science. This commensurability thesis, however, requires that two other conditions be met. First, we would have to accept a foundationist view that there is some objective reality, some absolute foundation against which we can compare the theories to determine their truth value. Ideally, this would be accomplished based on how well the theory captures and corresponds with the foundation of reality. Second, there would be a commitment that it is possible to disregard the context in which the theories were developed, including the viewpoints and judgments of the people involved, and to accept them as devoid of such influences, thus rendering them equal for purposes of comparison.

It does not require a lengthy argument to refute these claims—that we can capture reality with such accuracy and permanence and that human beings could engage in inquiry with freedom from bias. Nowhere are such limitations more evident or more troublesome than in sciences that deal with human beings. At one time, we might have been able to accept that a foundation of truth existed, against which we could compare our knowledge claims on at least a basic physiological level. Surely there were truths that would provide the definitive answer to why a particular disease occurs in an individual, for example. But recent history is full of situations that show that even on this level such a foundation may be unreasonable. One particularly striking example concerns how the long-standing *germ theory* for the origin of disease has given way to environmental, sociobehavioral, chemical, and genetic conceptions of disease.

Problem Solving as a Process of Knowledge Development

Recognizing that our traditional views of science are not plausible, we are left with what is one of the primary questions confronted by philosophers of science: How does science work? What process is involved? In the philosopher's terms, what is responsible for scientists forming consensus, for supporting a particular approach or theory over competing ideas, and for continuing to pursue a particular line of inquiry? One potential answer found in writings in philosophy of science is this idea of problem solving—that it is the desire to solve problems that underlies knowledge development activity. It is the problem-solving value of the new knowledge that accounts for its support and acceptance in a discipline. This view of knowledge as problem solving can provide nursing with some different ways to view our own discipline and possibly enhance our own progress in developing our knowledge base.

Most of the writings that address problem solving and knowledge come from recent philosophy of science, particularly the writings of Kuhn (1962, 1970, 1977) and Laudan (1977). Laudan, in fact, points out that the idea of science as problem solving "is more a cliché than a philosophy" (p. 11). This interpretation, however, may be due to the lack of attention to this aspect of knowledge development, consequently the lack of focus to develop this point of view into what might stand as a distinct philosophy.

Kuhn (1962, 1970) deserves credit for introducing the perspective of problem solving in the contemporary literature, although problem solving, per se, was not a major focus of his work. Instead, his contributions have been invaluable in helping to move beyond the binds of modernist views of science and knowledge, particularly those of Logical Positivism. Kuhn's work was monumental in shifting the focus of discussion from the *prescriptive* ideas, those presenting how science *should* be done, to a *descriptive* approach, addressing how science works and what makes it work well. As a significant component of this thinking, Kuhn showed how individual as well as disciplinary values and judgments have an insurmountable role in scientific activity and progress. He argued that scientific activity does not consist merely of a narrowly cumulative and linear approach to development and expansion of existing theories. Rather science is focused on the articulation of a paradigm, a more complex constellation of facts, concepts, and values within a discipline.

In doing so, Kuhn helped to remove the emphasis on the *product* of scientific activity and placed it on the *process* by which scientific work was carried out. For Kuhn (1970), the process of science was a process of problem solving. Actually, Kuhn referred to the overall process as one of puzzle solving and made an interesting, but somewhat confusing, distinction between puzzles and problems. In looking at problem solving as a possible way of conceptualizing knowledge, the finer points of distinctions between puzzles and problems is of little significance. Kuhn's puzzle-solving phrase can be replaced easily by what is referred to here as problem solving without doing any injustice to Kuhn's work.

Laudan maintained a similar emphasis and addressed problem solving within science in very specific terms. Accordingly, "Science is essentially a problem-solving activity" (Laudan, 1977, p. 11). The measure of science that is of scientific progress and of rationality is not based on the theories or other products that result from scientific activity but is the contribution that is made to solving problems.

Views of historicists, such as Kuhn and Laudan, as well as those thinkers reflective of a Logical Positivist tradition, are often presented as comprising a stark dichotomy. However, on closer evaluation that dichotomy is not necessarily the case, especially where the implications for scholarly effort are concerned. On a purely philosophical level, there is little similarity between the two perspectives. In regard to the goals of science or knowledge development, it is worthwhile to note that a view of knowledge as problem solving does not require us to abandon the pursuit of theory development or truth or closer approximations of truth. It does mean, however, that we can be freer to pursue the forms of inquiry that are most appropriate in our discipline.

What Is a Problem?

Toulmin (1972) has a remarkably simple and concise way to explain what counts as a problem in this context. For Toulmin, a problem is the difference between the goals of the discipline and its current intellectual capabilities. This thinking is expressed in a simple formula:

Scientific Problem = Explanatory Ideals/Current Capabilities (Toulmin, 1972, p. 152)

A problem, therefore, can concern any knowledge that the members of the discipline believe they need to have, yet which they do not currently possess. According to Laudan, all that is necessary for something to be deemed a problem is for the situation to be *thought* to be an actual state of affairs and to reflect an area important to the discipline.

The problems confronted within a discipline "[arise] within a certain context of inquiry" (Laudan, 1977, p. 15). Problems will change, as they are defined by the current knowledge base of the discipline and new discoveries and procedures provide strategies to resolve the problem. Social and other situational factors as well can influence problem definition by calling attention to certain areas for inquiry and providing incentives for work in particular areas (Laudan, 1977; Toulmin, 1972).

An example of this thinking is currently taking place in nursing inquiry. After qualitative research being considered secondary for decades, there has been a significant increase in the use of qualitative methods. This development is explained easily in reference to problem solving and provides a good example in our own discipline of Laudan's and Toulmin's views of change. For some time, qualitative research methods were viewed by many scholars in a variety of disciplines as inconsistent with the primary disciplinary goal of developing a substantive, empirical knowledge base. Knowledge development continued using traditional, empirical approaches to inquiry, consistent with prevailing ideology over the last several decades. However, scholars began to recognize that potentially important elements were missing in this type of inquiry especially in the human sciences (Gadamer, 1975, 1976; Habermas, 1968). Nurses and others began to see problems in regard to people's experiences and perceptions of their situations, in addition to problems amenable to standard forms of research.

Problem Solving, Knowledge Developments, and Change

A variety of contextual factors seem to have stimulated changes in knowledge development and science. Members of technological societies began to recognize disparities between so-called high-tech and high touch. Their recognition provides an example of yearning for attention to aspects of existence such as quality of life and personal experience. At the same time, there was more work being done to understand qualitative methods and demonstrate their appropriateness and rigor. These efforts brought about methodological improvements in something that previously had survived based primarily on an oral tradition. Through this transition, problems defined by the discipline became redefined, and we took on new problems in our inquiry based on our developing knowledge base. We improved our capabilities through methodological advancements and also the "ripeness" (Toulmin, 1972) of problems as a result of societal and disciplinary influences.

The history of medical knowledge, as well, is replete with examples of how problems change in response to new knowledge, new methods, and changes in context. A number of changes in medical knowledge and practice can be traced from Empedocles' ancient humoral theory of illness; through changes in anatomical knowledge contributed by such a diverse group as Aristotle, Galen, Harvey, and Boyle; through alchemy, the development of the microscope and the discovery of microorganisms.

It is interesting to note that what followed in some respects reverted to ideas that resemble earlier sets of beliefs and practices such as the current emphasis placed by some practitioners on chemical or other imbalances as the source of illness. There are significant examples of how changes in our ideas about problems and especially what we might count as solved problems do not happen quickly or easily. The recommendations regarding asepsis were ridiculed by American and European physicians for more than 20 years, even though Semmelweiss was able to reduce the maternal mortality rate from childbirth fever by more than 90%. The problem of childbirth fever was not considered solved until Pasteur demonstrated the bacteriologic basis for the recommended aseptic techniques, thus converting Semmelweiss' success from a mere anomaly, as Kuhn might have called it, into a solved problem.

This example also shows how naïve it is to think of problem solving on a functional level, as merely achieving a desired outcome, as a matter of doing, rather than as a matter of knowing. The sophistication of a problem-solving approach is evident in that solving problems entails not just achieving a desired outcome, alleviating an existing troubling situation, but in understanding why the change occurred. Problem solving should not be misconstrued as a matter of application; it is the attendant increase in knowledge and understanding that contributes to a solved problem.

Similar changes in nursing's values, capabilities, and knowledge have created a situation where many nurses reading Nightingale's (1860/1969) *Notes on Nursing* for the first time are inclined to be struck by how right she may have been all along. Clearly, Nightingale was not subjected to the same ridicule as Semmelweiss when her ideas first were published more than 140 years ago. However, as a discipline, nursing did drift away from these core beliefs, in search of other answers and solutions. Only later did nurses recognize some of Nightingale's ideas with renewed credibility because of other changes in thinking.

The processes of knowledge development involve problems of all types; that is, empirical, conceptual, and what might be called perceptual problems. What constitutes a problem ultimately stems from a complex of intersecting values, beliefs, and current capabilities and knowledge. None of these elements was static. Disciplinary goals and values may change in response to the contexts in which the knowledge development activities take place (Laudan, 1984); changes in intellectual capacities occur as a result of new knowledge that is generated as well as developments in methodology that make it rational to expect new things from our knowledge development efforts. Consequently, the problems at the forefront of inquiry in a discipline change along with these intertwined elements, and what will be considered a solved problem will change as well.

Validity of the "Problem-Solving" Approach

In addition to reviewing various elements of a problem-solving approach, consideration must be given as to whether this approach constitutes a valid epistemic viewpoint. One approach to examining epistemic validity is to look at whether the idea of problem solving is consistent with what is known about science. The description so far shows considerable similarity between the history and processes of science and the notion of problem solving. Additional credibility is given to this position by observing that even the long-standing emphasis on theoretical products as the measure of "good" science could be explained by this idea of problem solving. Laudan (1977) pointed out that

> theories matter, they are *cognitively important*, insofar as—and only insofar as—they provide adequate solutions to problems ... the function of a theory is to resolve ambiguity, to reduce irregularity to uniformity, to show that what happens is somehow intelligible and predictable. (Laudan, 1977, p. 13)

Thus, the focus on theoretical products that has characterized much of philosophy of science in modern times could itself be a reflection of the problem-solving emphasis of scientific activity.

Descriptive credibility in evaluating a philosophical position regarding science can only go so far. One of the difficulties with such an approach concerns the fact that historical accounts of science are inherently biased by the perspective of the writer of that history. If the history of science is viewed with an eye toward whether or not a problem-solving approach accounts for much of the activity, chances are we will find problem solving in that account. Lacking any objective criterion to evaluate the credibility of this approach, we need to ask different questions. The question to be asked is whether or not such a view can provide a positive heuristic, consistent with nursing's perceived needs for a knowledge base. Will this approach help us to develop the knowledge we need to do what it is that we need to do? Will it further our own epistemic and intellectual goals? What would it mean for nursing if we were to view knowledge development as problem solving?

What "Knowledge as Problem Solving" Means for Nursing

The effects of using knowledge as problem solving as an approach for nursing knowledge development activities span the philosophical and applied aspects of our discipline. On a basic philosophical level, a problem-solving approach is quite consistent with the in-ternalized values of the discipline. Although nurses may disagree about some aspects of our discipline and clinical practice, there can be little argument that nurses value human beings in their entirety. We believe that people are holistic beings constituting multiple facets, including the physical, mental, spiritual, social, and ethical realms of existence. Nurses value human beings as individuals, subject to their own unique backgrounds and experiences. As scientists and practitioners, we espouse an ontology, or view of reality, as changing the world we live in, the people in it, and the application of knowledge; that is dynamic as well as diverse (Donaldson & Crowley, 1978; Flaskerud & Halloran, 1980; Schultz, 1987).

These goals demand flexibility and openness to new ideas. In nursing educational programs, we need to move beyond the psychomotor skills lab and the belief that there is one, and only one, right way to perform some intervention. Nurses are taught that what we do is based on principles, and the value in our doing comes from our ability to act on those principles in a way that is flexible, consistent with our aim to individualize the care we provide. The situations in which we provide that care are as diverse as the recipients of that care, including people on individual, family, community, and population levels. Often, we act on their environments as well.

A problem-solving approach to knowledge does not require a change in nursing's values and convictions. This approach is consistent with the flexibility needed to remain responsive and relevant in changing contexts and with changing disciplinary aims. It also is consistent with nursing's need to work on development in many areas. An emphasis in nursing knowledge development activity on a singular theory, or on a narrow set of concepts or phenomena, as advocated by philosophers in the 20th century, could constrain our knowledge development efforts and compel us to focus on a constricted part of the world to satisfy these externally imposed requirements. Problem solving, however, allows us to have multiple focal points for our energies, as scientists cluster together to pursue similar interests for the sake of producing the knowledge needed within the discipline.

Problem Solving and Emerging Science

It is reasonable, for example, for us to pursue inquiry and develop taxonomies, such as those represented by Nursing Diagnosis (NANDA, 2005–2006), the Nursing Interven-tion Classification System (Dochterman & Bulechek, 2004), and the Nursing Outcomes Classification (Moorhead, Johnson, & Maas, 2004), to provide language needed to de-scribe nursing's thinking and acting. In addition, nursing's participation in the develop-ment of critical pathways and desired outcome criteria for common conditions provide opportunities to articulate nursing problems, interventions, and outcomes attributable to nursing knowledge. Concurrently, nurse-scientists can use phenomenological or critical approaches to capture other aspects of these conditions. In fact, if a problem identified within the aims and values of our discipline includes subjective, individual experiences as important components of the illness experience, then nursing protocols and clinical pathways will include such experiences. If this does not occur, then outcomes or results of nursing care will be limited and fail to reflect problem-solving effectiveness. Nursing must remain cognizant of its own purposes, values, aims, and goals as we identify and define disciplinary problems and responses. Working with members of other disciplines to take advantage of alternate perspectives may assist us as we *study* solutions to our most pressing problems.

In the past we might have considered such a scenario to be laissez-faire. It might seem to lack the focus and clarity consistent with real science. Certainly, it does not match the dichotomies that we often rely on to discuss science such as art and science, borrowed and unique knowledge, "hard" and "soft" forms of research.

The development of nursing knowledge, however, presents us with anything but these either or situations. Nursing values and intellectual aims are not consistent with efforts toward dichotomization. There are problems associated with classifying what we do, particularly as computer technology is now prevalent in our practice. There are also additional problems related to the broader empirical realm, as well as perceptual realms of nursing and of knowledge in general. Nurses are working to develop effective roles in situations as diverse as violence, teen pregnancy, chronic illness, cardiovascular disease, and environmental health. As nurses we also confront problems associated with access to care and determining what constitutes quality care. At the same time, we strive to develop a broad understanding of the experiences of people who live with these situations. Far from a laissez-faire approach, using a problem-oriented approach to develop our knowledge base offers nursing scholars and scientists an opportunity to relieve deficits in our knowledge according to the situations that are most pressing at any time. To do otherwise—to focus only on theory building, increasing observational evidence, testing of interventions, or on description alone—would ignore a large part of what we do, what we need to know, and what society expects from us.

Problem Solving and Knowledge Development—Future Directions

Although this discussion may be progressive from a heuristic standpoint, it does present us with some new challenges. The knowledge developers in nursing, the researchers and scholars, need a readily available repertoire of skills and perspectives and a diversity of methodological and theoretical tools in order to provide the diversity needed as we develop and expand nursing's knowledge base. This, in turn, places demands on research and educational institutions to provide the support and preparation needed to meet our problem-solving goals. This approach also calls for maintaining a strong linkage between research and nursing practices, as problems emerge within nursing practice. There is also a need to develop linkages with people outside of our own discipline, who are consumers of our knowledge. Because every discipline has some realm in which the members practice or apply the knowledge generated, we avoid the term *practice discipline*. Our knowledge needs to be returned to settings in which they are used for purposes of evaluation and further refinement. We cannot begin to deal with questions about whether, or how well, a problem has been solved until that new knowledge is evaluated in the situation from which the problem was derived.

It is important to recognize that all of nursing's problems do not arise only from practice. Work needs to continue on a philosophical level as well. A problem-solving approach means a reframing of our questions along the lines of disciplinary aims, knowledge-development goals, and determining what problems are most appropriate and fruitful for us to pursue—in Toulmin's (1972) words, those problems that are "ripe" for us to confront. There needs to be disciplinary consensus around what will count as adequate "solving" of our problems, a challenge that requires continuous reevaluation of our goals and aims as a discipline and what our inquiry into defined problems can contribute to overall health care. This effort will require nurses to be flexible and open to new ideas and new ways of seeing. Our aims, capabilities, and the problems we pursue and seek to solve will continue to change.

A problem-solving approach offers a solid philosophical foundation to support continuing development of knowledge in nursing. With this approach, nurses can work to develop knowledge in multiple areas, through diverse strategies, and with collaborative and cooperative arrangements that can help advance our work. Use of a problem-solving approach to knowledge development presents some unique challenges to our usual ways of thinking about knowledge and to our ways of thinking about nursing as a discipline. The end result can be development of the knowledge essential to confront effectively some of the many needs for knowledge we face in our discipline to effect the needed changes in health care delivery.

REFERENCES

Ayer, A. J. (Ed.). (1959). *Logical positivism*. New York: Free Press.

Bowers, R., & Moore, K. N. (1997). Bakhtin, nursing narratives, and dialogical consciousness. *Advances in Nursing Science, 19*(3), 70–77.

Carnap, R. (1956). *Meaning and necessity*. Chicago: University of Chicago Press.

Dochterman, J. M., & Bulechek, G. (Eds.). (2004). *Nursing interventions classification* (4th ed.). St. Louis, MO: Elsevier.

Donaldson, S. K., & Crowley, D. M. (1978). The discipline of nursing. *Nursing Outlook, 26*, 113–120.

Flaskerud, J. H., & Halloran, E. J. (1980). Areas of agreement in nursing theory development. *Advances in Nursing Science, 3*(1), 1–7.

Gadamer, H. (1975). *Truth and method* (G. Barden & J. Cumming, Trans. and Eds.). New York: Seabury Press.

Gadamer, H. (1976). *Philosophical hermeneutics* (D. E. Linge, Trans.). Berkeley: University of California Press.

Habermas, J. (1968). *Knowledge and human interests* (J. J. Shapiro, Trans.). Boston: Beacon Press.

Harden, J. (2000). Language, discourse and the chronotope: Applying literary theory to the narratives in health care. *Journal of Advanced Nursing, 31*, 506–512.

Harding, S. (1991). *Whose science? Whose knowledge?* Ithaca, NY: Cornell University.

Hemple, C. (1966). *Philosophy of natural science*. Englewood Cliffs, NJ: Prentice-Hall.

Horkheimer, M., & Adorno, T. W. (1972). *Dialectic of enlightenment* (J. Cumming, Trans.). New York: Herder & Herder.

Moorhead, S., Johnson, M., & Maas, M. (Eds.).(2004). *Nursing outcomes classification*. (3rd ed.). St. Louis, MO: Mosby.

Kuhn, T. S. (1962). *The structure of scientific revolutions*. Chicago: University of Chicago Press.

Kuhn, T. S. (1970). *The structure of scientific revolutions* (2nd ed.). Chicago: University of Chicago Press.

Kuhn, T. S. (1977). *The essential tension.* Chicago: University of Chicago Press.

Laudan, L. (1977). *Progress and its problems: Towards a theory of scientific growth.* Berkeley: University of California Press.

Laudan, L. (1984). *Science and values: The aims of science and their role in scientific debate.* Berkeley: University of California Press.

NANDA (2005–2006). *North American nursing diagnosis association: Definitions and classification.* Philadelphia, PA: Nursecom, Inc.

Nightingale, F. (1969). *Notes on nursing: What it is, and what it is not.* New York: Dover. (Original work published 1860)

Popper, K. R. (1976). *Conjectures and refutations.* London: Routledge & Kegan Paul. (Original work published 1963)

Popper, K. R. (1979). *Objective knowledge.* Oxford: Oxford University Press. (Original work published 1972)

Rodgers, B. L. (1991). Deconstructing the dogma in nursing knowledge and practice. *Image: Journal of Nursing Scholarship, 23,* 177–181.

Schultz, P. R. (1987). Toward holistic inquiry in nursing: A proposal for synthesis of patterns and methods. *Scholarly Inquiry for Nursing Practice: An International Journal, 1,* 135–146.

Toulmin, S. (1972). *Human understanding.* Princeton, NJ: Princeton University Press.

Experiencing the Whole: Health as Expanding Consciousness (State of the Art)*

8

Margaret A. Newman
Dorothy A. Jones

N ursing claims to be a discipline dedicated to understanding and relating to the health of the whole person, not just to the pathology that often brings the person to the attention of health care professionals. The preponderance of nursing research, however, fails to focus on this commitment. In an effort to be scientific, we have allowed our vision to be bluffed by the paradigmatic demands of objectivity and control. In an attempt to be predictive, we have divided the person into parts. My theoretical and research pursuits reflected these demands for a while but gradually they became consistent with a paradigm of wholeness. I want to share the major turning points of this journey and where I think it leads us as a discipline.

*From, Experiencing the Whole: State of the Art by Newman, M., (1997), *Advances in Nursing Science* *20*(1), p. 34–39. Reprinted with permission.

The Journey

My research interest has always stemmed from the experience of the person involved. I had observed the problems associated with restricted movement in relation to the time and space of one's life. I had experienced it personally in the care of my mother, who was paralyzed by amyotrophic lateral sclerosis. I had worked with persons in rehabilitation settings where their movement was restricted by other forms of paralysis and trauma. I could envision it in the lives of new parents who find the movement–time–space of their lives restricted by their responsibilities to their newborn infants.

I turned to the literature and found a basic theory of time perception as a function of movement and from there designed an experimental study manipulating movement and measuring time (Newman, 1972). The research design was the epitome of manipulation and control, so much so that the natural effects of movement were lost. The participants, however, described their response to the manipulation of their rate of movement and how they had consciously compensated for this factor. That experience was an important lesson in how the human being interacts with the research process. This way of approaching nursing knowledge did not fit the reality of the life situation and revealed little about how to practice nursing.

Bit by bit I relinquished some of the control I thought I had under experimental conditions and began to focus on the natural characteristics of movement and time in relation to age and other factors. The changing perception of time across the life span revealed a seemingly developmental phenomenon of expanding consciousness (Newman, 1982) and supported my proposed theory of health as expanding consciousness (Newman, 1979). Still, this interactive, integrative approach was locked into the scientific expectations of objectivity and control. The findings were enlightening but too static and particulate to provide a comprehensive guide for nursing practice.

Finally, seeing that these ways were not working, I let go of the research expectations of objectivity and control and allowed the tenets of my theory to guide the methods of study (Newman, 1990). These tenets included:

- Mutuality of interaction between nurse and client.
- Uniqueness and wholeness of pattern in each client situation.
- Movement of the life process toward higher consciousness.

I began to see more clearly the core of pattern and process as the reality of nursing practice. I equated the evolving pattern with the meaning of the whole. This view required the letting go of the concept of observer-observing-the-observed and demanded an approach of mutual process.

The research that emerged from these beliefs focused on the unfolding pattern of a person's life (Endo, 1996; Jonsdottir, 1995; Lamendola & Newman, 1994; Litchfield, 1993; Moch, 1990; Newman, 1994; Newman & Moch, 1991). To my surprise the pattern revealed evidence of expanding consciousness in the quality and connectedness of the relationships portrayed. It also pointed to the nurse-researcher's creative presence as important in revealing the participant's insight.

The theory of health as expanding consciousness became evident in the unfolding lives of the client-participants as they found new, loving connections with the people in their lives and were able to see openings for action that brought about increasing alternatives and greater freedom of movement. The theory was alive! Not just theoretical propositions linking the concepts in fixed patterns, but meaningful, moving relationships. Bernstein (1983), citing Gadamer, emphasized that it is in the performance of a play or music that we encounter the work. And so it was in the experience of a theory that its power became a reality.

A theory must be judged in terms of its evolvement through various stages (Bernstein, 1983). The stages of understanding of the theory of health as expanding consciousness unfolded through these six stages:

1 Identifying the underlying assumptions, key concepts, and axiomatic relationships among movement, space, time, and consciousness as relevant to patterning of health (Newman, 1979).
2 Seeing these concepts emerge from the implicit grasp of the total pattern of the person (Newman, 1986a, 1994).
3 Moving from identifying the pattern of person-environment at a point in time, as was done in the early days of nursing diagnosis, to seeing the pattern as sequential configurations evolving over time, like waves of explicit-implicit phenomena, unfolding-enfolding (Newman, 1984, 1986b, 1987).
4 Seeing the insights that occurred in the process as choice points of action potential (Endo, 1996; Newman, 1990, 1994).
5 Realizing that both the client and the nurse mutually participate in a process of expanding consciousness (Newman, 1990).
6 Experiencing the pattern unfolding (Endo, 1996; Litchfield, 1993).

The evolution of the theory moved from a linear explication and testing of general principles to an elaboration of interacting patterns as manifestations of expanding consciousness. Litchfield's (1993) work shifted the emphasis to the evolving dialogue of the researcher and participant in the process of health patterning. The dynamic, holistic nature of the experience is consistent with a unitary, transformative view.

Reality and How We Know It

Newman, Sime, and Corcoran-Perry (1991) sought to eliminate some of the confusion regarding the nature of the discipline of nursing by identifying the focus of the discipline and the prevailing paradigms of science. In declaring "caring in the human health experience" the focus of the discipline, we considered it to be at the metaparadigm level, a level beyond the disparate paradigms. We thought the focus should be paradigm-free. Because we saw ourselves as each coming from different paradigms, we proceeded to try to illustrate how the focus could be addressed from each of the prevailing paradigms of the day. Trying to be inclusive, we stated that knowledge emanating from the particulate-deterministic and interactive-integrative paradigms is relevant to nursing but asserted that knowledge from the unitary-transformative paradigm is essential to our discipline. In retrospect, if this type of knowledge is essential to the discipline, then is it not the knowledge of the discipline?

Since airing that all-inclusive view, I have had doubts about trying to establish the focus of the discipline as paradigm-free. The act of doing so may be merely academic: When one attends to the focus from a particular view, it takes on the characteristics of that view. A paradigm consists of the coming together of the focus, philosophy, and theory of the discipline. These elements must be consistent with each other. Otherwise, as a discipline with a professional commitment, we are offering an incoherent message to society.

The paradigm of the discipline is becoming clear. We are moving from attention to the patient as an object to attention to the we in the relationship, from fixing things to attending to the meaning of the whole, from hierarchical one-way intervention to mutual process partnering. It is time to break with a paradigm of health that focuses on power, manipulation, and control and move to one of reflective, compassionate consciousness. The paradigm of nursing embraces wholeness and pattern. It reveals a world that is moving, evolving, transforming—a process.

If one can accept that the reality of our world of nursing practice is process, it is incumbent that our emphasis is in the present, not holding onto the past, and not looking to prediction of the future. Attachment to the past, such as in searching for causal explanations, hinders movement. Focusing on the future, as in predictive relationships, channels our vision, possibly occluding important elements of the present complexity. Only as we immerse ourselves fully in the present can we follow the direction of the process. That means relaxing into the uncertainty and unpredictability of this process.

We are at a choice point. We can no longer equivocate with "everything goes." Bernstein (1983), harking back to Thomas Kuhn and others, raised the question of whether there are incommensurable paradigms. In our efforts to try to create unity within the discipline, we have overlooked the incommensurable paradigms existing under the rubric of nursing. Our history of alignment with medical science and later social science has made it difficult for us to grasp and embrace the reality of our own science. Nursing scholars should be able to articulate the focus, philosophy, and theory of the discipline. Nursing scholarship should have a ring of coherence about it.

The nature of nursing is a dynamic, relational process, and to understand it we must engage in the experience of it. We must study the process of our relationships with clients from within, as part of the process. We are embedded in what we want to study. We cannot step outside the process. The nature of reality is not outside ourselves.

Unbroken wholeness is what is real—not the fragments we devise with our way of describing things. And the wholeness is in continual movement. Bohm (1980) referred to this phenomenon as the "holomovement"—the flowing movement of an undivided whole. We do not stop the movement when we take a picture of it in an observer–observed mode; we simply miss the continuity of the flow, the evolving pattern. We must be fully present in the moment as it unfolds. Individual consciousness cannot be separated from the web of things and events. We are manifestations of an infinite whole. We need to study the meaning of the whole.

Study Consistent With Reality

The nature of wholeness is such that it cannot be addressed by the scientific method as currently conceived. It cannot be observed, named, or manipulated. The whole cannot be found in summation or integration of the parts. But the parts are manifestations of the whole. The whole is always present everywhere and, as in a hologram, is experienced by going into the parts. Bortoft, in explicating a science of wholeness, had this to say: "We understand meaning in the moment of coalescence when the whole is reflected in the parts so that together they disclose the whole" (Bortoft, 1996, p. 9). "Thus the whole emerges simultaneously with the accumulation of the parts, not because it is the sum of the parts, but because it is immanent within them" (p. 12). He compares the whole to the essence of a play: Actors "enter into a part in such a way that they enter into the play. . . But actors do not encounter the play as an object of knowledge over which they can stand like the lines they learn. They encounter the play in their part as an active absence which can begin to move them. . . An actor starts to be acted by the play" (p. 15). In addition, he observed, "their awareness being occupied with the lines to be spoken, they encounter the whole which is the play—not as an object but as an active absence" (p. 15).

So, too, as a nurse by necessity attends to the parts, the meaning of the whole will emerge. We come to the meaning of the whole not by viewing the pattern from the outside, but by entering into the evolving pattern as it unfolds.

It has been difficult to switch from ways of conducting research in which objectivity and control prevail to a participatory, open-ended unfolding that is innovative and unpredictable and brings about changes in the lives of those participating. In the beginning, even Rogers (1970, 1990) advocated empirical approaches based on probability and predictability but later rejected those concepts as inconsistent with her vision of homeodynamics and the innovative nature of human becoming.

Research in a paradigm characterized by pattern and process is participatory research. If the way we know this reality is by experiencing it, then to study it we must engage in the process of practice. We are seeking knowledge that illuminates transformation from one point to another. Morgan (1983) equated the quest for knowledge with transformation: "When we engage in research action, thought, and interpretation, we are . . . involved in . . . processes through which we actually make and remake ourselves as human being" (p. 373).

The researcher participates in the research to help the participants understand the meaning of their situations and with it potential for action. I have found Wheeler and Chinn's (1984) definition of praxis meaningful: "thoughtful reflection and action that occurs in synchrony, in the direction of transforming the world" (p. 2). The content of nursing practice is process wisdom, evolving insight, occurring in the midst of chaos. The specifics are not predictable. The process of the nurse's interacting with participants (clients) involves interpretation of each person's perspective in a hermeneutic dialectic mode.

In this type of research the researcher becomes the practitioner. In like manner the reciprocal is also true—the practitioner can be the researcher. The research is reality based. It involves questioning the nature of nursing, enhancing the meaning of the experience, and enriching the theory. The insight gained by adopting this method applies equally to practice. Brink (1990) once proposed that a discipline and its method are one and the same. As I contemplate the praxis nature of nursing research, I tend to agree. The knowledge of nursing is an immanent, transforming process of unfolding pattern.

Epilogue: Impact and Future Considerations

In a recent publication entitled *Giving Voice to What We Know: Margaret Newman's Theory of Health as Expanding Consciousness in Nursing Education, Practice, and Research* (Picard & Jones, 2005), a number of nurse scholars using the work of Newman in research, theory development, education, and practice wrote extensively about impact of health as expanding consciousness (HEC) on nursing. The authors agreed that the theoretical perspective provided by Newman was a useful framework to guide research as praxis (hermeneutic dialectic), nursing innovation within the environment of care and curriculum development. For many, HEC articulates the essence of nursing as the relationship between the nurse and the patient. Within this relationship "lies opportunity for discovery, awareness, choice, and transformation for the patient (family and community) as well as the nurse" (Jones, 2005, p. 219).

Expanding of Theory, Practice, Research: An Iterative Process

HEC recognizes knowledge development as an iterative process. Within HEC, the interrelationships between and among theory, research, and practice relate to one another in a "reciprocal, cyclical and interactive way" (McEwen & Willis, 2002, p. 80). HEC has been used to guide research (i.e., research as praxis), which in turn has generated new knowledge that has informed nursing education and practice. Basic assumptions underlying the theory have been tested and refined through research and theory has been enhanced, supported, and validated by the process. The numerous examples contained within the publication (Picard & Jones, 2005), as well as the emerging research investigations continue to support HEC as an iterative process reflecting the development of theoretical knowledge to shape nursing practice, education, and research.

Application of HEC in Research, Practice, and Education

"Knowledge developed using HEC as a framework for research has been found to uncover information that helps illuminate the meaning of the person's present situation within the context of the past and future and stimulates new insights that lead to clarity of action" (Jones, 2005, p. 222). In research as praxis, the participant is invited to share meaningful persons and experiences in their lives. The researcher embodies HEC, and, along with the participant uncovers new understandings, illuminates patient experiences, and uses knowledge to guide actions.

Examples of research to date have generated new understandings around meanings associated with achieving a peaceful death (Barron, 2000), self-growth in women (Picard, 2000), wound healing (Capasso, 2005), sustaining weight loss (Berry, 2004), addressing loss and disconnections early in childhood (Novolesky-Rosenthal, 1996), illuminating life choices for women with ovarian cancer (Endo, 2000), and as healing for patients with rheumatoid arthritis (Neill, 2002). Pharris (2002) reported on the effectiveness of pattern analysis to describe the impact of life disruptions and transformations in individuals and family members as a whole.

Investigations exploring the influence of HEC on education also revealed interesting changes in students regarding self-growth, reflection, and discovery. Novolesky-Rosenthal & Solomon (2001) developed selected learning experiences designed to link HEC with patient interactions and enhanced student sensitivity to patient experiences and the therapeutic role of the nurse engaged in patient care. Picard & Margolis (2002) used HEC as a framework to guide the teaching of psychiatric nursing.

Within clinical practice, clinicians have found HEC a useful framework in the redesign of patient care environments for individuals and families. Ruka (2005) introduced changes in a nursing home setting to create a model of care that was responsive to residents experiencing dementia. Within the new model, families were invited to tell stories to the nurse about their loved ones. This new knowledge was integrated into patient care plans and guided interventions that were more sensitive to the individual resident's evolving pattern.

Flanagan (2002) used a HEC-oriented framework to redesign nursing practice for patients during the preadmission visit prior to surgery. The physical space where the nurse–patient encounter occurred was intentionally recreated. A planned increase in attention to the nurse's intentional presence with the patient enhanced the patient's sense of self and promoted actions designed to optimize choice and promote change. In another study, the use of the dialogue within the patient care experience enhanced the presence of the nurse and promoted patients' comfort (Lee, 2005). These studies showed that pattern analysis provided opportunity for meaningful reflection, discovery, and actions that supported change and personal transformation.

Health as Expanding Consciousness: Future Considerations

"Nursing theory expresses the values and beliefs of the discipline, helps to frame the human experience and guides the caring process" (see the Consensus Statement, chapter 1, this volume). HEC is a dynamic theory, supported by research and useful to clinicians in practice and to educators as an important way to articulate and build nursing knowledge.

Continued evaluation of the theoretical perspective offered within Newman's theory of HEC will further explicate elements of the theory related to such concepts as presence, intentionality, and caring. Research investigations using the phenomenological hermeneutic dialectic methodology will be enhanced by the recruitment of larger sample sizes of subjects that represent increased diversity of the population overall and add new knowledge about the human experience. Extending the use of pattern appraisal beyond the two encounters suggested by Newman will help illuminate both the impact of the dialogue over time as reflected in life choices and by sustained changes made by participants. Increased use of aesthetic expression, as used by some researchers (Picard, 2000) may increase nurses' and patients' understanding of the total experience. Although "similarities of pattern among participants of a study may be designated by themes and stated in propositional forms" (Newman, 1994, p. 149), there is a need for further study of the usefulness of pattern manifestations across populations to uncover new knowledge. This may provide new insights for the educator and practitioner by enhancing understanding of patient experiences.

Pattern appraisal and recognition help differentiate the focus of nursing from other disciplines, require a specialized body of disciplinary knowledge, and lead to a practice in which outcomes are responsive to nursing actions. "Guidelines for the creation of theory-based, practice models, especially HEC, need to be developed to guide clinicians in the development, preparation, implementation and evaluation of these models of care across settings" (Jones, 2005, p. 226). Practice settings using a HEC framework require continued evaluation to describe the patient-nurse experience with care, as well exploring linkages to selected organizational outcomes, such as length of patient stay, healing and recovery, and professional growth, as well as achievement of organizational goals and cost savings.

As faculty use principles and assumptions embedded in HEC, they can help students articulate the contributions of nursing to care outcomes. Within academic settings, HEC can be a useful framework to guide curriculum development as well as teaching learning experiences. Use of HEC can help the learner understand the linkages between theory and practice, theory and research, and research and theory and more readily link nursing knowledge with patient care.

Summary Thoughts

HEC focuses on knowing the person and his or her experiences. The encounter between the nurse and patient in mutual partnership can be a life changing experience. Application of this theoretical framework in practice, education, and research can provide new understandings about health and illness; promote growth and personal transformation; illuminate the meanings, choices, and actions of individuals, families, and groups; and guide the redesign of nursing and health care globally.

REFERENCES

Barron, A. M. (2000). Life meanings and the experience of cancer. *Dissertation Abstracts International, 54* (UMI No. 30-08589).

Bernstein, R. J. (1983). *Beyond objectivism and relativism.* Philadelphia: University of Pennsylvania Press.

Berry, D. (2004). An emerging model of behavior change in women maintaining weight loss. *Nursing Science Quarterly, 17*(3), 242–245.

Bohm, D. (1980). *Wholeness and the implicate order.* London: Routledge & Kegan Paul.

Bortoft, H. (1996). *The wholeness of nature.* Hudson, NY: Lindisfarne.

Brink, P. J. (1990). Editorial. *Western Journal of Nursing Research, 12,* 279–281.

Capasso, V. (2005). The theory is the practice: An exemplar. In C. Picard & D. Jones (Eds.), *Giving voice to what we know: Margaret Newman's theory of health as expanding consciousness in nursing education, practice and research* (pp. 65–72). Sudbury, MA: Jones and Bartlett.

Endo, E. (1996). *Pattern recognition as a nursing intervention with adults with cancer.* Unpublished doctoral dissertation, University of Minnesota, Minneapolis.

Flanagan, J. (2002). Nurse and patient perception of the pre-admission practice model: Linking theory to practice. *Dissertation Abstracts International, 56* (UMI No. 30-53657).

Jones, D. (2005). The impact of HEC: Concluding thoughts and future directions. In C. Picard & D. A. Jones (Eds.), *Giving voice to what we know: Margaret Newman's theory of health as expanding consciousness in nursing education, practice and research* (p. 219). Sudbury, MA: Jones and Bartlett.

Jonsdottir, H. (1995). *Life patterns of people with chronic obstructive pulmonary disease: Isolation and being closed in.* Unpublished doctoral dissertation, University of Minnesota, Minneapolis.

Lamendola, F., & Newman, M. A. (1994). The paradox of HIV/AIDS as expanding consciousness. *Advances in Nursing Science, 16*(1), 13–21.

Lee, S. (2005). Exemplar: Transformation of the patient-nurse dyad. In C. Picard & D. A. Jones (Eds.), *Giving voice to what we know: Margaret Newman's theory of health as expanding consciousness in nursing education, practice and research* (pp. 187–202). Sudbury, MA: Jones and Bartlett.

Litchfield, M. C. (1993). *The process of health patterning in families with young children who have been repeatedly hospitalized.* Unpublished master's thesis, University of Minnesota, Minneapolis.

McEwen, M., & Willis, E. M. (2002). *Theoretical basis for nursing.* Philadelphia: Lippincott Williams & Wilkins.

Moch, S. D. (1990). Health within the experience of breast cancer. *Journal of Advanced Nursing, 155,* 1426–1435.

Morgan, G. (1983). Toward a more reflective social science. In G. Morgan (Ed.), *Beyond method: Strategies for social research* (pp. 368–376). Beverly Hills, CA: Sage.

Neill, J. (2002). Transcendence and transformation in the life patterns of women living with rheumatoid arthritis. *Advances in Nursing Science, 24*(4), 27–47.

Newman, M. A. (1972). Time estimation in relation to gait tempo. *Perceptual and Motor Skills, 34,* 359–366.

Newman, M. A. (1979). *Theory development in nursing.* Philadelphia: Davis.

Newman, M. A. (1982). Time as an index of expanding consciousness with age. *Nursing Research, 33,* 290–293.

Newman, M. A. (1984). Nursing diagnosis: Looking at the whole. *American Journal of Nursing, 84,* 1496–1499.

Newman, M. A. (1986a). *Health as expanding consciousness.* St. Louis, MO: Mosby.

Newman, M. A. (1986b). Nursing's emerging paradigm: The diagnosis of pattern. In A. M. McLane (Ed.), *Classification of nursing diagnoses: Proceedings of the seventh conference of the North American nursing diagnosis* (pp. 50–60). St. Louis, MO: Mosby.

Newman, M. A. (1987). Patterning. In M. Duffy & N. J. Pender (Eds.), *Conceptual issues in health promotion: A report of proceedings of a Wingspread conference* (pp. 36–50). Indianapolis, IN: Sigma Theta Tau.

Newman, M. A. (1990). Newman's theory of health as praxis. *Nursing Science Quarterly, 3,* 37–41.

Newman, M. A. (1994). *Health as expanding consciousness* (2nd ed.). New York: National League of Nursing.

Newman, M. A., & Moch, S. D. (1991). Life patterns of persons with coronary heart disease. *Nursing Science Quarterly, 4,* 161–167.

Newman, M. A, Sime, A. M., & Corcoran-Perry, S. A. (1991). The focus of the discipline of nursing. *Advances in Nursing Science*, *14*(1), 1–6.

Novolesky-Rosenthal, H. T. (1996). *Pattern recognition in older adults living with chronic illness.* Unpublished doctoral dissertation, Boston College, Massachusetts.

Noveletsky-Rosenthal, H. T., & Solomon, K. (2001). Reflections on the use of Johns' model of structures: Reflection in nurse practitioner education. *International Journal for Human Caring*, *4*(2), 21–26.

Pharris, M. D. (2002). Coming to know ourselves as community through a nursing partnership with adolescents convicted of murder. *Advances in Nursing Science*, *24*(3), 21–42.

Picard, C. (2000). Pattern of expanding consciousness in middle life women: Creative movement and narrative modes of expression. *Nursing Science Quarterly*, *13*(2), 150–158.

Picard, C., & Jones, D. (2005). *Giving voice to what we know: Margaret Newman's theory of health as expanding consciousness in nursing education, practice and research.* Sudbury, MA: Jones and Bartlett.

Picard, C., & Margolis, T. (2002). Praxis as a mirroring process: Teaching psychiatric nursing grounded in Newman's health as expanding consciousness. *Nursing Science Quarterly*, *15*(2), 118–122.

Rogers, M. E. (1970). *An introduction to the theoretical basis of nursing.* Philadelphia: Davis.

Rogers, M. E. (1990). Nursing: Science of unitary, irreducible, human beings: Update 1990. In E. A. M. Barrett (Ed.), *Visions of Rogers' science-based nursing* (pp. 5–11). New York: National League for Nursing.

Ruka, S. (2005). Creating balance: Rhythms and patterns in people with dementia living in a nursing home. In C. Picard & Jones D. A. (Eds.), *Giving voice to what we know: Margaret Newman's theory of health as expanding consciousness in nursing education, practice and research* (pp. 95–104). Sudbury, MA: Jones and Bartlett.

Wheeler, C. E., & Chinn, P. L. (1984). *Peace and power: A handbook of feminist process.* Buffalo, NY: Margaret-Daughters.

Poststructuralist Feminist Analysis in Nursing

9

Janice Thompson

Nursing ethics is hardly a recognized field of inquiry, even for academics. Books on nursing ethics typically borrow the principles of medical ethics and apply them to nursing situations, with little recognition that the nurse's situation is profoundly different than that of the doctor. The prototype medical ethics scenario presented to conference participants, as often happens involved a dramatic case, choices of heroic intervention, a situation of crisis—and now the doctor must choose. Medical ethics is thus characterized by dilemmas in which the lone individual must decide the right thing to do. Philosophical medical ethics largely assumes this freedom of the practitioner to choose; the ethical problem lies in deciding what choice is morally right. But in nursing, the problems are frequently those over which nurses have no control: They are not dilemmas, in the sense of an individual's quandary, at all, and the language of ethical dilemmas hardly works for a profession whose work is so determined by the choices of other, more powerful actors (Chambliss, 1996).

The task of presenting a discussion of a poststructuralist feminist perspective on nursing and knowledge development is an ambitious project. Although I will sketch some characteristics of this perspective, I need to say that a poststructuralist feminist position is not one that I entirely endorse. I don't agree with many of its political commitments and remain more interested in critical theory and feminist analysis as discourses for nursing practice. I have some ambivalence because I have come to understand the critique of critical theory articulated by poststructuralists. Although there are many insights from poststructuralist feminist analysis that are useful to nurses, there are also risks in this position. I have come to believe that many assumptions can lead in the long run to dead ends.

This philosophical position combines some assumptions of poststructuralist theory with some assumptions of postmodern feminist analysis. As a result, a feminist poststructuralist position rejects many assumptions of modernity and yet stands in agreement with others. As a philosophy or, more accurately, as a discourse, poststructuralist feminist work is a complex hybrid. It is a position that is critical of power but one that does not promise to correct power structures.

This chapter (a) reviews some basic characteristics of poststructuralism; (b) reviews convergences between poststructuralist and feminist theory; (c) briefly reviews some recent trends in nursing literature, particularly related to ethics, which have relied on feminist poststructuralist analysis; and (d) suggests some effects for nursing practice and knowledge development that might warrant attention. In this analysis, I am positioned and I choose to position myself as a specific intellectual (Foucault, 1980) and as an organic intellectual (Gramsci, 1971). The contradictory location is an issue that is troubling and is a topic that deserves examination. Therefore, I will offer closing remarks about the role of specific intellectuals in nursing that present new challenges.

Poststructuralism

Poststructuralist theory emerged in Western Europe and the United States as an important intellectual influence in the 1970s. Although it is frequently associated first with literary theory, as an intellectual practice, it might best be understood as a reaction against both the literary theory of structuralism in France and the political discourses of Marxism (Sarup, 1989). With its greatest strength first in France, poststructuralism comprised a variety of critical perspectives that displaced structuralism from its prominence as the radically innovative way of dealing with language and other signifying systems (Abrams, 1993, p. 258). Most accounts of poststructuralist theory review the thinking of Lacan, Derrida, and Foucault as the most influential early theorists in the field. These three theorists are seen as carving out locations that are poststructuralist. They are positioned after the structuralism of Saussure, a prominent literary theorist whose work was influential between 1913 and 1960.

In addition, poststructuralists also were reacting against the work of other prominent modern theorists, especially Marx and Freud. As poststructuralism spread in the West following the 1970s, its influence appeared mostly within academic disciplines. No longer restricted to literary studies, poststructuralist assumptions now occupy most interdisciplinary landscapes. Feminist poststructuralist work is a complex hybrid in that it combines some dimensions of poststructuralist theory with oppositional feminist politics. So what are the most salient characteristics of poststructuralism?

Language to Signify Reality

As in most continental philosophies, in poststructuralist work there is an explicit focus on the primacy of language in the construction of human reality. Poststructuralists do not begin with individuals. They insist that social identities, individual subjectivity, and the social world are all products of signifying activities. This explicit focus on language and the way it constructs the social world is usually critical of the politics and power relations involved in such signifying activity. For poststructuralists, language operates to create the objects that it names and of which it speaks. Usually the signifying activities that are creating these human realities function in more or less invisible ways. When poststructuralists make language explicit, we experience the effects of the "specific" intellectual. Foucault (1980) coined the term *specific intellectual* as one who conducts local and context specific work to open up meanings and insights that were previously unnoticed.

A brief detour into Saussurean linguistics is important here. Thanks to Saussure, literary theorists after World War I recognized that meanings are not inherently located within particular terms or words. Within structuralist linguistics, the meaning of a term such as *nurse* is understood as a function of two interrelated dimensions, which together create the sign *nurse*. The sign comprises the sound-image *nurse*, which Saussure called the *signifier* and the concept *nurse*, which he called the *signified*. Saussure argued that the relationship between signifier and signified is not inherent but is rather more or less arbitrary. Although the sound image and the concept function together to create the meaning of the sign, this meaning is based not on an inherent link between sound image and concept but rather on exclusions and discriminations made from chains of other signs whose meanings the sign nurse does not match.

Saussure allowed us to see that the concept of a nurse—the signified, concept of the nurse—is structurally linked to chains of other signs. Such structural linguistics emphasizes this structural relationship, with stress on the concept and its linkages with other concepts, such as nurse, woman, body, nature, pollution, sacred, and so forth (Wolf, 1988). Exclusions are important here, for example, the maneuver that recognizes the meaning of nurse as not mother, lover, witch, and others. Although Saussurean structuralism discovered the structural relations between chains of signs, structuralism's emphasis on the signified, the concept, encouraged an ahistorical perspective regarding meaning.

Later poststructuralists, especially Derrida, rejected Saussure's emphasis on the stable sign as well as his preoccupation with the signified or the concept. Both Derrida and Foucault focused instead on the unstable signifier, the word-image and the signifying activities that construct chains of signs. For both Derrida and Foucault, it became important to notice the ways in which meanings are always constructed and therefore always fluid, the concept sliding under the signifier in an endless process of deferring closure on meaning. For a review of these ideas, works by Sarup (1989) and Weedon (1997) provide essential and comprehensive details.

Psychoanalytic applications of poststructuralist theory retain an emphasis on signifying practices and argue that there can be no self independent of language. Further subject positions are fragmented by competing discursive practices and the myth of wholeness of a unified self is an invention of ego psychologists. Perhaps most controversial was Lacan's belief that the power of the signifier is located in a phallic order and that power of the unconscious resides in a presyntactical order. These theoretical positions have created important openings for criticism and reversal among feminist poststructuralist theorists, notably Kristeva, Cixous, and Irigaray. Tong (1989) and Weedon (1997) provided a detailed discussion of these theorists and their resistances to Lacan.

Rejecting Assumptions of Modernism

All of the early poststructuralist theorists (Derrida, Lacan, and Foucault) held in common their focus on language, signifying activity and its role in the construction of human realities. Additionally, all rejected the Renaissance notion of humanism and the human as an autonomous, free, and rational individual. Poststructuralists instead emphasized that the social world, or in phenomenological terms the *lebenswelt*, as a product of signifying activities that "are both culturally specific and generally unconscious" (Sarup, 1989, p. 2).

> In this emphasis on the hidden role of signifying practices, poststructuralists criticize important modern assumptions, positioning their work as opposition and challenging central values of modernity. The critique of humanism and the suspicion of humanist tendencies occur in poststructuralist work because their approach de-centers the human subject. The poststructuralists focus not on the autonomous knower but rather on the discourses and signifying practices that position the knower as a subject in a whole world of contested meanings. It should come as no surprise then to see that most poststructuralists are deeply suspicious of scientific discourse and frequently have been radically antiscientific. (Sarup, 1989, p. 2)

Beyond this critical emphasis on signifying practices, a second prominent feature of poststructuralist work is its rejection of modern assumptions about history. Specifically, poststructuralists reject the notion that there is some overall pattern in history and especially reject the notion that such a pattern would involve progress, freedom, or enlightenment. They are particularly suspicious of grand stories or meta-narratives regarding oppression, freedom, progress, or civilization. As a result, most poststructuralists reject modern revolutionary theories and politics. This political commitment has earned many poststructuralists the label of *neoconservative*. From the standpoint of leftist politics, the absence of alignment with political commitments, or the insistence on apolitical commitments by many poststructuralists is seen as functioning in the service of the status quo (Bernstein, 1985; Habermas, 1988; Habermas & Kelly, 1994).

Ambiguity of Political Commitments

The preceding characteristics lead to another dimension of poststructuralist work that has important consequences for poststructuralist feminists in nursing. The ways in which poststructuralists attend to signifying activity and the ways in which they reject modern assumptions and politics lead to a certain ambiguity regarding their political commitments. Whereas many view poststructuralism as thoroughly conservative, others maintain that it is consistently radical and critical work. This suggests a third characteristic of poststructuralism, its ambiguity regarding politics.

Many nursing scholars are drawn to poststructuralism, especially to the work of Michel Foucault (1980), because of its critique of power in contemporary society. Foucault, in fact, rejected Lacan's psychoanalytic position and argued instead for a focus on the specific practices, disciplinary techniques, discourses, laws, and institutions that constitute and regulate individuals. Generally, Foucault's work is used in nursing to critique specific apparatuses of power, including science, that operate as disciplinary techniques both within and outside nursing. His work and subsequently the works of the "new" poststructuralist theorists (Deleuze, Guattari, and Lyotard) have been influenced largely by Nietzsche, and this lineage, it seems to me, is extremely important. Sarup (1989) has commented in helpful ways on Nietzsche's influence.

> Many of the fundamental beliefs of post-structuralism have their roots in Nietzscheanism. . . . They share with him an antipathy to any "system." Secondly, they reject the Hegelian view of history as progress. Thirdly, they are aware of the increasing pressure toward conformity and are highly critical of this tendency. Fourthly, their obsession with the subjective and the "small story" has led them to affirm the anti-political individual. . . . Post-structuralism is largely a product of 1968. . . . it is not just an aberration of a few intellectuals but must be seen as mirroring a widespread mood of disorientation among the generation of '68. The "new philosophers" believe that human society is permanently and inherently oppressive; but domination is no longer conceived of in class terms. They uphold various forms of romanticism and individualism. They denounce "science" and any totalizing beliefs in the name of the spontaneous and the particular. . . . These ideologues combine an odd idealization of rebellion with an ultimately passive pessimism and acquiescence in the status quo. This is not surprising, as they have no conception of historical advance or permanent transformation. (Sarup, 1989, pp. 115–116)

Poststructuralist Feminist Theory

Poststructuralist feminist analysis is probably best understood as something other than the kind of theory we have come to think of in the West. In fact, it would be ironic to characterize poststructuralist feminist theory as a single, seamless discourse. Certainly poststructuralist feminist thinkers have warned against the kind of universalizing analysis that applies a grand or metatheory to any and all social phenomena (Sawicki, 1991). But we can offer some sketches of poststructuralist feminist positions and notice how these accept some of the premises of poststructuralism and where there are important corrections and divergences.

Signifying Practices and the Poststructural Feminists

Poststructuralist feminist analysis shares with Foucault a rejection of many assumptions of modernity. Like Foucault, poststructural feminists decenter the Enlightenment subject, rejecting the notion of an enlightened, autonomous knower who acquires true concepts through reasoned knowledge. Feminist poststructuralists emphasize instead the signifying practices that constitute the human world and the human subject. They focus on discourses that position the knower in the social world and that subsequently constitute an individual's subjectivity, particularly in regard to gender, class, race, and sexual identity. For poststructuralist feminists, women's identity and subjectivity emerge within the interstices of powerful discourses, languages, and vocabularies that operate subtly to mold gender, race, class, and sexual identity (Weedon, 1997).

In this emphasis on signifying practices, Foucauldian feminists privilege the notion of the discourse. Discourses are social practices that create objects of knowledge. They include many forms of signifying activity such as laws, policies, collected literature, institutional practice, techniques, concepts, and vocabularies. Discourses both create and transform the objects and subjects of which they speak. Scientific discourses can be examined by focusing on their eruption at specific historical moments and by noticing that the objects and subjects that they create are the product of historically specific practices. The disciplines of psychiatry and evolutionary biology can, for example, be located historically by focusing on the beginnings of their respective discourses, by tracing their lines of descent, not back to one single origin, but rather back through various divergences and ruptures to the emergence of specific institutional practices that made these disciplines possible.

Poststructuralist feminists excavate such discourses as a way of showing that sexist and racist meanings are contingent and that they have emerged in specific historical contexts and are therefore vulnerable to change (Flax, 1990). Such an approach to excavating the history of disciplinary power comprised an analytic technique that Foucault called genealogy, a term borrowed from Nietzsche. Feminist poststructuralists have appropriated this approach from Foucault, writing genealogies from specific feminist commitments. Like other genealogists, feminists have used this analytic approach to reverse the effects of Enlightenment historiographies.

Genealogical analysis, then, differs from traditional forms of historical analysis in several ways. Whereas traditional or total history inserts events into grand explanatory systems and linear processes, celebrates great moments and individuals, and seeks to document a point of origin, genealogical analysis attempts to establish and preserve the singularity of events, turns away from the spectacular in favor of the discredited, the neglected, and a whole range of phenomena that have been denied a history. According to Foucault, there has been an insurrection of subjugated knowledges of a whole set of knowledges that have been disqualified as inadequate, naive knowledges located low down on the hierarchy, beneath the required level of scientificity (Sarup, 1989, p. 64).

Many poststructuralist feminists are actively committed to deconstructing the discourses that shape women's identity. In doing this, Foucauldian feminists help women to see that their subjectivities have been shaped by powerful signifying practices whose influences are frequently invisible. Additionally, poststructuralist feminists work actively to invert the effects of these powerful metadiscourses by revalorizing lost or buried knowledges that have been discredited in patriarchy.

Poststructualist Feminists' Rejection of Modern Assumptions

Poststructuralist feminists also reject modernist assumptions. Like other poststructuralists, they are suspicious of grand narratives of oppression, liberation, and freedom or the modern assumption that progress is an overall pattern in history. A skepticism regarding modern revolutionary politics (Marxist and Neomarxist) is therefore frequently a part of feminist poststructuralist analysis and political commitments. On this issue of the politics of liberation, important divergences are created between the position of the feminist political commitments and other poststructuralist commitments that create an uneasy alliance with poststructuralism.

Related Ambiguity of Political Commitments

Skepticism regarding large stories of oppression and other assumptions of modernity is a characteristic of poststructuralism that complicates the picture for many feminists. Those who share poststructuralist commitments argue that feminism can no longer tell grand stories about the oppression of all women and the liberation of all women. White, middle-class, heterosexual feminists have been reminded of this by minority women, who legitimately criticize the grand scale, totalizing, and essentialized metanarratives of women's liberation. Poststructuralist feminists instead focus on the specific and local stories of women's resistances, emphasizing both the differences and continuities in women's lives.

Feminists with poststructuralist commitments, especially Foucauldian feminists, have wrestled extensively with the political implications of this issue. Many have insisted that feminist corrections can form the basis of different political commitments within poststructuralist feminist analysis (Flax, 1990; Fuss, 1989; Hekman, 1990). These hybridized uses of feminist poststructuralist analysis include an ongoing tension. Recognizing the power of discursive practices to constitute subjectivity, feminists still insist on the agency of women to resist oppression and to take up multiple ways of being in the world. Additionally, feminists have rejected the passivity and pessimism of much avantgarde white, elite, male work. Whereas they acknowledge the limitations of essentialized feminist politics, they nevertheless insist on the importance of feminist commitments, recast in the notion of many diverse forms of struggle and resistance (Grosz, 1990, 1994; Sawicki, 1991; Weedon, 1997).

This last characteristic of poststructuralist work then, its ambiguity about political commitment, is the pivot point for a hyphenated, hybridized theoretical position in poststructuralist feminist analysis. For this version of feminist theory, political agenda or rather political agendas are still important. Poststructuralist work and poststructural feminist work differ in this one important dimension. In poststructural feminist analysis, a no-nonsense commitment to work against the oppression of women and in support of women's resistance(s), does constitute a political commitment. This commitment exists even given the poststructuralist sensibilities to and suspicions regarding grand narratives of oppression and liberation (Ramazanoglu, 1989).

Poststructuralist Feminist Analysis in Nursing

Most recent poststructuralist feminist work in nursing has borrowed and adapted methods and assumptions from Michel Foucault (1980). Foucauldian feminist discussions have appeared in nursing literature with increasing frequency since a few early articles in both the United States and in the United Kingdom particularly in the journals *Advances in Nursing Science*, *Nursing Inquiry*, and the *Journal of Advanced Nursing*. This is not surprising because Foucauldian approaches achieved ascendancy in many disciplines during the 1990s. The similarities in perspectives were noted above in the discussion of signifying practices.

In nursing, Dzurec (1989) argued that the discourses of empiricism and phenomenology were both essential for knowledge development. Doering (1992) argued that knowledge and disciplinary power cannot be separated and that discourses function as apparatuses of power. Henderson (1994) argued that disciplinary techniques in nursing that produce knowledge function normatively as a "gaze" to regulate and control patients.

Poststructural Feminist Perspective and Biomedical Ethics

As one example of the role of poststructural feminist analysis, we can examine issues of biomedical ethics. It seems likely that it may take several more years, perhaps more than a decade, to create a new and different discourse regarding the complex moral problems surrounding patient's requests such as action at the end of life. This might be compared to the process outlined by Chambliss (1996) regarding the institutionalization of Do Not Resuscitate (DNR) orders. In the United States, the practice of DNR took roughly 10 years to emerge as a discursive entity and to become a routine part of hospital practice. Perhaps we are living through a time ripe for another similar discursive eruption. It seems that a different discourse and different disciplinary techniques regarding heroic measures are needed and that their absence will continue to be problematic in practice.

Currently, what we frequently rely on to examine these situations is the language of bioethics. When bioethicists examine different life stories, they deploy the vocabularies, principles, and concepts of bioethics, applying these in such a way as to suggest that the murkiness of the story can be clarified through the concepts of utilitarian theory or deontological theory or through the use of principles such as beneficence, justice, self-determination, informed consent, or cognitive competence. It goes without saying that bioethicists provide significant insight and assistance to individuals during times of conflict and dilemma. But it has been argued recently that the discourse of bioethics is only one field of signifying activity available to nurses.

More important, bioethics, as a discourse, may be only marginally meaningful to the majority of nurses. The discourse of biomedical ethics is characterized by rules that govern who may speak and from what institutional sites they may speak. Unless they have been trained in applied ethics, and unless they occupy positions of privilege, nurses usually do not speak in the language of autonomous, principled, ethical decision making.

Biomedical Ethics and Its Adequacy for Nursing

There has been a remarkable recognition that when nurses speak in morally problematic situations, they do so primarily in the language of care and compassion (Bishop, 1991,

1996; Bishop & Scudder, 1990). Nurses know the ethics of care. They use and need another language to express it.

This point about the discourse of biomedical ethics being inadequate for nursing practice has been made frequently by nurses and philosophers who focus on the social and political organization of ethics in practice. Two decades ago, E. Joy Kroeger Mappes, noted that ethical problems in nursing practice are a function of the social and political contexts in which nurses practice.

> The tension that exists for nurses in (morally problematic) situations is not really that of a moral dilemma, but rather, a tension between doing what is morally right and what is least difficult practically, a tension common in everyday life. The problem is not that the nurse's obligation is unclear, but that in actual situations, fulfilling this moral obligation is extremely difficult. . . . It is the classist and sexist economic and social context of the physician–nurse relationship that often inhibits the nurse from effectively functioning on behalf of the patient. Nurses have a moral responsibility to act on behalf of the patient, but in order to expect them to carry out that responsibility, changes must be made in the workplace. (Mappes, 1981, pp. 99, 101)

Similarly, Dan W. Brock also argued that

> [F]ocusing on the nurse–patient relationship. . .has the effect of ignoring at least one extremely important aspect of most nurses' overall moral situation. Specifically, most nurses now work in hierarchic, institutional settings in which they are in the employ of others, hospitals, physicians, etc. Many of the most important moral uncertainties and conflicts nurses experience concerning their rights, duties and responsibilities derive from their role in the hierarchical structure, and from questions about the consequent authority to decide and act in particular matters. (Brock, 1981, p. 94)

More recently, Richard Chambliss made this point again explicitly in his ethnography of hospital nursing practice.

> The nurse's role in the hospital is shaped by multiple, sometimes contradictory, imperatives. The nurse is a paid employee of the hospital, but she is more than that. She is actively encouraged to be simultaneously, a caring person, a committed professional, and a loyal subordinate. Obviously, these components of her role frequently conflict with each other. Ethical problems in nursing primarily reflect conflict between nurses and other constituencies in the hospital. In this sense, the "shape" of an organization, especially its division of labor, creates conflicts. When these conflicts are described in moral terminology, they become 'ethical problems' for the staff. But more often they face political difficulties in dealing with physicians, administrators and others which they experience as moral conflicts. More generally, it seems that the idea of "dilemmas," so central to our usual language of ethics, is appropriate primarily for actors who are relatively autonomous or powerful. Subordinates (such as nurses, or most people) are less concerned with dilemmas than with practical difficulties of working with, or under, other people. (Chambliss, 1996, pp. 181–182)

To summarize these thoughts, Chambliss noted that nurses face political conflicts, not logical quandaries.

To a feminist poststructuralist, the discourse of bioethics is inadequate; that is, the language of bioethics is incapable of constituting the complexity of moral practice in nursing. Bioethics is a language that works for powerful decision makers, but it does not offer a great deal of meaning to nurses. Further, it does not address political dimensions of the social organization of ethics, those contextual characteristics that position nurses as agents of compassion and care.

As Chambliss and others indicate, the social and political organization of ethics is a structural issue that bioethicists have consistently ignored. The language of bioethics itself encourages a neoconservative focus on logical, psychological, and moral quandaries, deflecting attention from the political organization of care and the divisions of labor that create political conflicts for patients, their families, and nurses. In the language of bioethics, nurses have very little to say about this macro level of constraint, except to wait and to be "in-between" (Bishop & Scudder, 1990) with their compassion and care.

Phenomenologic Contributions to Complex Use of Moral Dimensions of Nursing Practice

In recent years, nursing scholars have initiated a different conversation about the moral tensions and dilemmas of practice. Recognizing the limits of both bioethical and postpositivist discourse, nursing intellectuals have insisted that the moral dimensions of nursing practice can best be understood within the discursive formation of phenomenology. Benner (1996) has done much to reverse the effects of scientism and bioethics and their superficial understandings of nursing skill and expertise. Benner and her colleagues have explicated the complexity of practical knowledge through phenomenologies of nursing care. Because of the work of these scholars, nursing as a discipline has been reminded that clinical expertise is a very complex kind of knowledge, one that carries within it complicated and sophisticated moral judgments. As the discourses of empiricism and postpositivism have been supplemented with complex phenomenologies of practice, nurses have witnessed the effects of a new discursive formation. The phenomenologies of care have demonstrated that clinical expertise is a kind of practical knowledge that is significantly more complex in terms of its embodied knowledge and wisdom than can be explained by scientific theory.

In many ways, the phenomenologies of practice have functioned much like genealogies: They have celebrated subjugated knowledges in nursing, valorizing a whole set of practical knowledges that have been denied authority during the ascendancy of science. To see the phenomenologies of care as genealogies would be to suggest that nursing scholars have been involved in Foucauldian feminist work, perhaps without acknowledging Foucault's direct influence. I want to suggest here that the discourses of practice do provide an alternative language for nursing ethics and that, as such, they might be seen as a form of poststructuralist feminist work. Were they to contain specific historical analysis, they would, in fact, function explicitly as genealogies. In examining components such as ethical comportment, embodied knowing, and context-specific practical knowledge versus theory, one finds that the narratives of caring are far more descriptive than the language of bioethics.

Over the last 15 years, nursing scholars have, in fact, performed this function of retrieving lost or subjugated moral knowledge in nursing practice. Like other feminists (Dalmiya & Alcoff, 1993), phenomenologists have suggested that the discourse of bioethics, such as the discourse of empiricism, operates as only one kind of knowledge. This discourse may frequently conceal or cover up a whole other set of subjugated knowledges, located beneath the level of bioethics or beneath the level of science. Over recent decades, we have seen a blossoming of narratives regarding the complexity of practical knowledge, a virtual insurrection of practical wisdom, all valorizing the sophistication of *clinical know-how*. These discourses have offered an alternative language for the conceptualization of ethics in nursing.

All too frequently, these interventions—the phenomenologies of practice—have remained silent on the social and political issues addressed by earlier critics of bioethics. If the discourse of bioethics has been recognized as inadequate for the practical and moral wisdom of nursing, the new phenomenologies of clinical ethics in nursing are even less focused on those social and structural forces that position nurses as conflicted moral agents. Instead, the new discourses of practical knowledge focus almost exclusively on the valorous position of the nurse. The nurse's subordinate status is seen as a privileged standpoint within the hierarchy of complex medical bureaucracies.

Limitations Lead to Larger Call for Change

It may be strategically important to valorize the practice of nurses who have come to disbelieve the complexity of their own knowledge. However, it is not enough to celebrate the identity of nurses and leave unnoticed the structural forces that are problematic for their moral practice. I suggest that there is a need for a different kind of genealogy of moral expertise in nursing than that which has been provided by the phenomenologies of care. More radically critical and feminist genealogies of practical knowledge would be openly critical of the power structures of corporate health care and would not disguise these political commitments (Reverby, 1987). Theses sorts of feminist genealogies, I suggest, would open up different discursive spaces for practice and for practice outcomes in the future.

Unless phenomenologies of nursing practice make explicit the social and political nature of moral conflicts in nursing practice, and unless they explicitly address structural transformation of the health care industry in terms of class struggle, gender, and race relations, they, in fact, function as neoconservative interventions that do very little to transform the landscape of burned out, alienated, and routinized hospital practice.

Although remaining committed to the political struggles of women, poststructuralist feminist analysis rejects the possibility that all women have the same interests or that all women share common experience or that all women are similarly oppressed. Whereas a poststructuralist feminist analysis would resist the grand narrative of women's oppression at large, it would nevertheless search for the continuities as well as the discontinuities in women's experiences. For example, do lay women caregivers and professional women caregivers share common suggestions about the transformation of organized care?

Although such an analysis rejects the assumptions of grand revolutionary transformation, we might ask whether it nevertheless remains committed to the politics of liberation, searching for different languages, different structures, and different models for the organization of care.

If we notice that nurses are constrained by the context in which they work, then it might behoove us to pay close attention to those social forces that organize ethics and their issues in complex hierarchies. Again, Chambliss and others have reminded us that ethical problems are usually more a function of the sociopolitical context than they are a function of nurses' moral judgment. For a discipline as context oriented as nursing purports to be in its metaparadigm, it seems quite remarkable that our analyses frequently conceptualize context in apolitical or less than critical ways. Although the phenomenologies of practice claim that it is important to recover the complexity of moral practice in clinical contexts, this conceptualization frequently happens in neoconservative descriptions that valorize the in-between position of nurses, never providing any critique of the oppressive conditions or the hierarchical structuring of nurses' work. This tendency in the phenomenologies of care makes them vulnerable to criticisms regarding their conservative political commitments.

When the phenomenologies of nursing remind us of the complexity of our moral practice, they function as powerful tools of empowerment, building subjectivity and identity within the profession. This use of genealogies and phenomenologies is crucial, and it should not be underestimated as a discourse of resistance. But when stories of clinical expertise are used in the absence of any structural or historical analysis of power and domination, their political effects are open to criticism. In particular, without an explicit focus on the structural organization of the health care industry and without an explicit critique of power relations, including race, class, and gender, the discourses of clinical expertise and practical knowledge function as ideologies that valorize the in-between location of nurses. Such valorization is dangerously neoconservative because of its silences. In this apolitical but really exquisitely political maneuver, the phenomenologies may offer nurses a powerful new language for docility, encouraging nurses never to press for the kinds of structural transformation that would democratize the industry and never to examine our own complicity in a system that perpetuates corporate profit and its ethical problems. As a result, I find that the political commitments of the new phenomenologies are dangerously ambiguous.

The Challenge for 21st Century Knowledge for Practice

From Patricia Benner (1996) and her colleagues, we have learned that nurses are exquisitely moral in their practice. Yet much of the new material available to nurses concerning the ethics of nursing practice remains silent regarding the social and political origins of ethical dilemmas in nursing. I believe that we ought to ask, "To whom the good?" Who benefits from academic work that mystifies or hides the social and political constraints on nursing practice? The answers we provide to this question will have much to do with outcomes for nursing in the 21st century. From a future historical point, we will be looking back on nearly 20 years of identity politics in nursing practice. If we come at this question from a neoconservative feminist position, we might believe that the phenomenologies of practice will continue to empower nurses, by disclosing the moral complexity of practical know-how. Then we could hope to see individual nurses with exquisitely shaped subjectivity, keenly aware of the complexity of their knowledge base and self-confidently using this knowledge. This is the new class of professionals, a new "subaltern" professional, which many nursing intellectuals see on the horizon.

In this feminist position, there is no place for revolutionary politics, at least not in the typical modern sense of revolutionary politics. The liberation of nurses does not require a radical transformation of class structure or racist institutions. The resistance of women is narrated in this discourse at the micro level. The empowerment of nurses is a local, small story. In fact, larger issues, especially the class structure of advanced postindustrial capitalism, is assumed as given and as a standard dimension of future contexts. On the issue of other structural questions (e.g., concerning racism, homophobia, and other power relations) the phenomenologies of practice remain largely silent. Again, the subjectivity of nurses in *small stories* does not require a look at larger-scale or macro-level realities.

In this neoconservative position, the only liberatory commitment required is the reversal of subordinate identities among nurses. This can happen, without any significant transformation of the political economics of the health care industry and without any large scale corrections for racism and other structural power relations. All that is necessary is to insert another professional constituency, by socializing subalterns to take power within the existing structures.

These are the political strategies of a partial or tactical identity politics (West, 1993). The outcomes of this political intervention are by now predictable. The liberatory commitment within this kind of feminist discourse is wholly ambiguous. As has been the case in many neoconservative examples of feminist work, the outcomes of new discursive formations are likely to benefit a relatively small percentage of privileged experts. Large scale, democratic transformation of the conditions of nurses' work is not likely within this feminist perspective. We might ask Foucauldian feminists where they fall out on this question.

The presence of critical or rather radical intellectual work in nursing is raised by the question, "To whom the good?" Foucauldian feminist academics usually position themselves as specific intellectuals, working in local ways and resisting grand narratives. After 30 years of this work, we might ask the old Marxist question, "To whom the good?" If we are to do this sort of work in nursing, then it will be necessary for us to engage with other feminist poststructuralist workers in asking such questions regarding the effects of our academic practice. For example, Sawicki (1991) discusses the need to "discipline" Foucault.

Will the outcome of feminist poststructuralist criticism be the kind of elite and ironic analysis that is resigned to endless power struggles and increasingly individualistic responses? Or does this position move out of partial tactical identity politics and into more radically democratic politics (Mouffe, 1992; West, 1993) forging coalitions with other communities who are also struggling for the democratization of the health care industry? To ask this question is to wonder about the political commitments of organic intellectuals (Gramsci, 1971; Said, 1994) in nursing.

Are the moral responsibilities of intellectuals in nursing limited to the production of discourses that position nurses increasingly as in-between agents of biopower in the health care industry? Does our knowledge also have the moral responsibility to make explicit the ethical contradictions of a practice that is driven by the interests of corporate capital?

The outcomes of this academic debate, it seems to me, will have important implications for nursing practice in the 21st century. We ask that our specific intellectuals in nursing engage in a kind of reflexivity that struggles with the structural contradictions of the question, "Who benefits from our intellectual work?"

REFERENCES

Abrams, M. H. (1993). *A glossary of literary terms.* Fort Worth, TX: Harcourt, Brace Jovanovich.

Benner, P. (1996). *Caregiving: Readings in knowledge, practice, ethics and politics.* Philadelphia: University of Pennsylvania Press.

Bernstein, R. (1985). *Habermas and modernity.* Cambridge, UK: Polity.

Bishop, A. (1991). *Nursing: The practice of caring.* New York: The National League for Nursing Press.

Bishop, A. (1996). *Nursing ethics: Therapeutic caring presence.* Sudbury, MA: Jones and Bartlett.

Bishop, A., & Scudder, J. (1990). *The practical, moral and personal sense of nursing: A phenomenological philosophy of practice.* Albany, NY: State University of New York.

Brock, D. W. (1981). The nurse–patient relationship. In T. Mappes & J. Zembaty (Eds.), *Biomedical ethics* (pp. 90–94). New York: McGraw-Hill.

Chambliss, D. (1996). *Beyond caring: Hospitals, nurses, and the social organization of ethics.* Chicago: University of Chicago Press.

Dalmiya, V., & Alcoff, L. (1993). Are "old wives tales" justified? In L. Alcoff & E. Potter (Eds.), *Feminist epistemologies* (pp. 217–244). New York: Routledge.

Doering, L. (1992). Power and knowledge in nursing: A feminist poststructuralist view. *Advances in Nursing Science, 14*(4), 24–33.

Dzurec, L. (1989). The necessity for and evolution of multiple paradigms for nursing research: A poststructuralist perspective. *Advances in Nursing Science, 11*(4), 69–77.

Flax, J. (1990). *Thinking fragments: Psychoanalysis, feminism and postmodernism in the contemporary west.* Berkeley: University of California Press.

Foucault, M. (1980). *Power/knowledge: Selected interviews and other writings, 1972–1977* (C. Gordon, Ed.). Brighton, UK: Harvester Press.

Fuss, D. (1989). *Essentially speaking: Feminism, nature and difference.* New York: Routledge.

Gramsci, A. (1971). *Selections from the prison notebooks.* New York: International.

Grosz, E. (1990). A note on essentialism and difference. In S. Gunew (Ed.), *Feminist knowledge as critique and construct* (pp. 332–334). London: Routledge.

Grosz, E. (1994). *Volatile bodies: Toward a corporeal feminism.* Bloomington: Indiana University Press.

Habermas, J. (1988). *The philosophical discourse of modernity.* Cambridge, UK: Polity.

Habermas, J., & Kelly, M. (1994). *Critique and power: Recasting the Foucault/Habermas debate.* Cambridge, MA: MIT Press.

Hekman, S. (1990). *Gender and knowledge: Elements of a postmodern feminism.* Cambridge, UK: Polity Press.

Henderson, A. (1994). Power and knowledge in nursing practice: The contribution of Foucault. *Journal of Advanced Nursing, 20,* 935–939.

Mappes, E. J. K. (1981). Ethical dilemmas for nurses: Physicians' orders versus patients' rights. In T. Mappes & J. Zembaty (Eds.), *Biomedical ethics* (pp. 95–101). New York: McGraw-Hill.

Mouffe, C. (1992). Feminism, citizenship and radical democratic politics. In J. Butler & J. Scott (Eds.), *Feminists theorize the political* (pp. 369–384). New York: Routledge.

Ramazanoglu, C. (1989). *Feminism and the contradictions of oppression.* New York: Routledge.

Reverby, S. (1987). *Ordered to care.* Cambridge, UK: Cambridge University Press.

Said, E. (1994). *Representations of the intellectual.* New York: Pantheon.

Sarup, M. (1989). *An introductory guide to poststructuralism and postmodernism.* Athens: University of Georgia Press.

Sarup, M. (1996). *Identity, culture and the postmodern world.* Athens: University of Georgia Press.

Sawicki, J. (1991). *Disciplining Foucault: Feminism, power and the body.* New York: Routledge.

Tong, R. (1989). *Feminist thought: A comprehensive introduction.* Boulder, CO: Westview.

Weedon, C. (1997). *Feminist practice and poststructuralist theory.* New York: Routledge.

West, C. (1993). The new cultural politics of difference. In C. McCarthy & W. Crichlow (Eds.), *Race, identity and representation in education* (pp. 11–23). New York: Routledge.

Wolf, Z. (1988). *Nurses' work: The sacred and the profane.* Philadelphia: University of Pennsylvania Press.

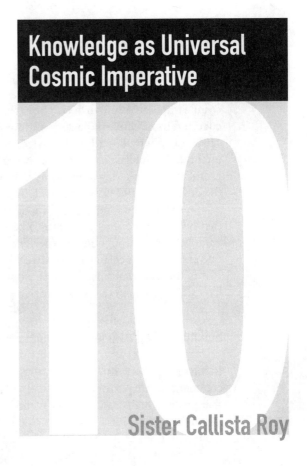

Knowledge as Universal Cosmic Imperative

Sister Callista Roy

The scientific world was abuzz with reports of evidence suggesting microscopic life on the planet Mars. Likely, we have never before in history had such a resplendent example of the impact of knowledge. Commentators searched for words to describe the stunning, yet inconclusive discoveries pointing to the first direct sign that life may be ubiquitous in the universe. Apparent fossils of ancient microbial life inside tiny cracks of a rock from Mars will change our science, our history, our philosophy, our theology, most of all our beliefs about persons and environment. Many were quick to anticipate the implications and to raise questions as to whether our particular human species on earth is ready for this. I submit that one group of persons that are most likely ready for this are the nurse scholars. As a group, we have opened ourselves to the rich ontological and epistemological explorations into understanding person and environment relations the past 20 years. As the great universe story unfolds nurses are in the position of being shapers of the next human era.

An Alternative Approach to Nursing

The challenge of nursing science today is to envision the impact of nursing knowledge in the 21st century. My goal is to take the position that knowledge is rooted in a universal cosmic imperative and to derive from that statement the links between theoretical knowledge and its effective impact on our nursing practice in the rapidly changing health care scene. I begin by describing knowledge as a universal imperative. This position is based on three characteristics of a cosmic perspective, unity, purposefulness, and promise. Each characteristic will then be explored in broad outline linking this philosophical stance with the development of nursing knowledge and its impact on nursing practice.

In recent years, nurse scholars have made great efforts to steer clear of any position that hints at there being a truth to be discovered. We are rightly concerned about the realities created from human experience. However, consider the possibility that there is a universal truth, a cosmic imperative. What possibly could convince us of such a reality? If it is the case that knowledge is a universal imperative, what does such a reality look like? Can the characteristics of such a perspective be described?

Setting up the Position: A Personal Journey

In setting up this position of *Knowledge as Universal Cosmic Imperative*, it will be useful to comment on my personal journey related to perspectives on knowledge. I have often said that professionally, my primary commitment is to nursing knowledge. The Roy Adaptation Model of nursing has provided particular strategies for developing knowledge. Examples from the Roy model are used to illustrate the points about my beliefs about the nature of nursing knowledge development, my main focus.

As an undergraduate nursing student, I was totally enamored with new knowledge in every form. I read everything I could to be prepared to care for patients assigned to me, skipping ahead in my anatomy and physiology book, and asking the faculty for references on psychoanalytic personality development. Also, I signed up for Saturday courses so I also could study poetry and French political science. However, amidst this broad and general excitement, three specific encounters with knowledge left a deep impression. First, I was fascinated with the study of the function of the human nervous system. Even with what we knew then, it seemed to me to be the greatest proof for the existence of God, a truly awesome human capacity. Second, I loved philosophy, particularly metaphysics. Questions such as *What is reality?* and *What is the meaning of existence?* were vitally important to me. I wanted to know what every great mind had said about them. Third, there were some very progressive faculty at my home institution, Mount St. Mary's College in Los Angeles, who planned a series of lectures on the work of Pierre Teilhard de Chardin. The Christian paleontologist's insights and the strategies he used to take the findings of science and grasp the essence of the universe provided a lasting foundation for both the approach to and content of my epistemological thinking. By completion of the baccalaureate degree, I viewed knowledge as exciting and immense, but I also was convinced that it could be discovered.

After a year of clinical practice, I accepted the assignment from my religious community to begin graduate studies. Working with the great thinker and mentor, Dorothy

E. Johnson, I become convinced of the importance of describing the nature of nursing and of identifying the knowledge required for practice. In addition, studying in related disciplines, particularly social psychology, at the University of California at Los Angeles (UCLA) in the later 1960s served to further establish my epistemological position. It seemed clear that building a body of knowledge and describing nursing's unique perspective were at the top of the agenda for nursing as a profession and as a scientific discipline. Describing nursing's distinct way of viewing phenomena would provide the outline for knowledge for nursing.

The body of knowledge for nursing science, I believed, would be developed by nurse scholars' observations and classification of facts and establishment of verifiable theories and general laws about the phenomena outlined by discipline of nursing. The work of nurse theorists and the identification of commonalties, such of those noted by Donaldson and Crowley (1977) helped to shape a vision that seemed quite promising. I participated in discussions around having laws of order and laws of disorder (Johnson, 1968; Roy, 1983). Completing a doctoral degree in sociology in the 1970s contributed valuable content and some new skills as I studied self and role theories and theory construction as a field.

Building Nursing Knowledge: Gaining Insight

Building knowledge using what has been called traditional science, worked well for me during the years of undergraduate curriculum development and consultation, writing theory books, and speaking about the accountability of nursing for its scientific and professional development. I was for a time a great skeptic of the process as content approach.

However, something happened on our way to building this grand structure of knowledge. Margaret Newman (chapter 8, this volume), and like thinkers, provided new insights into the view of process as content. This thinking along with gradual responses to developments in philosophy and science raised questions about our views of knowledge. Kuhn (1970) let us know that knowledge was not necessarily cumulative. Gortner (1990) summarized efforts by nurses to include values in their view of science. Further, nurses became aware that physics had moved beyond relativity theory to a new worldview called quantum physics.

Amid rapid progress in the biological, behavioral, and physical sciences, the era called postmodernism was upon us. I generally do not find this term useful. However, the meaning of it, as discussed by Watson (1995), provides a bridge here. She uses Lather's (1991) definition of postmodern as a response across disciplines to the contemporary crisis of profound uncertainty brought about by the crash of modern hope of rationality and technology to solve human dilemmas.

I have noted elsewhere (Roy, 1997) two relevant influences from my work in the 1980s and 1990s. First was a 2-year Robert Wood Johnson postdoctoral fellowship at University of California, San Francisco, with Dr. Connie Robinson as mentor in neuroscience nursing. From this experience, I gained sensitivity to the immense potential of the human body and spirit to adapt to major neurologic injury. In addition, this opportunity provided access to scholars and literature in the neurosciences with insights into current study of brain and mind functions, including human consciousness.

A second major project involved celebrating the 25th anniversary of the first publication on the Roy Adaptation Model. Eight members of the Boston Based Adaptation in Nursing Research Society (BBARNS) embarked on a project to critically analyze and synthesize 163 published studies, dissertations, and theses based on the model between 1970 and 1995 (BBARNS, 1999). The group identified and retrieved studies from 46 English-speaking journals, representing three countries in North America, two in South America, Australia, two countries in Asia, seven countries in Europe, and one in Africa. In addition, dissertations and theses were retrieved from 30 schools of nursing in 20 states in the United States and from Canada. Two distinct impressions came to me from these two foci of my work. First, they are a rich source of knowledge for clinical nursing that we have only begun to tap adequately. At the same time, the inevitable limitations of both the process and content of the work were a haunting reality for me.

Other professional experiences include teaching epistemology of nursing courses with wonderful, inquiring women and men in the PhD program in nursing at Boston College and participating in a series of Knowledge Colloquia at Boston University, the University of Rhode Island, and Boston College. These significant contacts served as catalysts for fruitful insights about knowledge and practice. On a personal level, I had opportunities for relating my spirituality to developments in science. It has been clear that my life commitments include a religious faith within family and religious community that is philosophically and theologically based. Ongoing spiritual development opportunities provided key resources in my search to identify issues and approaches for adequately describing person and environment interactions within my personal belief system.

Additionally, retreats focusing on the work of Pierre Teilhard de Chardin provided the opportunity to explore further Teilhard's primal intuition of what he called the law of progressive complexity and increasing consciousness, that is, the problem of the relation between spirit and matter (de Chardin, 1966). Other significant retreat experiences were at Genesis, a Spiritual Life Center in Westfield, Massachusetts, committed to cultivating an integrated spirituality emerging from the creative and natural environment that surrounds us and including programs by Diarmuid O'Murchu and Thomas Berry.

This story has been used to set the stage for taking the position that knowledge is a universal cosmic imperative. In the process, my thinking has come full circle, from a rationalist view of science to holding open numerous options of realism, constructivism, and interpretism, hermeneutic human science, and critical theory. The discussion to follow reflects my justified beliefs on the nature of knowledge. Ewing (1951) described justified beliefs as another form of knowledge.

Articulating A Position on Knowledge Beliefs

In the post-Kuhnian era, it is clear that new developments do not have to be either revolutions or totally accumulations. Growth can occur by building new insights upon foundational assumptions and thus maintaining some continuity of beliefs. In a 1988 publication on the philosophical assumptions of the Roy Adaptation Model, three worldviews were presented and contrasted. These views can be considered ways of knowing: (a) rationalism, in which the scientific mode is used to know truth by empirical fact; (b) relativism, whereby fact is known to exist only in relation to the thinking person; and (c) veritivity, in which the highest form of knowing is integration with the unity of truth. The term *veritivity* was coined to identify a philosophical assumption that connotes the richness of rootedness in an absolute truth that leads to values of conviction, commitment, and caring.

It is this third worldview that I am explicating in this discussion. The goal is to expand the philosophical assumption of veritivity to explore the ontological and epistemological perspective of *knowledge as universal cosmic imperative*. Knowledge as universal cosmic imperative can be understood by identifying its major characteristics. At this point I base this position on a cosmic perspective that includes the characteristics of unity, purposefulness, and promise.

Unity and the Universal Imperative

The unity of knowledge is supported by both philosophical arguments and scientific evidence. Our very notion of science originates in Greek ontology. True knowledge is knowledge of essences. And the essence, in logical terms, is the universal. Aristotle is credited with the famous line, "All knowledge is of the universal." There are degrees of the doctrine of monism. The extremist's version is that everything is just *one* and there is nothing more to be said about it. Another extreme, pantheism, claims that a creator God actually includes in himself everything that is.

Spinoza was less extreme, but asserted that everything is one substance, though with different attributes. Absolute idealism spoke of a single experience, and coherence theory purports one logical system. Kant formulated the principles of the permanence and unity of substance and of a priori knowledge to guide moral judgments. Russell, who at times asserted extreme pluralism, also said that everything we know is made of one kind of stuff.

Ewing (1951) summarized three bases for the resurgence of ideas of the unity of knowledge at most periods in history. First, to believe in one God is itself to adopt a fairly monistic view of the universe, and this belief generally occurred in most periods of time. Second, theories of causation often include assumptions of logical necessity that are argued by philosophers and that are closely akin to commonsense views. This is also known as entailment theory; that is, if two things entail each other, they necessarily belong together and cannot be separated. Although everything does not itself cause every other particular thing, everything we know is in some way directly or more or less indirectly causally connected.

Even if we are not so enamored with causality language, we can relate to the contention that the flutter of the butterfly's wings in a South American forest has an influence on everything in the universe. The third rationale Ewing discussed is that there simply is a natural tendency, very strong in some people, and present in some degree in most, to regard it as intellectually, and in other ways too, more satisfying to think of the universe as a unity rather than as a plurality. Ewing noted in particular that the great mystics have claimed that they could be immediately aware of an enormously greater unity between things than any which appears through intellectual reasoning or nonmystical forms of religion.

In their powerful book *The Universe Story*, Swimme and Berry (1992) noted that cosmogenesis is organized by communion:

To be is to be related, for relationship is the essence of existence. In the very first instance when the primitive particles rushed forth, every one of them was connected to every other one in the entire universe. At no time in the future existence of the universe would they ever arrive at a point of disconnection. Alienation for a particle is a theoretical impossibility. For galaxies too, relationships are the fact of existence. Each galaxy is directly connected to the hundred billion galaxies of the universe, and there will never come a time when a galaxy's destiny does not involve each of the galaxies in the universe. Nothing is itself without everything else. The universe evolves into beings that are different from each other, and that organize themselves. But in addition to this, the universe advances into community—into a differentiated web of relationships among sentient centers of creativity. (p. 77)

From another perspective, Zohar (1990) provides a wonderful illustration of how the human being is a microcosm of cosmic being. The author noted that the mind/body, or mind/brain, duality in the human person is a reflection of the wave/particle duality in quantum physics. Specifically, we are in our essential makeup, composed of the same stuff and held together by the same dynamics as those that account for everything else in the universe. And equally, which brings out the enormity of this realization, the universe is made of the same stuff and held together by the same dynamics as those, which account for us (Zohar, 1990, p. 101).

Zohar argued that if we interpret consciousness in this way, as a particular kind of creative relationship made possible by quantum wave mechanics, then we can combat materialism and the whole reductionist tendency. This insight allows us to argue that the mind is not merely an offshoot of brain function. In the words of de Chardin:

We must accept what science tells us, that man (person) was born from the earth. But more logical than the scientists who lecture us, we must carry this lesson to its conclusion: that is to say accept that man (person) was born entirely from the world not only his flesh and bones but his incredible power of thought. (1969, p. 20)

Expanding on the image, Houston discussed the metaphor of the hologram and quoted a description in the 2nd-century Buddhist Avatamska Sutra:

In the house of Indra there is said to be a network of pearls so arranged that if you look at one you see all the others reflected in it. In the same way, each person, each object in the world, is not merely itself, but involves every other person and object and, in fact, is every other person and object. (Houston, 1982, p. 188)

This metaphor was made concrete by Gabor's 1947 invention of optical holography (Lerner & Trigg, 1991, p. 512). The unique characteristic of holographic imaging is the idea of recording both the amplitude and the phase of the light waves coming from the object. In information processing terms, the whole is in fact present in each part. Pribam (1971) developed a holographic model of memory storage in the brain. Neurophysiology continues to provide evidence that there is a sense in which the brain functions as a whole, with individual neurons behaving holographically.

A related scientific notion of unity of knowledge is Bohm's sweeping theory of the implicate order of the universe. Briggs and Peat (1984) noted that Bohm, a professor in theoretical physics, explored deep insights into traditionally nonscientific subjects such as truth, insight, and language, which he tried to show are as important to understanding the physical world as the classical concepts of momentum and change. This thinking offered a new map for a new universe. Bohm's writings (1951) present quantum theory in an orthodox form. This quote reflects the flavor of the authors' early thoughts on implicate order:

> Quantum concepts imply that the world acts more like a single indivisible unit, in which even the "intrinsic" nature of each part (wave or particle) depends to some degree on its relationship to its surroundings. It is only at the microscopic (or quantum) level, however, that the indivisible unity of the various parts of the world produces significant effects. (Briggs & Peat, 1984, p. 95)

We have seen, then, some highly suggestive, if not compelling, support for the first characteristic of knowledge as universal imperative, the cosmic notion of the unity of knowledge. Let me provide an image of the characteristic of unity of knowledge from Young's book *The Unfinished Universe* (1986). Figure 10.1, for example, depicts the North

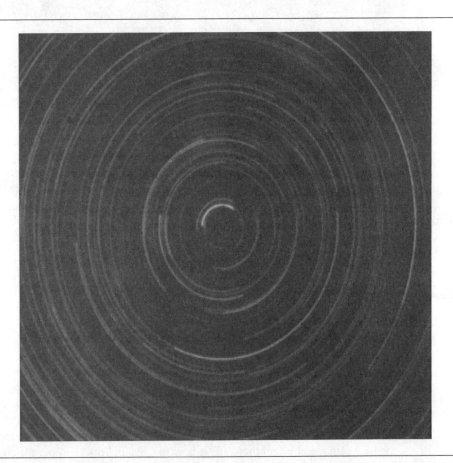

North Sky about the Pole Star: Eight-Hour Exposure. (Lick Observatory Photograph. Used with permission.)

Figure
10.2

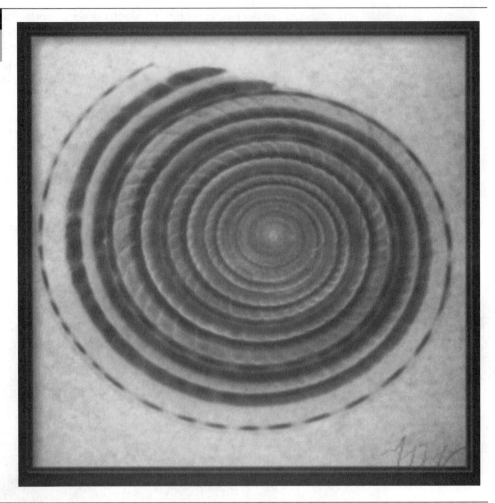

Sundial Shell.

Sky about the Pole Star and Figure 10.2 shows the comparable shape of a Sundial Shell to illustrate this point. Let us turn now to a somewhat more difficult characteristic to establish: that of the purposefulness of the universe.

Purposefulness and the Universal Imperative

The principles of classical dynamics, discovered by Galileo and Newton, postulated that immutable laws control the motion and interaction of material objects, large and small, everywhere in the universe. These concepts led to a mechanistic interpretation of the universe, with every piece of knowledge just another cog in the great machine. It was 20th-century physicists who demonstrated that some degree of indeterminism exists at the base of natural phenomena. The laws of physics appear to be ironclad only because large numbers of events are involved at the atomic and subatomic levels. A worldview emerges in which the universe is generated by chance. Randomness averages out and the laws that emerge are statistical in nature. This perspective denies the possibility of direction and leads to a nihilistic interpretation of nature.

Young (1986) noted that it is ironic that while the mainstream of scientific thought restates its denial of meaning or purpose in the cosmos, more and more remarkable facts have been emerging from cosmology, geology, and the study of life that seem to point to a purposeful and ordered universe. The author referred to Albert Einstein's famous quote, which says that he could not believe that God plays dice with the universe. Further, Young discussed a series of understandings that contribute to a cosmic view of order, form, change, and the creative forces in the universe. A new perception of the relationship of time and universal change is described. In addition, Young saw the emergence of a new evaluation of the role of chance in the birth of stars and the formation of the building blocks of life, a new understanding of the way complex organisms are constructed from simple ones and how communities of living things may be higher organisms in the process of becoming. Though no simple insight is enough to disclose the true nature of the universe, together they illuminate the dim outlines of an orderly design, suggestions of a work-in-progress, and make possible a new interpretation of an awesome, beautiful, but still unfinished universe. Young postulated that we are witnessing, and participating in, a creative act that is taking place throughout time.

One example among many discussed by Young (1986) is the synthesis of life. Theories about the origin of life have passed through several phases. Beginning in the 20th century, and well into the 1960s, most biologists believed that life was created by pure chance in the warm soup of the primordial seas. More recent discovery of the speed of evolution from inorganic matter, and geologic evidence, suggests that mechanisms other than the workings of pure chance were involved in the creation of life. A likely theory of the origin of life is that two evolutionary lines, related to nucleic acid and protein, fused. The process of fusion is ubiquitous throughout nature and provides a mechanism for rapid evolution. Young (1986) described life as a stage in the organization of matter.

Complexification, the same term used by de Chardin, is the process of organizing higher forms of life from ameba to fish, to amphibian, to mammal, to primate, and finally to the human person. The term *evolution*, coming from the Latin *evolvere*, to roll out or unfold, has come to mean more than the word implies, because it refers to a process with more emphasis on creativeness. In the natural world, errors are not as common as one would expect if chance alone were responsible for change; but the existence of tragic mistakes would not be expected at all if a pattern, already created, were simply being unrolled. The evolutionary process, then, is not entirely composed of an immense number of very small steps. Rather there is evidence today that creative leaps in the pattern have taken place. Two images illustrate these points. In this set, Figure 10.3 compares a snowflake with Queen Anne's Lace (Figure 10.4). In these images, I think we see both the unity and purposefulness of the natural world.

From another perspective, that of ecology and theology, Haught (1993) argued that a commonly held belief that the cosmos is a significant process, that it unfolds something analogous to what we call "purpose," an essential prerequisite of sustained global and intergenerational commitment to the earth's well-being. He noted that in a way that is entirely consistent with science, nature may plausibly be interpreted as purposeful in the sense that it holds a promise of ultimate meaning and beauty. Further, Haught explained that process theology reconciles the ideas of God and evolution in a uniquely reasonable way.

Figure
10.3

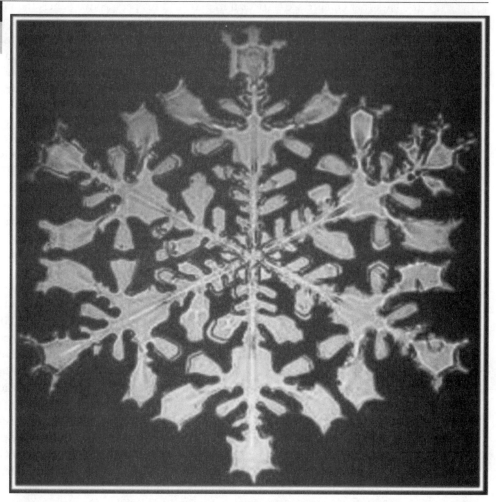

Snowflake.

Process theology understands God as the very source and stimulus of cosmic evolution. Instead of seeing evolution as an embarrassing scientific problem, it views God as intimately involved in, though still remaining distinct from, the cosmic process. God is the creative eros that arouses the world to evolutionary movement, to life, consciousness, and civilization. God is forever attracting the cosmos toward more complex levels of evolution. God is the source of the world's beauty and value, persuading the cosmos to body forth in its evolution. The evolutionary advance of the universe suggests a cosmic aim toward increasingly more intense forms of ordered novelty, that is, toward heightening the beauty and value of the universe (Haught, 1993, p. 33).

It should be noted that neither unity nor purposefulness necessarily includes certainty. Unity and purposefulness relate to the premise that laws of nature do hold, that intentionality and universal concepts make sense. However, these key notions do not apply to the content of laws, concepts, and experiences; they do not lock in a given direction or a given premise (von Weizsaker, 1971).

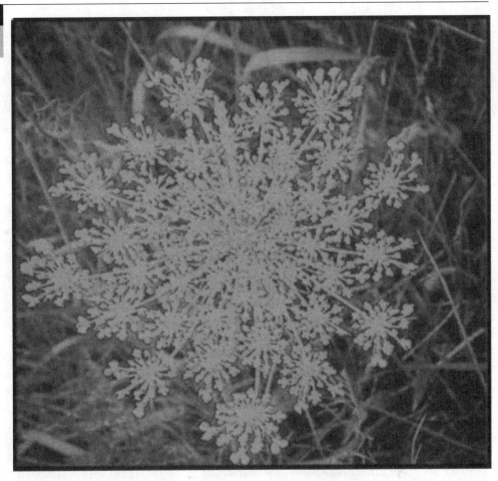

Figure 10.4

Queen Anne's Lace.

Ewing (1951) extended this notion to individual human freedom. He noted that a view of dependency on the universe as a whole is sometimes associated with exalting the state at the expense of the individual and decreasing freedom in political life. Again, the connection is not a necessary one. "We cannot, from a general proposition about the unity of everything that is, conclude that unity ought to be realized in a particular way in human life, thus deducing our politics from our metaphysics" (Ewing, 1951, p. 211).

I am also saying, then, that a purposeful universe does not negate, but rather emphasizes, individual human freedom. Therefore, a second major assumption upon which I base my position about the nature of knowledge comes from a broad view of the purposefulness of cosmic reality. If the universe is purposeful, then I argue that this characteristic can be applied to knowing the universe. Knowledge itself has meaning and purpose. The characteristics of unity and purposefulness give rise to the third point, a cosmic perspective evokes a promising future.

Promise and the Universal Imperative

The new millennium brings a time of transition and likely radical change. Authors such as Davies (1988) and Swimme & Berry (1992) have been sounding the alert that current changes in the life systems of the earth are so extensive that a major epoch is ending. The names of the eras are conceptual expressions invented to enable us to think about the larger patterns of functioning of the biosystems of the planet. The Paleozoic, the Mesozoic, and the Cenozoic eras covered about 550 million years. During the 67 million years known as the Cenozoic era, expansive life processes developed on the earth. It is significant that the great creativity of this era emerged without human influence. Rather, humankind appeared late in the era, actually having no say about their appearance upon the earth. The next era will be different. Swimme and Berry (1992) noted that we are entering into a new period of creativity participated in by the entire earth community. They identify this new period as the Ecozoic era, a fourth biological era. The authors highlighted the central commitment of the emerging Ecozoic as an era of communion of subjects rather than a collection of objects. Together people will decide what kind of a universe we will inhabit.

The promise for the future that is characteristic of the cosmic imperative is based upon understanding time and timelessness, the omega point, and human participation in transformation. Recent writings have dealt with the issue of time in a way that demonstrates that the commonsense view of time agrees with the most advanced scientific theory. Time does in fact move like an arrow, shooting forward into what is unknown (Coveney & Highfield, 1990). We witness time moving in one direction, from the past to the present, to the future. If you drop a cup, it shatters and does not reassemble itself. The leaves fall from the trees and shrivel and die. Young (1986) suggested a view of time that is consistent with the cosmic perspective being described. Within this context, time can be perceived as a way of measuring the progressive change that is building the universe even while we live and take part in it.

Time is cosmic and time is spiritual. Pope John Paul II (1994) helped the Catholic Church prepare for the new millennium by proclaiming that the Year 2000 be celebrated as the Great Jubilee. He noted: "In Christianity, time has a fundamental importance. Within the dimension of time the world was created; within it the history of salvation unfolds, finding its culmination in the fullness of time of the Incarnation and Resurrection" (Pope John Paul II, 1994, p. 17). He further stated, "The Church respects the measurements of time: hours, days, years, and centuries. She thus goes forward with every individual, helping everyone to realize how each of these measurements of time is imbued with the presence of God" (Pope John Paul II, 1994, p. 23).

This brings us to a profound concept in considering the promise of the future, the *omega point*. Thought-provoking discussions of this element of the future are found in two very different sources, the Christian Paleontologist de Chardin and the Atheist Physicist Tipler.

Tipler (1994) wrote on the physics of immortality and concluded that the omega point and the physical universe necessarily exit. He based his thinking on proof provided by metaphysical implications of modern computer science and modern cosmology. Tipler offered the argument, and some scientific consensus, for the validity of a theory of the branching of universes according to the Many-Histories Interpretation. He considered the vertical axis as the radius of the universe and the horizontal axis as time. A measurement early in time causes the universe to split into Many Histories, and the end point is final singularity, for which he borrows the term omega point from de Chardin.

De Chardin (1964) provided both a definition of omega point and his basis for postulating it with one simple statement: "At the heart of the universe prolonged along its axis of complexity, there exists a divine centre of convergence . . . and in order to stress its synthesizing and personalizing function, let us call it the point *Omega*" (de Chardin, 1966, p. 127). In other publications (Roy, 1988, 1997), I have referred to the promising future of convergence by citing the elegant verses of the medieval poet Dante, who wrote about three states of the afterlife and expressed a belief in the final coming together of persons, creation, and God in the image of a rose in Paradisio.

We further our understanding of the cosmic characteristic of a promising future by emphasizing something alluded to several times in this discussion. Human participation in transformation is key to our future. Human consciousness, the thinking and feeling person is at the heart of the emerging universe, as knower and known, and as creator.

Zohar (1990) provided one view of the chain of evolving consciousness. *Termions* (or matter fields) and *bosons* (or force fields) give rise to the world of living things from which emerged our species of human beings. Individuals then, with personal psychologies, develop relationships involving personal and cultural morality, aesthetics, concepts, and so forth. From this emerges what the psychologist Jung calls a *collective unconscious*. Our religious awareness and experience derive from the collective unconscious. Zohar described the evolution of consciousness in religious categories. For myself, it is easy, and necessary, to use such terms. The role of person in the universe has shifted as we have shifted from an old cosmology to a new cosmology.

De Chardin put the challenge to us this way: "The whole future of the Earth, . . . seems to me to depend on the awakening of our faith in the future" (1962, front page). In writing nearly three decades ago, Bronowski (1977) made our human responsibility even more specific. He noted that continued absence after the Renaissance of free inquiry in the field of ethics has contributed to moving us backward. Further Bronowski contended that we are responsible for increasing our understanding of moral behavior in the same way we increase our understanding of nature, by the use of the human mind in scholarly inquiry.

Ferris, in an August 19, 1996, editorial in *The New Yorker* magazine on the report of evidence of microscopic life on the planet Mars said this: "Our creativity and our future are now one, our fate less certain than that of any wayward meteor" (p. 5). The only thing that is uncertain is what kind of future we will create. The opportunities and promise lie before us. As put by Swimme and Berry (1992), human participation in the universe is a sequence of irreversible transformations. I believe that the promise of the future is a characteristic of cosmic reality, and thus a characteristic of knowledge. In spite of a common cynicism in America, in the words of the social justice movement, nurses are countercultural. We believe in the promise of the future.

The Imperative

As the final step in describing knowledge as universal cosmic imperative, the term *imperative* requires clarification. Imperative, within the context of this discussion, refers to a fact that compels attention or action, an obligation or need (Stein & Urdang, 1967).

The assumptions of a cosmic perspective—unity, purposefulness, and promise—act as the facts that compel us. Our attention is inescapably drawn to developing knowledge of person and environment within the view of a purposeful unity that has a destiny. From this stance, nursing is in a position to shape the future stage of evolution of the universe. The kind of knowledge that nurses develop is immediately relevant to impact upon practice.

To derive the linkages of the philosophical stance of knowledge as universal cosmic imperative to impact on nursing practice calls for forging a new conceptual structure that identifies nursing's view of person and environment within the challenges of modern science and the values of the discipline. Our sequence of knowledge development for impact on practice can be described by a worldview leading to a paradigmatic definition of nursing, from which derives the conceptual structure. The conceptual structure provides for specification of practice imperatives. The impact on practice results from these practice perspectives.

The Imperative and Linkages to Nursing Practice

In a paper focused on redefining adaptation for the 21st century, Roy (1997) outlined the assumptions about nursing knowledge derived from the philosophical position described here as the cosmic imperative. Nursing sees persons as coextensive with their physical and social environment. The discipline takes a values-based stance and believes and hopes in human persons as creators of the future. A conceptual structure is based on a redefinition of the term *adaptation*. Adaptation is defined as the process and outcome whereby the thinking and feeling person uses conscious awareness and choice to create human and environmental integration.

Briefly, then, the scientific assumptions for this view of nursing for the 21st century are

- Systems of matter and energy progress to higher levels of complex self-organization.
- Consciousness and meaning are constitutive of person and environment.
- Awareness of self and environment is rooted in thinking and feeling.
- Human decisions are accountable for integration of creative processes.
- Thinking and feeling mediate human action.
- System relationships include acceptance, protection, and fostering of interdependence.
- Persons and the earth have common patterns and integral relations.
- Person and environment transformations are created in human consciousness.
- Integration of human and environment meanings result in adaptation.

Based on the worldview taken here of knowledge as *universal cosmic imperative*, the philosophical assumptions for the 21st century emerge as:

- Persons have mutual relationships with the world and with a God figure.
- Human meaning is rooted in an omega point convergence of the universe.
- God is intimately revealed in the diversity of creation and is the common destiny of creation.
- Persons use human creative abilities of awareness, enlightenment, and faith.

■ Persons are accountable for entering the process of deriving, sustaining, and transforming the universe.

The foci of practice imperatives are on mutual complex person and environment self-organization and on the meaningful destiny of convergence of the universe, persons, and environment, in what can be considered a supreme being, or creator God. The thinking and feeling person assumes great significance in the processes whereby humankind carries out responsibility for the creation of a new epoch. Nursing practice will focus on decisions about persons' integral relationship with the earth and will shape the future stage of the evolutionary creativity.

Practice Imperatives: An Exemplar

The worldview of the universal cosmic imperative changes who I am, which in turn changes me as a nurse. As an example from my experience, when with a person who is dealing with responses to neurologic changes, as a researcher and as a clinician, I have a strong sense of connectedness with a person who shares a place in the universe. I trust in the meaningfulness of this life and the person's experience. I believe that as I speak, listen, and sometimes touch the patient, I communicate a sense of awe before the purposefulness and part mystery of the human journey. I hold a hope in the promise of the future that neuroscience may have knowledge to handle what it is that the person is dealing with. In the meantime, I am convinced that my nursing knowledge perspective is necessary in the immediate interpersonal situation.

In this example, I picture myself doing the initial neurologic assessment of a patient in the emergency room just admitted with a gunshot wound to the neck that has resulted in an as yet undetermined amount of spinal cord injury. It is only my sense of unity, purposefulness, and promise that provides the sensitivity with which I am present as the patient responds to feeling or not feeling pinpricks along given nerve pathways and to my requests to push against my hand with motor movement. I need the same broad perspective as I am with the patient in the intensive care unit as there is a dawning awareness of the parts of life that have changed and what abilities remain and grow. My perspective and beliefs take in the family members and other persons immersed in the meaning of the person's experiences, including legal concerns related to the shooting. Weeks later I am with the patient again in a rehabilitation setting with a strong emphasis on realizing human potential. Finally, many months later, I do another neurologic exam showing only minimal recovery from quadriplegia. I am present to the developing relationship of the patient to a full-time caregiver.

I am changed by the patient's and others' struggles through these stages. At the same time, a foundational perspective of the cosmic imperative provides rootedness for my growth, and hopefully this is what I share with the patient.

Conclusion

I suggest that the view of knowledge as universal cosmic imperative can provide nursing science with integration and comprehensiveness. This position is broad enough to include the other two perspectives on knowledge that we have explored by the discipline to date, including knowledge as problem solving (chapter 7, this volume) and knowledge as process (chapter 8, this volume).

Nursing will always have thinking and feeling women and men who will enter the practice situations of their time and be influential in building new visions of mutual complex person and environment self-organization and convergence. The *universal cosmic imperative* offers a broad perspective to view the global nature of health care while creating opportunities for professional nurses to use their science to advance health care and improve social conditions for all.

REFERENCES

BBARNS. (1999). *Roy Adaptation Model-based research: 25 years of contributions to nursing science.* Indianapolis, IN: Center Nursing Press.

Briggs, J., & Peat, F. (1984). *The looking glass universe.* New York: Simon & Schuster.

Bronowski, J. (1977). *A sense of the future.* Cambridge, MA: MIT Press.

Cohen, J., & Stewart, I. (1994). *The collapse of chaos.* New York: Penguin Books.

Coveney, P. & Highfield, R. (1990). *The Arrow of Time.* W.H. Allen, Ed. London.

Davies, P. (1988). The cosmic blueprint. New York: Simon & Schuster.

de Chardin, T. (1962). *Letters from a traveler.* New York: Harper & Row.

de Chardin, T. (1964). *The future of man.* New York: Harcourt Brace Jovanovich.

de Chardin, T. (1966). *Man's place in nature.* New York: Harper & Row.

Donaldson, S. K., & Crowley, D. M. (1978). The discipline of nursing. *Nursing Outlook, 26*(2), 113–120.

Ewing, A. C. (1951). *The fundamental questions of philosophy.* London: Routledge & Kegan Paul.

Ferris, T. (1996, Aug. 19). A message from Mars. *The New Yorker,* p. 5.

Gortner, S. (1990). Nursing values and science: Toward a science philosophy. *Image, 22,* 101–105.

Haught, J. F. (1993). *The promise of nature: Ecology and cosmic purpose.* New York: Paulist Press.

Houston, J. (1982). *The possible human.* New York: Jeremy P. Tarcher/Putnam.

Johnson, D. E. (1968). Theory in nursing: Borrowed and unique. *Nursing Research, 17,* 206–209.

Kuhn, T. (1970). *The structure of scientific revolutions* (2nd ed.). Chicago: University of Chicago.

Lather, P. (1991). *Getting smart: Feminist research and pedagogy within the postmodern.* New York: Routledge.

Lerner, R. G., & Trigg, G. L. (1991). *Encyclopedia of physics.* New York: VCH Publishers, Inc.

McDonald, F. J., & Harms, M. (1966). Theoretical model for an experimental curriculum. *Nursing Outlook, 14,* 48–51.

Pope John Paul II. (1994). *The third millennium.* Boston: Pauline Books & Media.

Pribram, K. (1971). *Languages of the brain: Experimental paradoxes and principles in neuropsychology.* Englewood Cliffs, NJ: Prentice-Hall.

Prigogine, I., & Stengers, I. (1984). *Order out of chaos: Man's new dialogue with nature.* New York: Bantam.

Roy, C. (1983). Theory development in nursing: Proposal for direction. In N. Chaska (Ed.), *The Nursing profession: A time to speak*. New York: McGraw-Hill.

Roy, C. (1988). An explication of the philosophical assumptions of the Roy Adaptation Model. *Nursing Science Quarterly*, *1*, 26–34.

Roy, C. (1997). Future of the Roy model: Challenge to redefine adaptation. *Nursing Science Quarterly*, *10*(1), 42–47.

Stein, J., & Urdang, L. (1967). *The Random House dictionary of the English language* (unabridged ed.). New York: Random House.

Swimme, B., & Berry, T. (1992). *The universe story*. San Francisco: Harper.

Tipler, F. (1994). *The physics of immortality*. New York: Anchor Books.

von Weizsaker, C. (1971). *The unity of nature*. New York: Farrar, Straus, Giroux.

Watson, J. (1995). Postmodernism and knowledge development in nursing. *Nursing Science Quarterly*, *8*(2), 60–64.

Wu, R. (1973). *Behavior and illness*. Englewood Cliffs, NJ: Prentice-Hall.

Young, L. B. (1986). *The unfinished universe*. New York: Simon & Schuster.

Zohar, D. (1990). *The quantum self*. New York: Quill/William Morrow.

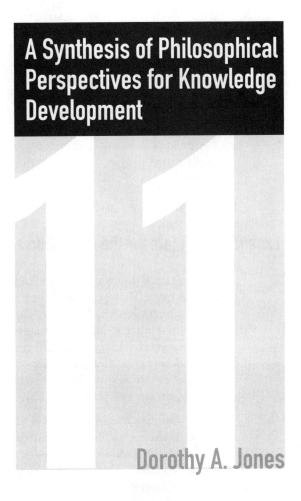

A Synthesis of Philosophical Perspectives for Knowledge Development

Dorothy A. Jones

The evolution of nursing knowledge has occurred in a variety of ways and has offered the scientist many strategies to know and understand the human experience. As nurses work to explore and develop knowledge, there is a continual struggle to find a shared vision around which nursing unites. One example of this search is found in the position paper in chapter 1. The success of reaching a broad consensus around a shared vision may ultimately rest with the ability of nurses to achieve unity around philosophical values and beliefs and consensus around the interface between knowledge development, use of knowledge, and refinement for application in practice.

The degree to which nursing practice is driven and informed by disciplinary knowledge will ultimately answer the question "why nursing?" and give voice to nurses' contributions to patient care outcomes. Achieving agreement on the basic philosophical assumptions that underlie knowledge development will continue to shape and inform disciplinary growth. As Redfield (1993) states, we must become part of a new spiritual awakening. "Whenever we doubt our own path, or lose sight of the process, we must remember what we are evolving toward, what process of living is all about . . . we know how it can . . . we know how it will be done" (p. 241).

The discussion to follow offers a synthesis of two of the philosophical perspectives discussed, namely, knowledge as problem solving—a postpositivist perspective— and knowledge as process, both from the Newman perspective and from a poststructuralist feminist perspective. The perspective of integrated knowledge, particularly the universal cosmic imperative is recognized as a developing perspective and is explored as such by other authors in this volume. This chapter will link philosophical perspectives to provide (a) an expanding view of nursing across the perspectives discussed, (b) a comparison of five practice constructs as operationalized within the perspectives, and (c) a synthesis of dominant themes from across perspectives and questions for further reflection and dialogue.

Expanded Mandate for the Discipline

Nursing knowledge development and related perspectives to date have helped to inform the discipline about content of nursing practice and the focus of the discipline. The current language of the American Nursing Association's *Nursing's Social Policy Statement* describes nursing in relation to society as a "pivotal health care profession, highly valued for its specialized knowledge, skill and caring in improving the health status of the public and ensuring safe, effective, quality care" (American Nurses Association, 2003a, p. 1). It continues by describing the values and assumptions that are inherent in the profession's social contract, which include:

- Humans manifest an essential unity of mind, body, and spirit.
- Human experience is contextually and culturally defined.
- Health and illness are human experiences.
- The relationship between the nurse and the patient involves participation of both in the process of care.
- The interaction between nurse and patient occurs within the context of the values and beliefs of the patient and the nurse.
- Public policy and the health care delivery system influence the health and well-being of society and professional nursing. (American Nurses Association, 2003a, p. 3)

Nursing as science is concerned with humans and how they live. Within this context, nursing knowledge emerges from within the partnership between the nurse and the individual (or groups), and these partnerships are central to the mission of nursing as a discipline. The intentional, authentic presence of the nurse helps create an environment of care that seeks to relieve suffering, promote healing, and be responsive to the life experiences of individuals and groups. Within the various philosophical perspectives being discussed, knowing the person is enhanced by partnerships that recognize persons beyond the experiences of their illnesses. This approach offers new opportunities for nursing to become a more central and visible force for social justice, and an advocate for justice.

As nurses seek to uncover meaning, foster new understandings about persons through research, monitor recovery, and provide new knowledge about human experiences, nursing knowledge grows and the science evolves. Through the nurse–client partnership, there is a personal unfolding and awareness that promotes choice, enables action, and sustains change. Exploration of multiple philosophical, as well as theoretical, perspectives around core values and beliefs of the discipline, can foster knowledge development and promote professional growth.

Philosophical Perspectives and Knowledge for Practice

Within the context of this discussion, five practice elements central to nursing have been selected for discussion from the philosophical perspectives identified earlier. These elements are (a) the nature of person; (b) the focus of nursing; (c) the language used to describe the human experience; (d) the nursing action; and (e) the care outcomes. Each element will be discussed within the various philosophical perspectives so that the reader can distinguish commonalities and differences among the philosophical points of view.

Definition of Person

The role of person (individual, family, or community) is the focus of nursing's concern (see Fig. 11.1). The following discussion depicts how each philosophical perspective being discussed addresses the nature of person.

The *problem solving perspective* (chapter 7, this volume) includes reference to humans as holistic, bio-psychosocial beings, interacting (functioning) within an environment with responses shaped by age, developmental stage, health status, and culture. Empirical (measurable and oberable) determinants (e.g., height, weight, crying) are often used to describe human responses and functional health. Definition of person is achieved through an organized systematic approach (e.g., clinical decision making; Gordon, 1994). The nurse obtains needed data through an organized assessment of the person and analysis of objective/subjective manifestations of the client experience. Using reasoning, analysis, and synthesis, a problem is identified, nursing outcomes are designed and interventions are selected to resolve the problem, improve function, and optimize health.

Within the perspective of *knowledge as process,* there are many distinct approaches (Table 1.1). One specific approach that is widely used is that of Margaret Newman (chapter 8, this volume). In this process-oriented perspective, the person is defined as unique, characterized by pattern (i.e., energy fields) continuously evolving and in rhythmical exchange with the environment (Newman, 1994; Rogers, 1970). The human experience is understood within a dynamic partnership between the nurse and person. Understanding and illumination of the human experience (Picard & Jones, 2005) is achieved through the dialogue. A process of human unfolding is manifested through storytelling and other modes of aesthetic expression such as art, music, or dance uncover meaning. Through mutual exchange with the nurse and personal reflection, the individual (or group) moves toward personal awareness and discovery, making new choices that expand the human experience and enhance well-being.

Another process approach to knowledge, the *poststructural feminist perspective,* places emphasis on the personal feelings of the individual as revealed through the "small" story. The focus is gender sensitive, with knowledge about person reflected within the social,

Figure 11.1

Process:
Newman
Emphasis on patient expression of
the human experience (the personal
knowledge of nurse and patient). View
persons as unitary and holistic energy
fields, identified by unique pattern in
rhythmical exchange with the environment. Humans move through time and
space toward a choice point where
the individual decides action.

Problem
Solving
Emphasis on observable, isolating
phenomena of concern. Individuals
seen as holistic bio-psychosocial beings,
functional status informed by variables
(e.g., health status, environment, culture,
age, development). Patient/family community assessments can reveal patient
perceptions through decisional
models and knowing the
patient.

Process:
Poststructural
Feminism
Emphasis on personal feelings of the
individual (nurse and patient); focus
gender sensitive with attention to specific
role of women. Person defined as individual
within the context of the collective whole
(i.e., women in society). Social position,
culture, economics, and race are variables that influence individual and
collective responses.

Person

Definition of Person.

cultural, economic, and racial influences that have an impact on the individual and collective responses. Improvements in the lives of the aggregate are believed to enhance the life potential of the whole.

Definition of Nursing

As the content of the discipline emerges and nurses respond to organizational and regulatory demands, the consumer is experiencing a "new wave" of health care. In a series of articles appearing in the *New York Times*, health care is described as "the degrading experience of entering a medical system, whether hospital, nursing home, or clinic" (Carey, 2005). The author of the series acknowledges the advances of medical science but also reports many examples of the consumer feeling less than human while being cared for within current health settings. Lack of communication by providers, uncertainty and fear for personal safety, and invasion of personal space by unannounced attendants are but a few of the violations described by the consumer.

Although improvements in curing disease have been impressive, the dissatisfaction remains with care, especially when hospitalized. Many current heath care delivery systems are impersonal, fast-paced businesses, designed to fix problems with little attention to the individual experiencing them. Nursing is a major professional group, able to use its knowledge to address these deficits of health care delivery. The focus, or goal, of nursing, as discussed across the philosophical perspectives, provides a position from which to improve care. In this way, nurses can bring knowledge, relief of suffering, realization of one's potential and can create a safe space for the person where the individual (group) is known and opportunities for personal potential for nurses and others are actualized (see Fig. 11.2).

Within the *problem solving perspective*, the focus of nursing is framed within a structure that enables the nurse to identify problems along with the individual's (family and community) strengths and weaknesses. Nursing's goal is to relieve the problem by linking clinical judgments to the selection of desired outcomes and interventions that restore function, promote comfort, and foster optimal health. This approach to knowing the patient allows for "the concept of therapeutic decision making . . . which is a cherished value in nursing practice . . . the individuation of patient care includes nurse experience, time and a sense of closeness between the nurse and patient" (Radwin, 1994, p. 142).

The focus of nursing within the Newman *process perspective* (Newman, 2002) is on the nurse's engagement with person in a reflective process. Within the dialog the authentic self is uncovered for both participants. The partnership between the nurse and the person is deliberative and requires knowledge. The nurse, intentionally present within the experience, seeks to embody the process, guiding the person through a journey of self-discovery, meaning, choice and actions to promote the human experience. The nurse creates an environment of care designed to promote healing and uses knowledge to enhance personal awareness and opportunities for change. The spiritual connectedness that is fostered by the nurse enables the person to transcend boundaries and give new meaning to life (Reed, 1992, p. 350).

The *poststructuralist feminist perspective* offers a view of nursing that focuses on the role of the nurse engaged in helping humans search for meaning and self-discovery. This is accomplished as the nurse participates in strategies that facilitate emancipation and freedom from social and political constraints. Nurses engage in activities beyond the individual encounter to liberate and reform those conditions that prevent communities and groups (women) from reaching their full potential. The use of personal stories helps uncover situations of oppression and compromise.

Language and the Human Experience

The use of language conveys a message and often represents the story of an individual or group (see Fig. 11.3). Within the *problem solving perspective*, the judgments or phenomena of concern to nurses are generated through clinical reasoning and are often described using standardized nursing languages. Since 1973 (Dochterman & Jones,

Process:
Newman

Through reflective dialogue, the
patient reveals a story. The nurse is a
partner in the unfolding of the patient's
authentic self. By being fully present to
the person, the nurse establishes trust and
promotes self-reflection. This interaction enables choice and self awareness.
"Health is expanding
consciousness." (Newman,
1994)

Problem
Solving

Identifies patient, family, and community responses across the health
continuum. Identifies phenomena of
concern; promotes optimal function and
symptom relief. Advocate for patient in
resolving dilemmas. Nurse identifies
patient problems and links judgments
to probable etiologies.

Process:
Poststructural
Feminism

Promotes the search for meaning and
self-discovery. Facilitates emancipation
and promotes freedom. The nurse engages
in dialogue with the individual to understand the lived experience unique to each
person. Nursing engages in activities
(political) to liberate and reform the
conditions that prevent individuals
(i.e., women) from reaching
their full potential.

Nursing

Focus of Nursing.

2003), developments in nursing language have generated classifications such as nursing diagnosis, interventions, and outcomes. The Nursing Practice Information Infrastructure of the American Nurses Association (2003b) is the national body designed to
approve nursing languages (e.g., data sets, nomenclatures, and classification systems) for
use by nurses. To date, there have been 13 language systems developed. Groups such as
the North American Nursing Diagnosis Association (NANDA 2005–2006), the Nursing
Intervention Classification (NIC), the Nursing Outcomes Classification (NOC), as well
as other classification system developers, for example, the Omaha Community Health
System (Martin & Scheet, 1992), have worked to design a unified structure to communicate nursing knowledge (problems, interventions, and outcomes) used by the discipline
to describe nursing practice and research (chapter 15, this volume).

Process: Newman

Phenomena of concern disclosed through nurse interaction with the patient. The patient's story (pattern appraisal) can be disclosed through multiple modes of expression (i.e., art, dance, the narrative). The nurse comes to know the human experience (pattern manifestation) and themes or phenomena can describe pattern (e.g., relating and communicating).

Problem Solving

Use clinical reasoning (judgment) process used to generate nursing problems; defining cues and probable related factors. Systems such as NANDA or the ICNP are used to name and classify Nursing Diagnoses. Issues related to the integration of problems from other classification systems (e.g., medicine) may be used to describe nursing actions.

Process: Poststructural Feminism

Through narrative dialogue, patients (women) describe the meaning associated with the personal, subjective experiences within the context of the lived experience. Through this process, phenomena are identified and described and become the focus of political reform and social change.

Language

Language and the Human Experience.

Newman's *knowledge as process* reveals the nurse–client experience expressed through the narrative, pattern appraisal, and reflective dialogue. Within this perspective, personal meanings unique to the individual and associated with life events and experiences are represented in a way that reflects the patterning of the human experience. Pattern representation is one example of displaying the individual's story in the person's own words. The pattern analysis occurs with the nurse in dialogue with the person and is validated by the individual. The nurse works with the person or group to illuminate life meanings, arrive at new insights, and identify how choices and decisions have impacted their life and health (Newman, 1994, 2002; Picard & Jones, 2005). Reflection on the pattern can lead to a personal discovery, awareness, and a decision to take action and make new life choices. The narrative is used to represent the story and display an individual's pattern and is derived from the individual's story, reflecting the language of the person's description of the experience.

Phenomena that emerge from within the *poststructural feminist perspective* provides a description of the personal, subjective experiences of individuals (e.g., women and groups) described in language that reflects their own exposure to a situation, event, or struggle. The phenomena that emerge from discussion and group dialogue can often result in isolating problems and revealing focal areas for social reform. The story is used to communicate issues of concern to groups and society as a whole. The language of the group promotes tangible evidence of injustice and compromise and the search for innovative strategies that relieve suffering and promote the good of all.

Knowledge and Action

Nursing is often defined by what it does rather than how nurses think about the actions needed to address the human condition within the context of cognitive processing or the knowledge needed to promote human wholeness. Therefore, there is a danger in operationalizing nursing by describing nursing actions or what nurses do (see Fig. 11.4).

Actions (interventions) used to treat or affect human responses or problems have been named within the *problem solving perspective* and classified in several systems. The most familiar is the Nursing Intervention Classification (NIC; Dochterman & Bulecheck, 2004). The NIC system uses problem solving to link the action (i.e., intervention) to the problem (i.e., nursing diagnoses) and the etiology in an effort to achieve the best outcome. Emphasis is placed on strategies or actions taken by the nurse and drawn from a body of knowledge that is research based and common to clinical practice. The identification of an etiology within the context of the nursing diagnosis guides the interventions or actions and increases accuracy. The knowledge within the NIC classification system describes actions taken by the nurse and becomes important content for curriculum development and clinical practice.

Nursing action within the context of Newman's *knowledge as process* places less emphasis on "the prescription" or actions performed by the nurse in response to an isolated problem. Instead, particularly from the Newman perspective the emphasis focuses on the interaction and the choices made by the individual to take actions that will lead to life changes, transformation and expanded consciousness. The nurse guides the person through a reflective dialogue that seeks to uncover meaning and promote personal discovery. The process illuminates past decisions and outcomes along with opportunities for action by an individual or group to achieve desired goals. The process perspective embodies the nurse within the experience. The intentional relationship experienced by both the nurse and the person is therapeutic and healing. Through continued pattern appraisal and reflection, the nurse can observe movement toward a desired goal and observe expressions of personal transformation and new awareness. The nurse uses theoretical and disciplinary knowledge to coach the person in seeking new options, while providing needed support and encouragement to sustain the desired change.

Action within the *poststructural feminist perspective* focuses on the removal of barriers that inhibit self-growth and limit personal knowing for individuals and groups. Interventions or actions are directed toward increasing freedom and emancipation from restrictions that will enable the individual or group to make the best choices to achieve desired goals. Nurses can become partners-in-action and develop and use knowledge that can inform groups and foster innovative strategies to optimize a group's direction.

Figure
11.4

Process:
Newman

Awareness and decision to select interventions that are based upon patient choices to act or change behaviors. Uniqueness of the individual is recognized as art and science blend. Creative practice initiatives move the person through transitions and toward personal transformation.

Problem
Solving

The NIC intervention classification system provides linkages between diagnosis/intervention and outcomes. Emphasis on both doing and knowing. Actions describe the work of nursing. Linkages can be interpreted as prescriptive.

Process:
Poststructural
Feminism

Where oppression is present, groups seek to increase freedom and ability to make "best choices" unopposed. Increased self-awareness to achieve personal and collective goals. Seek interventions that foster individual variation and uniqueness of person.

Knowledge and Action

Knowledge and Action.

Outcomes of Care

Outcomes of nursing care reflect achievement of a desired goal linked to intentional actions (see Fig. 11.5). Outcomes within a *problem-solving perspective* seek evidence that can be observed, described, and measured. They usually are seen as predictable and definable when adequate research evidence is available. The Nursing Outcome Classification System (Moorhead, Johnson, & Maas, 2004) is one system that contains research-based outcomes. The classification provides a language and measures that can be used to evaluate achievement of a desired goal. Assessment data used to identify the originating problem are analyzed, and specific criteria are identified as a standard against which an outcome is evaluated. As nursing research continues to develop, evidence to support the

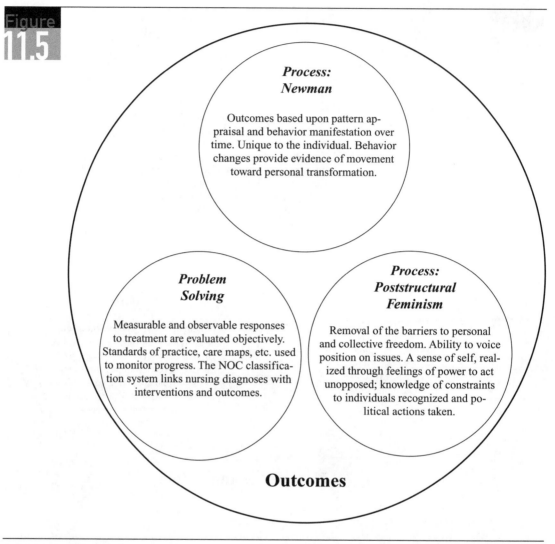

Outcomes of Care.

achievement of nursing outcomes will be integrated into existing databases and used to establish best practices within clinical practice.

Outcomes within the *process perspective* for Newman are determined in concert with the individual's perception of achievement and a sense of new awareness that emerges about the individual or group's personal perceptions. Pattern appraisals, conducted over time, along with personal dialogue can reflect the meaning of choices and changes made on behalf of personal decisions. New insights as perceived by the individual or group determine a personal triumph. In a number of recent studies (chapters 18, 19, 20, this volume; Picard & Jones, 2005), investigators acknowledge the development of new knowledge that emerges when an individual recognizes the impact of success. Data suggest that as one moves to make changes they appear to be increasingly open to other life changes (Berry, 2004).

When the obstacles or barriers that compromise personal and collective growth are removed and freedom from oppression is realized, outcomes within the *poststructural feminist perspective* are achieved. The accomplishment of group changes, complemented by a community's ability to voice an opinion on a topic without fear of reprisal, is motivating. Success is measured by feelings of empowerment of the individual, group, or community as they move toward a desired goal. Group success usually provides guidelines for ways to address future concerns and serves as an impetus to continue the quest for social action to achieve justice and the common good for all.

Future Perspective

The synthesis of the philosophical perspectives provides insight into nursing knowledge development, utilization, and evaluation in clinical and academic settings. It also offers a guide in determining strategies that require the development of new knowledge and reflects the presence of nurses within health care. Although no one perspective provides all of the answers, there is support for core beliefs and assumptions that guide the development and evolution of nursing science. Nursing as an unique discipline is realized in each perspective discussed and a synthesized knowledge perspective is offered. Each perspective supports knowledge rooted in core values and beliefs and is grounded in relationship with humans. Integrated knowledge perspectives are further explored in Part III, this volume.

Knowledge development in nursing continues to be an iterative process that occurs over time and is informed by strategies and methodologies that support growth and new understandings of the human experience (see Fig. 11.6). Nursing knowledge informs

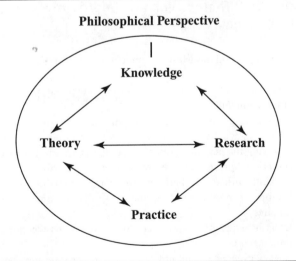

Philosophical Perspective

Knowledge

Theory   **Research**

Practice

Knowledge Development Iterative Process.

practice, is linked to outcomes, and generates new questions that help challenge and refine theory and move science forward. Roy asserts that "growth can occur while building
new insights" and that, in her perspective of, knowledge "veritivity was coined to identify a philosophical assumption that connotes the richness of rootedness in an absolute
truth that leads to values of conviction, commitment, and caring" (Roy, chapter 10, this
volume).

Concluding Thoughts

The exploration of knowledge development using different philosophical perspectives
(knowledge as problem solving and knowledge as process, from a Newman and a poststructuralist feminist approach) offers insights about how nurses think, make decisions,
evaluate care, conduct inquiry to guide care, and take actions that are part of their unique
scope of practice to improve health care for all. Table 11.1 synthesizes the language used
from these perspectives to describe the nursing and patient care.

Although there are some answers provided by this exploration, there are still questions that remain and challenge the evolution of nursing as a science. Table 11.2 provides
a list of some questions that have emerged from this discussion. The questions point to
opportunities for consensus and disciplinary clarity. They suggest directions for future
academic preparation, curriculum development, and research initiatives. They offer areas
for better articulation of nursing science, and ultimately they give voice to the unique perspective offered by nurses in the delivery of safe, efficient, timely, cost-effective, quality
patient care.

Table 11.1	Dominant Themes for an Emerging Focus of the Discipline Across Philosophical Perspectives

- Nursing is a relationship, a connection in partnership to understand the human experience.
- The essence of nursing is moving toward expanding conscious choice and mutual empowerment.
- Nurses solve problems and seek solutions.
- One is engaged in a process of discovery and uncovering personal meaning.
- Knowing the person through dialogue is central to practice.
- Intentional presence and knowledge both drive care.
- Seeking truth and authenticity are practice modalities.
- Promoting comfort and relieving physical, emotional, and spiritual suffering are goals of nursing.
- Creating a healing environment to promote self-reflection and pattern recognition is nursing care.
- Energy exchange, communication, choice, change and transformation are nursing processes.
- Nursing is a mutual, interactive process that has an impact on the nurse and the other.

Table 11.2	Future Questions to Consider in Development of Nursing Knowledge

- Is there agreement around the essence of nursing and the focus of the discipline? Should there be an overarching disciplinary focus? At a philosophical level?
- Is philosophical and theoretical pluralism needed to advance nursing science and knowledge development? Is there consensus around the values, beliefs, and assumptions of nursing?
- Is nursing a science? Is there consensus around the phenomena of concern to the discipline? Do we have the universal language to communicate this phenomena? Is the language of the discipline universal? And global?
- Do current research methodologies adequately address the issues of concern to the discipline and foster knowledge development? Are there new research methodologies that link nursing science and its disciplinary contributions to society?
- Are we committed to philosophical inquiry?
- Have we adequately described the essential/substantive knowledge of the discipline? Is it reflected across the research/education/practice perspectives?
- What role will informatics and the development and use of classification systems play in the development of knowledge and will it be clinically useful?
- Is nursing knowledge visible in practice? Are practice outcomes of care reflected in documentation systems that are nurse sensitive?
- What are the strategies currently used to isolate and research the ethical dilemmas in practice? How are they linked to knowledge development activities?
- How can nursing maintain and extend a disciplinary visibility within an interdisciplinary health care environment?

As we continue to seek disciplinary clarity, we also seek linkages among knowledge, research, and practice to enhance disciplinary visibility. Walker (1997) stated, "We can hope that by articulating our visions for the future and taking thoughtful actions, we can ensure that the vision will become a reality" (pp. 5–6).

REFERENCES

American Nurses Association (2003a). *Nursing's social policy statement* (2nd ed.). Silver Spring, MD: Author.

American Nurses Association (2003b). *Nursing practice information infrastructure.* Retrieved June 30, 2006 from http://www.nursingworld.org/npii/about.htm.

Berry, D. (2004). An emerging model of behavior change in women maintaining weight loss. *Nursing Science Quarterly*, *17*(3), 242–245.

Carey, B. (2005, August 16). In the hospital: A degrading shift from person to patient. *New York Times*, p. A1.

Dochterman, J. M., & Jones, D. (Eds.). (2003). *The unifying of nursing language: The harmonization of NANDA, NIC, and NOC.* Silver Spring, MD: American Nurses Association.

Dochterman, J. M., & Bulechek, G. (Eds.). (2004). *Nursing interventions classification* (4th ed.). St. Louis, MO: Elsiver.

Gordon, M. (1994). *Nursing diagnosis: Process and application.* New York: McGraw-Hill.

Johnson, M., Bulechek, G., Dochterman, J. M., Maas, M., & Moorhead, S. (2001).

Nursing diagnoses, outcomes, interventions: NANDA, NOC and NIC linkages. St. Louis, MO: Mosby Yearbook.

Martin, K. S., & Scheet, N. J. (1992). *The Omaha System: Application for community health nursing.* Philadelphia: Saunders.

Moorhead, S., Johnson, M., & Maas, M. (Eds.). (2004) *Nursing outcomes classification* (3rd ed.). St. Louis, MO: Mosby/Elsiver.

Newman, M. (1994). *Health as expanding consciousness* (2nd Ed.). (Pub. 14-2626). New York: National League for Nursing Press.

Newman, M. (2002). Caring in the human health experience. *International Journal of Human Caring, 6*(2), 8–12.

North American Nursing Diagnosis Association (NANDA) (2004). *Nursing diagnoses: Definitions and classification 2005–2006.* Philadelphia: Author.

Picard, C., & Jones, D. (2005). *Giving voice to what we know: Margaret Newman's theory of health as expanding consciousness in nursing education, practice and research.* Sudbury, MA: Jones and Bartlett.

Radwin, L. (1994). Knowing the patient: An empirically generated process model for individualized interventions. *Dissertation Abstracts International, B55*(01), 79. (University Microfilms No. DA 9414164)

Redfield, J. (1993). *The celestine prophecy: An adventure.* New York: Warner Books.

Reed, P. (1992). An emerging paradigm for the investigation of spirituality. *Research in Nursing and Health, 15,* 349–357.

Rogers, M. E. (1970). *An introduction to the theoretical basis of nursing.* Philadelphia: Davis.

Walker, L. O. (1997). *Challenge of creating impact: Linking knowledge to practice outcomes.* "Knowledge Impact Conference II: 1997 Proceedings." Ed. Roy, C. & Jones, D. Chestnut Hill, MA: Boston College Press.

Part

Integrated Knowledge for Nursing Practice

Introduction

This text explores the paradox that nursing knowledge has entered its greatest growth period and, at the same time, health care systems and care delivery have never been more lacking in meeting society's need for adequate health care. To provide a link to a preferred future where nursing knowledge provides new directions for clinical practice, part III addresses integrated knowledge for nursing practice. Building on discussions of the advances and visions in knowledge development and its philosophical basis, authors of this section derive the key elements of integrated knowledge for nursing practice. The notion of integrated knowledge for nursing has its roots in Carper's (1978) seminal work on identifying four ways of knowing in nursing: the empiric, personal, ethical, and aesthetic.

Through the years, nurse scholars have made attempts to realize the promise of nursing knowledge based on multiple ways of knowing. Notably, Chinn and Kramer (1999) "took a leap into territory that is not yet fully developed or understood" (p. viii). The authors made a commitment to address more fully each of the fundamental patterns of knowing, yet admitted that the development of the four ways of knowing was uneven. They viewed this edition of their book as a "bridge effort" in which they named the ideas and challenged the nursing community to share in the work of what they called integrated knowledge development. The following edition in 2004 had the new title of *Integrated Knowledge Development in Nursing*. Even with the authors' strong commitment and scholarly work over 2 decades, about three-fourths of the text reflects one way of knowing, an empirical approach. Attention to other approaches is given in the last 60 pages and to each, one at a time, in succession.

The current text links the challenge to create a new understanding of integrated knowledge to the important step of demonstrating its effect on the quality of health care. The verb "integrate" and the adjective "integrated" have several meanings (Barnhart & Barnhart, 1983, p. 1096) that can be useful in describing the focus of the chapters in part III and their place in this text. The first meaning of the verb is to make into a whole or to complete, as parts do, for example—various circuits of a computer are integrated to make a unified system. A related meaning is to put or bring together (parts) into a whole, such as a committee will try to integrate the different ideas into one position. In race relations, the common meaning is that to integrate is to make schools, parks, and all public places and facilities available to people of all races on an equal basis. As an adjective, integrated means entire and complete, or a composite, in particular, having all its parts combined into a harmonious whole.

Integrated knowledge for nursing can be described as knowledge that creates a complete, unified, and harmonious whole, representing various perspectives, with the value of meeting the needs of all persons. The authors of this part provide insights about how to achieve integrated knowledge and the authors of the final part offer examples of integrated knowledge for practice.

In chapter 12 Hesook Suzie Kim notes the need for pluralism and our inability to find a way to come to terms with how to deal with that pluralism. The author proposes critical normative epistemology as a framework for nursing knowledge that uses four separate but integrated spheres—human nature, human life, human agency, and practice.

The hope is that the framework can lead to engagement in integrative dialogues that move nursing closer to practice models. Yi-Hui Liu explores moderate realism, as proposed by Kikuchi, in chapter 13, to move discussion beyond competing worldviews that can lead to fragmentation. She proposed that this way of transcending paradigmatic positions can lead to an organized body of integrated knowledge for practice. Hesook Suzie Kim expands her epistemology of nursing in chapter 14 by connecting critical normative epistemology and critical narrative epistemology to explain fours spheres of knowledge within a structure that unifies rather than being merely eclectic. Given the importance of language in expressing integrated knowledge, in chapter 15, Joanne McClosky Dochterman and Dorothy Jones provide an edited version of the creation of a common unifying structure for the languages of the North American Nursing Diagnosis Association (NANDA), the Nursing Intervention Classification (NIC), and the Nursing Outcomes Classification (NOC). In chapter 16, Ruth Palan Lopez uses Roy's perspective of knowledge as a universal cosmic imperative to provide a philosophical foundation that supports multiple theories and research methodologies using the example of exploring of the complex concept of suffering. Finally, Carolyn Padovano extends the notion of integrated knowledge in chapter 17 to the examine how such knowledge is used to develop integrated ethical, educational, practice, and technological systems in nursing to create public policy that leads to integrated health care.

References

Barnhart, C. L., & Barnhart, R. K. (Eds.). (1983). *The world book dictionary*. Chicago: World Book.

Carper, B. A. (1978). Fundamental patterns of knowing in nursing. *Advances in Nursing Science, 1* (1), 13-23.

Chinn, P. L., & Kramer, M. K. (1995). *Theory and nursing: A systematic approach* (5th ed.). St. Louis, MO: Mosby.

Chinn, P.L., & Kramer, M.K. (1999). Theory and nursing: Integrated knowledge development (5th ed.). St. Louis, MO: Mosby.

Chinn, P. L., & Kramer, M. K. (2004). *Integrated knowledge development in nursing* (6th ed.). St. Louis, MO: Mosby.

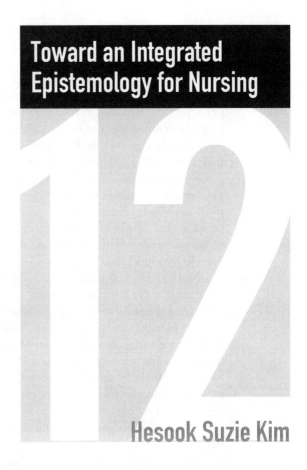

Toward an Integrated Epistemology for Nursing

Hesook Suzie Kim

As we reflect on the path nursing's knowledge development has taken during the past 20 years, we can acknowledge that nursing cannot succeed in its journey to develop a mature system of knowledge by emulating the modes taken either by the natural or the sociobehavioral sciences. However, as suggested at the conclusion of the series on Knowledge Development Symposium at the University of Rhode Island in 1994, nursing is in the throes of pluralism without having come to terms with how to deal with that pluralism. Because of this, it is essential that we come back to the issues of pluralism again and again until we can find ways to make sense of it both for the science and practice of nursing.

Modes of Inquiry and Pluralism

A cursory look at the recent copies of nursing's leading scholarly journals reveals the enduring commitment to the positivistic modes of inquiry, while at the same time suggesting that we are branching out into postmodern philosophies and epistemologic models with newer insights and awakenings. For example, experimental studies that test effects of interventional manipulations are abundant as well as those aimed at testing causal models and causal hypotheses. Specific illustrations include (a) the influence of symptoms, lung function, mood, and social support on level of functioning of patients with chronic obstructive pulmonary disease; (b) children's preoperative coping and its effects on postoperative anxiety and return to normal activity; (c) stress mediation in caregivers of cognitively impaired adults; (d) theoretical model testing; and (e) social support and patterns of adjustment to breast cancer.

Contained within *In Search of Nursing Science* (Omery, Kasper, & Page, 1995) are no less than nine different philosophical orientations identified by the editors as having some relevance to nursing knowledge development. These perspectives include empiricism, pragmatism, paradigmatic historicism, science as problem solving, feminism, phenomenology, hermeneutics, critical theory, and poststructuralism. Their authors' belief is that "a plurality of philosophies may be necessary to reflect the many facets of nursing science—that is, no one view may be sufficient to embrace or drive nursing knowledge in its totality" (p. x).

Nursing's ontological plurality is also evident, for example, when reviewing the program for the National Institute of Nursing Research's 1996 symposium program commemorating its 10 years at the National Institutes of Health. The symposium, "Advancing Health Through Science—The Human Dimension," offered program themes with a wide range of topics from "Translating Basic Science Into Clinical Care" and "Cognitive Impairment: Managing Behavior" to "Cultural Relevance: HIV/AIDS Prevention." Similarly, the nursing literature reveals many different ontological orientations, including, but not limited to, body/mind dualism, holism, cognitivism, cultural determinism, and so forth.

Pluralism is not only evident in nursing (Allen, Benner, & Diekelmann, 1983; Gortner, 1993; Kim, 1996a), but also in most scientific disciplines. Staats (1989) talks of psychology as having developed into fields of study identified as separate entities holding oppositional positions such as "nature versus nurture, situationism versus personality, scientific versus humanistic psychology, with little or no planning with respect to their relationships to the rest of psychology. Good (1994) also identified, for the field of medical anthropology, four different approaches to the anthropological study of illness and health. These include the rationalistic-empiricist tradition, the cognitive orientation, the "meaning-centered" tradition, and critical medical anthropology. Bhaskar (1986) suggests it inevitable that "on the new, integrative-pluralistic world-view which emerges, both nature and the sciences (and the sciences in nature) appear as stratified and differentiated, interconnected and developing" (p. 101).

Pluralism Within Nursing

Pluralism in nursing has resulted from the discipline's exposure to and experience with multiple sets of internal and external forces and events such as

1 The broader contextual forces depicting the 20th century
   • Two world wars.

- Scientific and technological developments.
- New physics and introduction of paradoxes in physical ontology and epistemology.
- Rise and fall of historical materialism (Marxism).
- Realization of the varied nature of human suffering and of multiple modes of social life.
- Realization of inequalities, hierarchies, and conflicts in human life.
- Realization of the limits of human rationality.

2 Various conceptualizations of human ontology—positivistic humans to existential humans to postmodern humans.
3 Changes in philosophy of science—demise of received view (logical positivism), and movement toward scientific realism, pragmatism, and relativism.
4 Various discourses on epistemology—interpretivism, constructivism, and postmodern critiques.
5 Various discourses on the nature of social and human sciences—especially those discourses that tried to differentiate social and human sciences from the natural sciences by
- Stressing the distinction of human phenomena and social life from those of the natural, physical phenomena.
- Specifying different ways of knowing about human conduct emphasizing the hermeneutical requirement for the human sciences from the arguments advanced by Dilthey, Gadamer, Ricouer, and Taylor.
6 Nursing's distancing itself from the medical model—the effort that began as a movement toward establishing nursing as a distinct profession now has come to encompass the antipositivistic stance.
7 Nursing's romanticizing of antiformalism, phenomenology, existentialism, and hermeneutics.

This has occurred as nursing scholars identified themselves with what James (1955) and Philips (1987) referred to as "the tender-minded." The descriptors for the tender minded are rationalistic, intellectualistic, idealistic, free willist, antinaturalistic, antirealist, hermeneutical/interpretative, relativist, qualitative, and epistemologically charitable.

On the contrary, "the tough-minded" are described as empiricist, sensationalist, materialistic, fallibilist, epistemologically uncharitable, and proscientific rationality (Philips, 1987, p. 84).

In addition, nursing's scientific activities are being carried out against an emerging scene of the philosophy of science that contains many new images such as
8 Postpositivistic versions of empiricism and scientific constructivism following the emergence of sophisticated realism and neo-Kantian alternatives (constructivism especially) to traditional empiricism.
- Alternative forms of scientific explanation resulting from the critique of the Hunean notion of causality and the covering-law model of explanation, which emphasizes *underlying* or *generative* mechanisms or heuristics as the bases for scientific explanation.
- Merging of *context of discovery* and *context of confirmation*.
- Acceptance of theory-dependence and theory-ladenness of scientific methodology.

- Nonreductionistic account of special sciences in their relations to physical and natural sciences, emphasizing the autonomy of biological, social, behavioral, and human sciences from physical sciences.
- Pluralism in knowledge as a philosophical position emerging with "the view that reality is multifarious, and that many rival theories can be true of it at the one time" (Phillips, 1987, p. 205).

Nursing's realization that scientism or the positivistic inquiry is limited to address its subject matter satisfactorily began in the 1980s (Meleis, 1991; Thompson, 1985; Watson, 1985). However, this debate continued into the 1990s and created a deep chasm between "the tough-minded" and "the tender-minded" among the scholars, and the discourse continues as though the two camps must be in opposition and an either/or position needs to be firmly established as the epistemological position for nursing. Emden (1991) suggests that there apparently is an increasing cross-camps discourse that may bring about a deeper understanding about what kinds of contributions the different types of inquiry make for the development of nursing knowledge. However, such discourse may not be enough without a unifying framework for epistemological discussions about nursing knowledge.

Images of Pluralism

We can conjure up two images of pluralism. One is described by Claxton and his colleagues as "We are like the inhabitants of thousands of little islands, all in the same part of the ocean, yet totally out of touch with each other" (Claxton, 1980, p. 15). Each has evolved a different culture, different ways of doing things, different languages to talk about what they do. Occasionally inhabitants of one island may spot their neighbors "walking up and down and issuing strange cries; but it makes no sense, so they ignore it" (p. 15).

Another image is that of a jigsaw puzzle that has been partitioned into pieces not randomly but around separate images. Although each piece depicts a specific part of the whole puzzle image, it would not make much sense if it is not put together with the rest of the puzzle. This image accepts the idea of what Good (1994) called, "heteroglossiac" (p. 62) as the matter of necessity, but the unification as a way of putting pieces together or constructing a net without tangles.

From this background, then, I propose a specific epistemology for nursing—critical normative epistemology—as a way of comprehending our knowledge both for knowledge development and for practice. This is based on aligning with the sentiment expressed by Good for medical anthropology that

disease and human suffering cannot be comprehended from a single perspective. Science and its objects, the demands of therapeutic practice, and personal and social threats of illness cannot be comprehended from a unified or singular perspective. A multiplicity of tongues is needed to engage the objects of our discipline and to fashion an anthropological, scientific, political, moral, aesthetic or philosophical response. (p. 62)

In addition, the position also reflects Bhaskar's idea that

any social science must incorporate a historically situated hermeneutics; while the condition that the social sciences are part of their own field of inquiry means that they must be self-reflexive, critical and totalizing in a way in which the natural sciences typically are not. But there is neither antimony nor unbridgeable chasm, nor the possibility of mutual exclusion between the sciences of nature and of (wo)man. (p. 101)

This discussion is an extension and elaboration of the ideas proposed in earlier writings (Kim, 1996a). What I am proposing certainly goes against those nursing scholars who insist on the necessity of a paradigm shift for nursing (for example, Plyle, 1995), as I believe that a one-dimensional view of nursing phenomena is certainly limiting in providing the knowledge for practice.

A Unifying Epistemology for Nursing

This position begins with the central concern for nursing: Human living centering on health, with implicit connections to disease, illness, sickness, disability, and dying. Second, nursing is a human practice discipline in which a social mandate is a necessary part. I emphasize *living* here in order to take issue with terms such as *human experiences* and *human responses* that are most commonly used in nursing as the focus of attention. I believe *human living* more fully expresses the central concern for nursing by emphasizing our everyday living with health/illness and in health/illness, while encompassing both *experiences* and *responses* but including the *living* of oneself, with others, and in situations.

Unavoidably, human living connected to health must be concerned with the empirical aspects of human nature, but at the same time it is necessarily tied to what Good (1994) refers to as the conscious, subjective, experiencing self. At the same time, nursing, in dealing with human living in this sense, must approach its work as a human engagement that is oriented to helping people with their living in the context of health. Under these considerations, then, the epistemology for nursing requires the following premises:

1 Human features, that is, states, conditions, experiences, processes, actions, and so forth, encompass both the empirical and the interpreted in an a priori sense pointing to an ontology that must address the complexity of human nature and of human living. Hence, there are aspects among the nursing's epistemic concerns that are knowable objectively and that are knowable only through subjective revelations and interpretations.

2 The reality, or the essence of reality, must be considered to exist prior to any science but is contextually (historically and socially) situated specifically to human agents who engage in producing knowledge (science) within any given hermeneutically

constrained horizon. Human practice requires mutuality that upholds emancipation of involved human agents. Human agents engaged in practice, both clients and practitioners must coordinate their freedom, meanings, and desires as a means of gaining emancipation and mutuality. Nursing work is founded on a normative, moral, and aesthetic grounding that is formulated through historical, social, and personal processes that go beyond the way scientific knowledge is produced. Nursing knowledge, thus, is oriented to developing understandings, explanations, and prescriptions rooted in the moral grounding and value orientations for ethical and aesthetic practice.

Given these premises for the critically normative epistemology for nursing as a human practice science, we are allowed to think about our knowledge development from four separate but integrated ontologies.

1 *Ontology of human nature* directs our attention to developing knowledge regarding human processes associated with health and nursing practice from the empirical and natural perspective. Under this ontology, human nature is considered in terms of humans' species-specific and group-specific features, characteristics, and aspects, such as the human phylogenetics.

2 *Ontology of human life* points to knowledge development for understanding human life in relation to how it is experienced, interpreted, and managed from the totality of the living self, the individual that is conscious, meaning-making, and reflexive all at once.

3 *Ontology of human agency* that directs us to develop knowledge about how clients' and nurses' coordinated engagement characterized by mutuality and emancipation could be achieved.

4 *Ontology of practice* that points to knowledge development associated with the moral (that is, goodness), ethical, and aesthetic grounding of nursing work.

This discussion of the premises and ontologies points to an epistemological framework for nursing that is organized into four specific knowledge spheres for nursing. The formulation can be thought of as an extension of Habermas's formulation of three aspects of human cognitive interests—the technical, practical, and emancipatory interests. Hence, this critically non-naïve epistemological framework for nursing encompasses the empirical sphere with a focus on developing generalizable knowledge regarding human processes, mechanisms, conditions, changes, and experiences. Further, the interpretive sphere has a focus on providing understanding, illuminations, and appreciation regarding human life as it is lived in a subjective, meaning-making, and contextually bound fashion. Third, the critical sphere develops knowledge as to how sensibility, emancipation, mutuality, and coordinated human living and practice can be achieved. Finally, the ethical/aesthetic sphere focuses on developing knowledge about the nature and processes of nursing's moral and value orientations and their development—that is, the ethics and aesthetics of practice. Such an integrative differentiation suggests that this epistemological framework enables us to integrate, make connections, and coordinate knowledge bits that are produced from various perspectives.

The Empirical Sphere of Nursing Knowledge

The empirical sphere of nursing knowledge may lead to the adaptation of various scientific methods in order to discover, identify, and develop generalizable theories (certainly in different levels of scope, depending on the problem and context), universalizing principles, or explanations. In nursing, there are many different paradigmatic orientations in developing such knowledge, including, but not limited to, the biobehavioral, holistic, systems, functional, and cognitive perspectives.

In addition, to generate knowledge in this sphere, one is not limited to the so-called quantitative methods but any empirical method that is oriented to discovering or developing general theories and explanations may be selected to produce such knowledge. Nursing knowledge in the empirical sphere provides the general foundations for thinking about and considering practice issues from the class-membership perspective. With its orientation toward objective validation and generation, such knowledge provides the grounds for identifying patterns, regularities, and tendencies that can be used to frame individual client's problems and experiences or the issues in nursing practice as a case in point. Thus, this sphere encompasses the knowledge regarding phenomena in the client, client–nurse, practice, and environment domains.

The Interpretive Sphere of Nursing Knowledge

Nursing knowledge development in the interpretive sphere focuses on humans' subjective experiencing, living selves in the context of everyday life and of practice. This sphere addresses nursing understanding from two directions. First, it focuses on ways that individuals make meanings and interpret their subjective experiences and how such meaning-makings and interpretations frame people's living in and with health/illness as well as nurse's practice. Second, it aims to reveal and arrive at theoretical understandings about how humans' hermeneuticity affect client–nurse engagement and nurses' practice. Various theoretical perspectives and methodological approaches are appropriate for the development of nursing knowledge in this sphere. Today, we are witnessing a growing number of works applying phenomenological hermeneutic, narrative, dialectic, and other interpretive methods as strategies to understand the human experience. It is hoped that results from these studies would thus be comparative, contrastive, and comprehensive understandings about the different and similar ways people, both clients and nurses, make meanings and coordinate those meanings with other interpretations in the context of nursing practice.

The Critical Sphere of Nursing Knowledge

The critical sphere of nursing knowledge development refers to the inclusion of knowledge necessary to bring about sensibility, mutuality, emancipation, and coordination for clients, nurses, and client–nurse engagement. The assumption is that health care situations and the context of nursing practice, as well as general life situations, are imbued with the possibility of "false consciousness," domination, and distortions. Hence, it is necessary to develop knowledge about such phenomena (a) in the context of clients who are ill and (b) in nursing practice.

Knowledge in the critical sphere also addresses the processes through which people can be emancipated from selves, others, and in situations. Thus, nursing knowledge needs to address such issues as how therapeutic alliances between clients and their significant others or between nurses and clients, can become established, or how nurses can become emancipated from their biases that can constrain clients' self-actualization. Various critical methods such as critical hermeneutics, critical ethnography, critical action research, discourse analysis, and critical phenomenology are applicable, and various perspectives ranging from feminism, the critical theory of Habermas, postmodernism of Foucault, Derrida, and Friere can be taken to develop nursing knowledge in this sphere.

The Ethical/Aesthetic Sphere of Nursing Knowledge

The ethical/aesthetic sphere of nursing knowledge development uses not only the general and specific normative standards of nursing practice but also values orientations associated with moral, ethical, and aesthetic practice. It provides the grounding for making connections between what is known and what must be done or is desirable to be done in nursing practice. Nurses must come to know what is desirable, beneficial, and creative in their practice. Thus, the knowledge development necessary for this sphere addresses what the nature of ethical/aesthetic frameworks for practice are; how they get established, generated, or changed; and their relationships to the larger culture and contexts. Philosophic analysis, dialectic analysis, historiography, and discourse analysis are examples of methods that can be used to generate knowledge for this sphere.

An Integrated Framework

This epistemological framework for nursing suggests that nursing is neither simply an empirical nor an interpretive science. It is a science that must be integrated from the four epistemological spheres, unique as a human practice science. What separates nursing knowledge from other human practice sciences must come from the substantive content that is placed within each sphere of knowledge as unique to nursing's epistemological concerns. Nursing practice requires a comprehensive knowledge base from all four spheres since each practice situation must be considered to encompass issues associated with four different orientations.

In confronting a situation or issue within clinical practice, the nurse must be able to draw knowledge from all spheres. This then means that the ultimate synthesizer of knowledge and its uses in practice must be the nurse. The nurse must be able to realize the critical aspects of her/his client and of one's own practice by dissecting each strata to view the clinical situation from one lens. At the same time, there must be layering of the multiple strata, bringing together the various perspectives and drawing from different spheres of knowledge and understanding to resolve issues and foster "human living." Nurses in practice have to be the final and ultimate synthesizers of knowledge. Because of this, nurses can contribute to producing knowledge by providing descriptions of synthesized information that inform the development of new practice models.

Conclusion

There is a danger, of course, in seeing such a framework as fragmenting nursing knowledge, a possible criticism from some holists. However, my belief is that nursing's subject matter cannot be comprehended or addressed from a unified, singular perspective both for the benefit of practice and for the advancement of nursing knowledge. The multifaceted nature of what we must address has to be integrated in this kind of framework so that we are not just shouting to each other without listening to other voices but engaging in integrative dialogues. The end products of such dialogue will move closer to practice models that can be readily translated into practice and make it easier for nurses' synthesizing burden.

The three perspectives addressed in this text reflect this proposed sentiment, and we should be able to discuss how knowledge as problem solving, as process, and as universal cosmic imperative are three different ways of viewing knowledge development for nursing, and how they can complement and coordinate with each other.

REFERENCES

Allen, D., Benner, P., & Diekelmann, N. L. (1983). Three paradigms for nursing research: Methodological implications. In P. Chinn (Ed.), *Nursing research methodology* (pp. 23–38). Washington, DC: Aspen Systems.

Bhaskar, R. (1986). *Scientific realism and human emancipation.* London: Verso.

Chinn, P. L., & Kramer, M. K. (1999). Theory and nursing: Integrated knowledge development (5th ed.). St. Louis, MO: Mosby.

Claxton, G. (1980). *Cognitive psychology.* London: Routledge.

Emden, C. (1991). Ways of knowing in nursing. In G. Gray & R. Pran (Eds.), *Towards a discipline of nursing* (pp. 11–30). Melbourne, Australia: Churchill Livingstone.

Good, S. J. (1994). *Medicine, rationality, and experience: An anthropological perspective.* Cambridge, UK: Cambridge University Press.

Gortner, S. R. (1993). Nursing's syntax revisited: A critique of philosophies said to influence nursing theories. *International Journal of Nursing Studies, 30,* 477–488.

James, W. (1955). *Pragmatism, and four essays from the meaning of truth.* New York: Meridian.

Kim, H. S. (1996a). Pluralism: Viable options for applying theory to practice. In *Invited papers of the 4th & 5th symposium for the knowledge development series: Building a cumulative knowledge base for nursing: From fragmentation to congruence of philosophy, theory, methods of inquiry and practice* (pp. 150–20). Kingston: University of Rhode Island College of Nursing.

Kim, H. S. (1996b). Nursing epistemology as a human practice science. In T. Bjerkreim, J. Mathisen, & R. Nord (Eds.), *Vision, viten, og virke* [Vision, knowledge and impact: (pp. 36–45)]. Oslo, Norway: Universitetsforlager AS.

Meleis, A. I. (1991). *Theoretical nursing: Development and progress* (2nd ed.). New York: Lippincott.

Omery, A., Kasper, C. E., & Page, G. G. (Eds.). (1995). *In search of nursing science.* Thousand Oaks, CA: Sage.

Philips, D. C. (1987). *Philosophy, science, and social inquiry: Contemporary methodological controversies in social science and related applied fields of research.* Oxford, UK: Butterworth-Heinemann.

Plyle, J. (1995). Humanism and positivism in nursing: Contradictions and conflicts. *Journal of Advanced Nursing, 22,* 979–984.

Staats, A. W. (1989). Unification: Philosophy for the modern disunified science of psychology. *Philosophical Psychology, 2,* 143–164.

Thompson, J. L. (1985). Practical discourse in nursing: Going beyond empiricism and historicism. *Advances in Nursing Science, 7,* 59–71.

Watson, J. (1985). Reflections on different methodologies for the future of nursing. In M. Leininger (Ed.), *Qualitative research methods in nursing* (pp. 343–349). New York: Grune & Stratton.

Moderate Realism as an Approach to Integrated Knowledge for Practice

13

Yi-Hui Liu

The development of knowledge as analyzed in this text reflects that nurse scholars have, for several decades, recognized that the questions "What is nursing?" and "How does nursing knowledge develop?" had to be answered if nursing was to become a discipline, a profession, and a science in its own right. Nurse scholars and theorists have continually sought answers to these questions within epistemology and the philosophical, conceptual, and theoretical perspectives of nursing. Kikuchi (2003), for example, identified several of these approaches. The author noted that Reed suggested that nursing adopt neomodernism. Wainwright proposed realism as a radically different paradigm, and Letourneau and Allen maintained that nursing knowledge stems from positivism. Each of these scholars recommended the adoption of worldviews that could lead to the development of the kind of nursing knowledge needed for nursing practice. Kikuchi believed that as long as nursing persisted in embracing the idea of worldviews as the bases of conceptions of nursing, nursing knowledge would be fragmented because of a plurality of conceptualisms of nursing. The author proposed that a philosophy of moderate realism could provide grounding for conceptions of nursing and nursing inquiry, while avoiding the idea of worldviews. This chapter explores moderate realism as an approach to developing integrated knowledge that is relevant for nursing practice.

Philosophy of Moderate Realism

Using worldviews is the initial point of inquiry when answering questions about knowledge in the discipline, and more particularly, knowledge for nursing practice, is commonplace. Leddy (2000) highlighted the fragmented state of nursing knowledge. The author proposed that we see worldviews as complementary in nature, theorizing that the present undesirable fragmentation of nursing knowledge is the result of viewing different perspectives as competitive. Kikuchi (2003) agrees with Leddy's belief about the fragmentation of nursing knowledge but disagrees with Leddy's solution and instead proposed exploring moderate realism.

Historical Background

Moderate realism reflects a more recent philosophical influence on nursing as compared with other philosophical perspectives used to guide theory development. Similar to other philosophies, moderate realism is influenced by the Greek philosophers. In particular, moderate realism is a form of realism in the Aristotelian sense of lying between extremes. That philosophy is one of the theories proposed as a solution to one of the most important perennial questions in philosophy—the problem of universals. The issue relates to the nature of knowledge—that is, how we know discrete things, as well as classes of things. This approach to resolving problems was a favorite topic for discussion in ancient times and again in the Middle Ages. Modern and contemporary philosophers continue to address the basic question of how we know universals and particulars.

Plato and the Idea

Among Greek philosophers, the issue was to reconcile the one and the many, the changing and the permanent, which leads to the problem of universals. Influenced by Socrates' thought, Plato provided the perspective that a concept represents all of the reality of a thing. Plato thought that if this was the case, then the reality must be something in the ideal order, not necessarily in things themselves, but rather above them, in a world by itself. For example, Plato substituted the *idea* for the concept.

The idea was viewed by Plato as absolutely stable and existed by itself isolated from the phenomenal world and distinct from the divine and from the human intellect. Following logically from the directive principles of his realism, Plato made idea an entity that corresponded to each of our abstract representations. This view was true not only for natural species but also for artificial products, not only for substances but also for properties and relations. Even negations and nothingness he proposed have a corresponding idea in the suprasensible world. "What makes one and one two is a participation of the dyad, and what makes one is a participation of monad in unity" (Plato, trans. 1999, p. lxix). The principal doctrine of Plato's metaphysics is the realism that invests the real being with the attributes of the being in thought (Mertz, 1998).

Aristotle and Moderate Realism

Aristotle formulated the main doctrine of moderate realism. Different from Plato's definition of philosophy as the science of *idea*, Aristotle defines philosophy as the science of
the *universal essence* of that which is actual. The real is not, as Plato says, some obscure
entity of which the sensible world is only the shadow. It lives in the midst of the sensible
world. Individual substance has reality alone and can exist alone. The universal is not a
thing in itself. It is immanent in individuals and is multiplied in all the representatives of
a class. As to the form of universality of our concepts, form is a product of our subjective
consideration. The objects of our generic and specific representations can certainly be
called substances, when they point out the fundamental reality with accidental deter-
minations. However, the objects of such representations are second substances. By this
Aristotle means precisely that this attribute of universality that affects the substance as
thought does not belong to the substance. It is the outcome of our subjective elaboration.
In this way this basic theorem of Aristotle is the antithesis of Plato's view of the idea
(Mertz, 1998).

Analysis by Porphyry

The Roman philosopher Porphyry (trans. 2003) divides the problem of knowing into
three parts:

1 Do genera and species exist in nature, or do they consist in mere products of the
   intellect?
2 If they are things apart from the mind, are they corporeal or incorporeal things?
3 Do they exist outside the (individual) things of sense, or are they realized in the
   latter?

These questions highlighted the philosophical issue of how the human mind can
know individual things as well as the classes of things.

Methaphysics in the Middle Ages

The metaphysical question of knowing the particular and the universal continued to
be debated in the Middle Ages. The discussion was focused on the elements of human
knowledge—that is, on ideas. Ideas as discussed during this period were seen as universal
and realities viewed as representations in our mind and represented there in a universal
manner. The question then was not only about the metaphysics of the individual and of
the universal. It also raises important questions in ideology, questions about the genesis
and validity of knowledge. In the Middle Ages, there were four possible doctrines about
universals and only one doctrine could be correct and true. It took the thinkers of the
13th century to establish the true doctrine—that is, Moderate Realism—to solve the
problem of universals ("Nominalism, Realism, Conceptualism," n.d.; "The perfecting
of philosophy in medieval times," n.d.).

Moderate Realism and the Mind

Moderate realism asserts that outside the mind only individual things exist. There is
no universal essence in the world of creatures. The mind, in forming its universal ideas,

does not have an inner drive to think in categories separate from the things it sees. Nor does it merely apply names to groups of similar things. The mind is able to see a plurality of things as one. The mind knows things really, according to the reality that is their essence, and the mind knows in a mode or manner that is its own. The mind's mode of knowing is the mode called universality. Hence, the universality of our ideas is in the mind and from the mind. It is based on reality because the essence that the mind knows universally is actually verified individually in each and every thing that has that essence (Mertz, 1998).

Contemporary Moderate Realism

Moderate realism today claims that reality consists of beings that are not only material in substance, nor only immaterial in substance, but are both material and immaterial in substance but in different respects. This perspective claims that people cannot attain complete knowledge of reality, given our human limitations, but we can know reality as it exists independent of the individual mind. Moderate realists believe that this is "a common-sense philosophy which attains its principles by reflecting on common-sense knowledge and reasoning there from in light of available evidence" (Kikuchi & Simmons, 1999, p. 44). Commonsense knowledge is described as judgments arising from our common sense that includes knowledge formulated from past experience, mere opinion, probable truths, and absolute truths. According to moderate realism, the object of inquiry is to attain knowledge of reality consisting of probable truths rather than of absolute truths, that is, opinion with evidence and/or reason to support it beyond a reasonable doubt.

Thus, moderate realism maintains that philosophy can attain probable truths about what exists and what happens in the world. The probable truths are attained by comparing our descriptive judgments against reality as it exists, independent of the individual mind and determining where the weight of the evidence falls. The truth about what we ought to do and to seek in human life is attained by comparing our prescriptive judgment against right desire. This view is proposed as the self-evident truth that we ought to want and seek that which is really good for us (Adler, 1990; Kikuchi & Simmons, 1999).

Contemporary moderate realism also holds that all human beings possess the same cognitive powers, material sensory powers, and immaterial intellectual powers. The degree of these powers is dependent on the circumstances under which each of us lives and is nurtured. The cognitive process is complex. Simply stated, it emerges from our sensory powers upon sensing object A, then a perception of object A is formed by our power of perception, in concert with our powers of memory and imagination. From the percept of object A, our power of conceptualization abstracts the concept of A. Thus, from this perspective we can say that concepts are attained by a grounding in reality—that is, they are empirically derived. We have only an understanding or conception of A by which we come to have knowledge of object A by the act of conceptualizing and assigning meaning. It is when we engage in the act of judging and make a claim about object A that we are operating at the level of knowledge. Engaging in the act of reasoning allows us to attain knowledge of object A (Adler, 1990; Wallace, 1983).

Moderate realism holds that reality exists outside and independent of the mind and that reality is knowable. However, the way in which we view things as they exist in reality is influenced by the different circumstances under which each of us lives and is nurtured. Objective reality with natural forms, boundaries, and orders, against which the truth of propositions can be tested, makes it possible to attain knowledge in the form of probable truth about reality. That is, we can compare our different views about something against an objective standard and through discussion, determine where the weight of the available evidence and reasons rests to ascertain objectively the probable truth of a matter under question.

Linking Moderate Realism to Knowledge for Practice

By standing in a position grounded in the moderate realist view of reality, Kikuchi (2003) argued that the aim of nursing as a discipline was to develop an organized body of knowledge for nursing practice that could be realized. She proposed that the starting point of this knowledge development must be as follows: reality exists in a way that is independent of the individual mind and is knowable—a starting point that is opposite to the idea of worldviews that says that reality exists as constructed by the mind. If conceptions of nursing are grounded in the idea of worldviews as has been the case in the past, we will continue to have a plurality of conceptions of nursing. Kikuchi pointed out that although a diversity of nursing views is essential for the healthy development of the discipline, the diversity of views that occur under the idea of worldviews presents several problems. In moderate realists' views, there is no need for, nor is there a place for, the idea of worldviews of reality preexisting our knowledge of it.

Applying Moderate Realism to Practical Knowledge

Moderate realists also hold that objects of thought enable us to attain knowledge, but they are not the objects of knowledge. The objects of knowledge are things as they exist in reality independent of our mind. Under moderate realism, the conduct of inquiry as a public enterprise is realizable, making possible the development of an organized body of knowledge by a discipline. In this way, all members of a discipline can work cooperatively when inquiry is conducted as a public enterprise (Adler, 1965, 1990; Kikuchi & Simmons, 1999). One example of how such knowledge is developed is in the naming and defining of a nursing diagnosis included in the nomenclature and classification of nursing diagnoses published by the North American Nursing Diagnosis Association (2004).

Maritain (1959, 1979) makes distinctions within moderate realism that are useful in exploring knowledge for nursing practice. The philosopher distinguishes between theoretical or speculative philosophy and practical philosophy. In speculative philosophy, knowledge is sought for the sake of knowing alone. In practical philosophy, knowledge is sought for the sake of acting or making. More specifically, in practical philosophy, human acting or the ultimate good of humankind is the concern of ethics or moral philosophy, and human making or a particular human good is the concern of the philosophy of art. Both branches of practical philosophy, ethics and the philosophy of art, consist of principles that are abstract and universal in nature. Maritain identifies these principles as speculatively practical in nature.

Clinical Judgment

The reasoning process reflects the application of practical principles and entails reasoning from the level of principles, to rules, to a decision in the particular case, according to Maritain. As one moves through the levels of reasoning, one takes into consideration increasing contingencies in order to arrive at a judgment that is principle based and also contextual and individual in nature (Kikuchi & Simmons, 1999; Maritain, 1959, 1979). Moderate realism can help the nurse to make the decisions that are principle based as well as contextual and individual in nature. An organized body of nursing knowledge provides nurses with principles for clinical judgment. In reasoning from principles to rules to the nurses' decision, nurses take into consideration the contextual circumstances of the situation in which they make their decisions. They recognize that context may shape the way the problem is manifested and therefore affect their clinical judgment.

Three key canons of moderate realism are applicable to such clinical judgment. The first is that which is good for us, meets our needs rather than our wants. The second is that despite an individual's experience and background, an objective view of reality is probably true. Last, we judge our personal views against reality using our natural powers to conceptualize and make judgments, basing our decisions on available reasoning and evidence, that is, our knowledge (Kikuchi, 2003; Kikuchi & Simmons, 1999).

A clinical example can be used to explain the movement from principle to rule to decision. The nursing goal is to maintain or promote the health of the patient. According to this goal, maintaining adequate oxygen saturation is the essential principle behind the goal. Based on this principle, nurses will draw upon knowledge about how to maintain oxygenation. From multiple ways of knowing, including theories and research, nurses develop a general rule: the first priority is to ensure a clear airway for the patient. The next step of decision making involves considering the immediate clinical situation and deciding what specific interventions to use to bring about the goal. In a given situation, the nurse may remove secretions by suctioning or may facilitate secretion flow by encouraging deep breathing.

Ethical and Cultural Implications

The underpinnings of moderate realism have the potential to help us understand the complexities of decision making by nurses and the moral/ethical dilemmas they face in the process. Further, this philosophical perspective can provide guidance in the moral issues among diverse cultures. The moderate realism conception of justice supports the thesis that "nurses must consider both perspectives (those subjective principles of both the nurse and the client) in light of objectively true principles related to the pursuit of happiness by human beings and must ground their nursing decisions in those principles" (Kikuchi & Simmons, 1999, p. 46). The objective principles of justice central to moderate realism are the following:

- Natural needs refer to those things in life we need rather than want and that are naturally good for us.
- Real goods are those goods that fill our needs rather than our wants.

■ Natural rights are those rights that we have by virtue of our humanness, rather than a legal right.

■ Duties or moral obligations require us to act in a just and fair manner to ourselves and to others as we aspire to that which is good rather than evil or unjust.

In order to make just decisions, knowledge of what is good for all humans is necessary, as well as knowledge of what natural rights and moral obligations we consider to be necessary (Kikuchi & Simmons, 1999).

In addition this approach to ethical reasoning can also provide a way to reach a solution for the dilemmas resulting from cultural diversity. Multiculturalists aim to respect the patient's cultural values and beliefs and not make any judgments about them. In the process, they tend to deny the existence of a specific common human nature, or what Roy (chapter 10, this volume) called "the common purposefulness of humankind." They assert that diversity is an absolute necessity of human behavior. Multiculturalists point out that the differences from culture to culture are language, eating utensils, health, religious practices, and so on. Following Hume, they also assert that moral or "ought" statements do not fall within the realm of objective truth in that there is no empirical way to establish the truth of "ought" statements. In denying the existence of a specific common human nature, proponents of multicultural ethics logically must deny the existence of unchanging common natural human needs (Kikuchi, Simmons, & Romyn, 1996, p. 160).

Under multicultural ethics, members of a culture decide what is good to do and seek what constitutes a good quality of life for members of that particular culture. However, dilemmas arise when the presuppositions and suppositions of multicultural ethics underlie orders that leave nurses unable to act responsibly as nurses (Kikuchi et al., 1996). In particular, when acting according to a cultural belief contradicts the ultimate good of humankind, as described in Maritain's practical philosophy noted above, then the nurse faces a dilemma.

Kikuchi (1996) brings up an alternative ethical basis for practice, a transcultural ethics grounded in moderate realism. This approach can provide a solution to many dilemmas because a transcultural ethics has principles that allow for responsible practice. Proponents of transcultural ethics agree with the proponents of multicultural ethics that human behavior varies widely. They assert that a specific common human nature underlies the observed diversity of human behavior, making such diversity possible. This common human nature is thought to consist of natural capacities or powers, by virtue of which humans have and can meet certain natural needs. Kikuchi noted that proponents of transcultural ethics agree with Hume's view. However, they also assert that "ought" statements can be derived from "is" statements with the use of the self-evident "ought" statement identified by Aristotle as the first principle of moral philosophy: "We ought to desire whatever is really good for us and nothing else" (p. 162).

In embracing transcultural ethics, nurses would know that judgments of good and bad and of right and wrong are inappropriate in multicultural matters—matters of taste, and that they are appropriate in transcultural matters—matters of truth. Therefore, under transcultural ethics, it would become appropriate for nurse researchers to pursue universal objective moral nursing truths and practice standards to guide nurses in their work (Kikuchi et al., 1996).

Clinical Research

Moderate realism provides a guideline to help develop an organized body of nursing knowledge through clinical research. If we take the position that reality is mind-dependent, all the truths we know and the universe we perceive are not objective but subjective. With this approach, building knowledge for a practice discipline is stymied. Quite the opposite, moderate realists acknowledge that if new evidence and better reasoning shows that propositions previously accepted as probably true to be really false, they are then rejected and new truths are sought that cohere internally and externally with those already established as probably true. Through this process, we would be seeking a better grasp of the truth in every pursuit of knowledge. Nursing inquiry would be dynamic in nature (Kikuchi, 2003).

Kikuchi (2003) points out that

> by grounding conceptions of nursing in moderate realism, we can work cooperatively and progressively to attain a common conception of the nature of nursing and of nursing knowledge with probable truth upon which we can confidently base our research studies and development of our disciplinary knowledge. (p. 14)

According to moderate realism, all members of the nursing discipline can work together as a community of scholars to develop a common conception of nursing. This could be accomplished by examining and discussing the soundness and adequacy of various conceptions of the nature of nursing and of nursing knowledge. The search for such a conception could be conducted as a public enterprise. Under a common conception of nursing and nursing knowledge, an organized body of nursing knowledge for practice can develop. Knowledge development results from an ongoing progressive approach based on a sound philosophical stance (Kikuchi, 2003).

Conclusion

Nurse scholars have put forth one worldview or paradigm after another in order to provide a basis for developing knowledge for practice in nursing. The position of moderate realism offers an alternative beyond worldviews, either multiple or individual. Some may say that moderate realism is just another worldview. Kikuchi (2003) defends moderate realism as follows. First, she noted that the idea of worldviews and worldviews themselves have arisen from and are dependent on the notion that reality conforms to the mind. Secondly, she pointed out that moderate realism holds the opposite to be the case—the mind conforms to reality. Whether we know it or not, the philosophy of moderate realism is operative in our daily lives and is present within nursing practice. We can possess knowledge of reality as it exists independent of our individual minds. When we are in doubt about what it is we perceive, we can use our powers of reasoning and discussion to help us reconcile the matter. Knowledge for the future of nursing can be grounded in the philosophy of moderate realism, and nurses will be able to develop an organized body of nursing knowledge for nursing practice.

REFERENCES

Adler, M. J. (1965). *The conditions of philosophy: Its checkered past, its present disorder, and its future promise.* New York: Atheneum.

Adler, M. J. (1990). *Intellect: Mind over matter.* New York: Macmillan.

Kikuchi, J. F. (2003). Nursing knowledge and the problem of worldviews. *Research and Theory for Nursing Practice: An International Journal, 17*(1), 7–17.

Kikuchi, J. F., & Simmons, H. (1999). Practical nursing judgment: A moderate realist conception. *Scholarly Inquiry for Nursing Practice: An International Journal, 13*(1), 43–55.

Kikuchi, J. F., Simmons, H., & Romyn, D. (Eds.). (1996). *Truth in nursing inquiry.* Thousand Oaks, CA: Sage.

Leddy, S. K. (2000). Toward a complementary perspective on worldviews. *Nursing Science Quarterly, 13*, 225–233.

Maritain, J. (1959). *The degrees of knowledge* (G. B. Phelan, Trans.). New York: Scribner's.

Maritain, J. (1979). *An introduction to philosophy.* London: Sheed & Ward.

Mertz, D. W. (1998). *Moderate realism and its logic.* New Haven, CT: Yale University Press.

Nominalism, realism, conceptualism. (n.d.). Retrieved November 17, 2004, from Catholic Encyclopedia Online, http://www.newadvent.org/cathen/11090c.htm.

North American Nursing Diagnosis Association. (2004). *Nursing diagnoses: Definitions and classification 2003–2004.* Philadelphia: Author.

The perfecting of philosophy in medieval times. (n.d.). Retrieved November 17, 2004, from The Radical Academy, http://radicalacademy.com/adiphilperfecting1.htm.

Plato. (1999). *Phaedo* (D. Gallop, Trans.). Oxford, UK: Oxford University Press. (Original work, n.d.)

Porphyry introduction (J. Barnes, Trans.), 2003. Oxford, UK: Oxford University Press. (Original work, n.d.)

Wallace, W. A. (1983). *From a realist point of view. Essays on the philosophy of science* (2nd ed.). Lanham, MD: University Press of America.

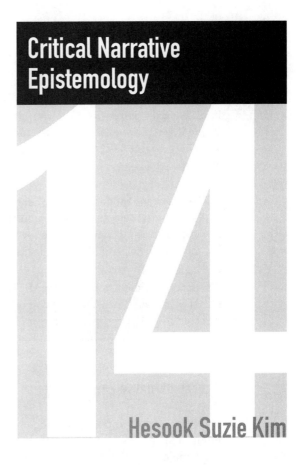

Critical Narrative Epistemology

Hesook Suzie Kim

I n this articulation of critical narrative epistemology I have expanded my perspective regarding nursing epistemology one step further. I began serious thinking regarding the notion of nursing epistemology in the context of pluralism in the mid-1990s. As noted in chapter 12, pluralism had become the position from which we were dealing with knowledge development in nursing. It was the subject of interest for philosophical dialogues that occurred at the University of Rhode Island's Knowledge Development Conferences from 1990 to 1994 and was well reflected in the nursing literature. My initial thoughts were presented at the first Boston College Knowledge Development conference in 1996 and were edited for chapter 12. There I state my notion of nursing epistemology as undergirded by critical normative epistemology. This continues to be the philosophical stance with which I view nursing knowledge and its development. My ideas regarding nursing epistemology have gone through several generations of development during recent years and have culminated into the current proposal. Here, through the model of nursing epistemology, I make a connection between critical normative epistemology and critical narrative epistemology.

Background

There is one premise that is critical to my thinking on nursing knowledge and its development. My key premise is that pluralism must be embraced as a necessary approach to knowledge development. However, pluralism must be organized into a system of unification if we do not wish to remain stuck in "eclecticism" rather than a true pluralism. As I noted in chapter 12, this is in the spirit of Good (1994) who stated regarding medical anthropology,

> Disease and human suffering cannot be comprehended from a single perspective. Science and its objects, the demands of therapeutic practice, and personal and social threats of illness cannot be comprehended from a unified or singular perspective. A multiplicity of tongues is needed to engage the objects of our discipline. (p. 62)

The same sentiment was expressed by Bhaskar (1986). This stance addresses the cognitive needs of nursing as a discipline. Today, nursing requires a knowledge system that is directed toward a comprehensive understanding of its subject matter and that points to different sorts of knowledge required for nursing practice.

Critical Normative Epistemology

To elaborate on this position, I begin with critical normative epistemology as the starting point. This philosophy is an integrated view combining critical realism, emancipatory epistemology, and a normative perspective of human practice. The critical realism of Bhaskar (1986) provides a beginning point for this epistemology. As noted in chapter 12, Bhaskar proposed critical realism for social sciences emphasizing the incorporation with situated hermeneutics, noting the reality that the social sciences are part of their own field of inquiry. This position means that the social sciences must be self-reflexive, critical, and totalizing. This approach is contrary to what is typical of the natural sciences. Bhaskar feels that the chasm between the natural and human sciences can be bridged.

Emancipatory Epistemology

I see emancipatory epistemology as two pronged. The first is oriented to what Habermas calls "emancipatory cognitive interest" with a focus on critical sciences. The other prong is oriented to the need for knowledge production to engage in continuous reflection and self-critique so that we are fully cognizant of *relativistic* and *perspectival* biases that are embedded in knowledge development. Critical realism and emancipatory epistemology for nursing thus point out that we are seeking knowledge of humans, human living, and human practice that is fundamentally contextualized. The agencies of the context include our language, language use, and history agents in producing knowledge within given hermeneutically located horizons. Hence, knowledge development must be framed within continuous reflection and self-critique.

In addition, nursing knowledge needs to be considered as knowledge that provides the foundation on which the practice must be shaped for the discipline and for individual practitioners. Nursing practice must be guided by normative foundations that are framed by the discipline's focus on people's health—effecting changes and prescribing for desirable outcomes. At the same time, the basic form of practice for nursing is human-to-human engagement. Nursing knowledge must be concerned with the nature of normative foundations and how moral and value structures for what is good or desirable are determined. Further, it is essential that the processes for such determination within the discipline be articulated. Critical normative epistemology for nursing can direct us to a view of nursing knowledge development that is a fundamental way to shape nursing practice.

Nursing Epistemology

As presented in my writings (Kim, 1997a, 2000a, 2000b), nursing epistemology specifying four spheres of knowledge is an appropriate structure for thinking about what types of knowledge should be developed in nursing. Fours spheres of knowledge for nursing within this epistemological structure refer to different types of knowledge, each sphere having a specific epistemic focus. These spheres expand on the views presented in chapter 12 and are specified as

1 The *generalized* knowledge with an inferential focus.
2 The *subjective hermeneutic* knowledge with a referential focus.
3 The *critical hermeneutic* knowledge with a transformative focus.
4 The *ethical/aesthetic* knowledge with a desiderative focus.

Cognitive Needs for the Discipline

These epistemic foci identified are based on my conceptualization of human rationality in relation to knowledge development in nursing. This view directs us to different sorts of cognitive needs or *knowing*. I differ from Barbara Carper when I say knowing or cognitive needs. Here as I am referring to the knowing in the discipline, rather than knowing in individual human beings. It is collective knowing for the discipline. This conceptualization may be contrasted with the ideas proposed by Habermas (1986). He distinguished three forms of human cognitive interests as technical for empirical science, practical for hermeneutical sciences, and emancipatory for critical sciences. It also differs from Bhaskar (1986) who specified seven levels of rationality in social sciences. Bhaskar's levels included:

■ Technical rationality for Level I and contextually situated instrumental rationality for Level II, both specified as instrumental reason.
■ Practical rationality for Level III and explanatory critical rationality for Level IV, both specified as critical reason.

Table 14.1	Cognitive Needs for Nursing Epistemology Contrasted With Habermas', Bhaskar's, and Carper's Formulations			
Four Cognitive Needs for Nursing Epistemology	**Three Forms of Cognitive Interests (Habermas)**	**Four Types of Reason (Bhaskar)**	**Four Patterns of Knowing in Nursing (Carper)**
• Inferential Needs • Referential Needs • Transformative Needs • Desiderative Needs	• Technical Interest • Practical Interest • Emancipatory Interest	• Instrumental Reason • Critical Reason • Emancipatory Reason • Historical Reason	• Empirics • Aesthetic Pattern of Knowing • Personal Knowledge • Ethics

■ Depth-explanatory-critical rationality for Level V and depth-rationality for Level VI, both specified as emancipatory reason.
■ Historical rationality for Level VII specified as historical reason.

I believe that three of the four cognitive needs identified in my thinking align with Habermas's and Bhaskar's ideas, with the addition of the desiderative needs that I think is specific to a practice discipline, as depicted in Table 14.1.

Cognitive Needs and Practice

My specification of cognitive needs is oriented to differentiating knowledge for nursing practice in terms of their cognitive utility. Cognitive rationality for nursing knowledge (Fig. 14.1) development encompasses (a) the inferential cognitive need that is oriented to the knowledge of generalizations, both broad and narrow, from which an understanding, explanation, and/or prediction of specific events can be derived; (b) the referential cognitive need that is oriented to the knowledge of situated hermeneutics for which depth-understanding about situated, specific events (phenomena) can be gained; (c) the transformative cognitive need that is oriented to the knowledge of critical hermeneutics through which mutual understanding and emancipation can be pursued in human life, including that of practice; and (d) the desiderative cognitive need that is oriented to the knowledge of ethics and aesthetics with which nursing practice can be grounded in norms, values, moral sensibility, and creativity.

Developing Knowledge for Practice

The four cognitive needs as discussed provide the basis for developing knowledge for practice. Each one further defines the focus of knowledge needed within each sphere and implies approaches that can be used for developing knowledge.

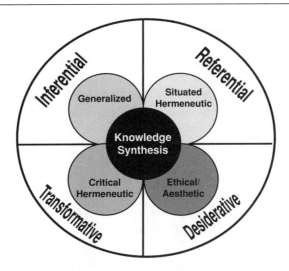

Schema for Nursing Epistemology.

Inferential Focus

Nursing knowledge with an inferential focus provides the knowledge to base inferences about specific situations drawing from various levels of generalized understanding, explanation, and prediction. Knowledge in the sphere of generalized knowledge is developed under the assumption of human patterns. That is, there are certain sets of human phenomena that are to be understood, explained, and predicted because there are features, underlying processes, and mechanisms that are relatively regular and patterned. To the extent that patterns exist, it may be possible to draw generalizeable conclusions as theories. Generalized theories of description, explanation, prediction, and prescription are the key features of knowledge in this sphere. However, generalization does not necessarily mean universal generalizations, but refers also to the context-specific and limited scope generalizations.

Systematization of knowledge in the generalized sphere must be oriented to refining ways to identify and delineate the nature of regularity and patterning in human phenomena of interest to nursing. Recently, chaos theory has aroused some new insights into the patterning in human phenomena of interest to nursing. In addition, there must be further clarification regarding how context-specified and scope-limiting nursing theories can be advanced in the emerging scientific culture in which scientific realism, relativism, and pragmatism are paradoxically juxtaposed.

Referential Focus

The need for knowledge with the referential focus is most apparent because nursing practice involves individual engagements of clients and practitioners. Situated hermeneutic knowledge is identified as critical for nursing under the premise that human beings are experiencing, subjective entities that are involved in creating and attaining meanings of their experiences. Each individual experiences occasions of his or her life through specific meanings. These meanings are created and attained uniquely in given situations. Although each human experience can be viewed as unique, human beings also share certain affinities that can be used for referential understanding. Hence, knowledge with a referential focus provides the referential points for understanding given situations through illumination, elaboration, depiction, and enlightenment gained from subjective experiences. The key method of knowledge development for this sphere is interpretation of meaning. Unlike generalized knowledge, the focus of referential knowledge is not regularity and patterning but is singularity, variation, and situatedness.

The knowledge in this sphere can provide nursing with an enrichment of understanding that is necessary to individualize nursing practice. The major problem faced with knowledge development in this sphere has been the lack of models for cumulating knowledge of this type. With the assumption that human empathy is the basis for understanding unique events and situations, nursing can develop ways to systematize referential knowledge so as to accentuate variations and differences in human experiences.

Transformative Focus

Nursing knowledge with the transformative focus addresses knowledge regarding human life as a form of social praxis. This perspective acknowledges that individuals engaged in coordinated living experience various forms of struggles, constraints, dominations, and disharmony. The critical hermeneutic sphere of knowledge refers to the knowledge of interpretation, critique, and emancipation regarding human's intersubjective and contextual coordination. It aligns with the critical scientific knowledge specified by Habermas (1971) and encompasses the postmodern critique of human life.

Knowledge with this focus is necessary for nursing because (a) human living in the context of health and illness does not involve only one's self-specific experiences but also experiences associated with living with other people in social contexts and (b) nursing is a form of social practice that involves human-to-human engagements—that is, between clients and nurses, and nurses with other nurses or other health care practitioners. The transformative focus refers to knowledge about the nature of social praxis in the context of health and nursing. The orientations are related to understanding, interpretation of meanings, and identification of distortions and disharmony in social praxis of health and nursing. The approach specifies forms of emancipatory projects oriented toward increasing autonomy and responsibility and eliminating, or decreasing, distortions and domination. This knowledge gives the base from which the coordinated work of practice, of getting well, and of living together can be formulated for nursing.

Desiderative Focus

Nursing knowledge with the desiderative focus is oriented to develop knowledge about how the discipline of nursing should be guided as a professional practice. It refers to *ethical and aesthetic knowledge* regarding normative ideals, ethical standards, value orientations, and aesthetic expectations. These foci need to be developed for the discipline to ensure that practice is quality oriented, ethically based, and aesthetic in its presentation. The knowledge from this focus provides the grounding for making individual nursing practice oriented to the professional values of ethics and aesthetics. Theories for this sphere of nursing knowledge need to be developed through philosophic analysis, dialectics, consensus building, and discourse analysis. Values and value standards are not only embedded in our practice but need to be formulated through an understanding of contextual requirements within which various forms of practice come to be designed. Hence, the knowledge in this sphere not only addresses the nature of ethical and aesthetic frameworks for nursing practice but also acknowledges how they become established, generated, or changed, and what the relationships are among such frameworks and larger culture, society, and context.

Summarizing the Four Spheres

These four spheres of knowledge are viewed as necessary for providing the foundation from which nursing practice is shaped for the discipline and for individual clinicians. Although it is possible to identify theories that exist currently in nursing according to these four spheres of nursing knowledge, their development has not been guided by the unifying epistemological position undergirding this framework. This schema of nursing epistemology (see Figure 14.1) moves the nursing discourse beyond debating about whether a nursing knowledge system should be positivistic, humanistic, or hermeneutical to the critical issue of what sorts of knowledge are required for nursing practice. It is a framework to view knowledge in terms of the epistemological requirements of nursing for inference, reference, transformation, and desirability/normativity. This understanding of four epistemological orientations as the necessary requirement for nursing knowledge directs pluralism to be viewed in a complementary perspective. At the same time, through this schema, pluralism in nursing knowledge can be examined systematically for significance in terms of heuristics and practice.

Synthesis of Knowledge in Practice: Critical Narrative Epistemology

Knowledge in these four spheres is critical as it is the comprehensive, unifying base from which nurses must draw knowledge that is applicable and useful in singular, clinical situations. The conclusion reached here is the same as noted at the end of chapter 12. This approach means that the ultimate synthesizer and knowledge generator must be the nurse in practice. Practicing nurses must be able to come to know the critical aspects of their client, the situation, and their own practice. The nurse alternatively dissects each stratum to view from one lens and, at the same time, layers and knits together the multiple strata in order to produce her or his practice.

Types of Syntheses of Nursing Knowledge

Synthesis can be viewed from two dimensions: (a) synthesis of the knowledge of the public domain into the private domains and (b) synthesis of knowledge in practice. The synthesis of knowledge of the public domain into the private domain is the process of *knowledge assimilation* that must occur before the public domain knowledge is used in

Table 14.2	Types of Knowledge in the Public and Private Domains in Four Knowledge Spheres		

| | | The Private Domain | |
Knowledge Sphere	The Public Domain	Declarative (Formal) Knowledge	Experiential (Procedural) Knowledge
Generalized Knowledge	• Descriptions, explanations, and predictions • Prescriptive theories • Propositional research		• Generalized schemas of clinical encounters • Experiential typologies and models • Experience-based propositions
Situated Hermeneutical Knowledge	• Situational theories • Situated hermeneutics analysis • Narratives and discourses		• Clinical stories and scripts • Clinical impressions • Clinical narratives
Critical Hermeneutical Knowledge	• Critical hermeneutic analysis • Critiques, deconstruction, discourse analysis • Emancipatory projects and theories		• Self-reflective critiques • Emancipatory experiences • Personal transformations
Ethical/Aesthetic Knowledge	• Formal values, norms, standards, and consensus • Ethical theories • Aesthetic practice theories		• Personal beliefs and preferences • Value commitments • Situational guidelines • Experiential scripts of creativity

practice. Types of knowledge may be specified analytically for the public and private domains according to the structure of nursing epistemology proposed as shown in Table 14.2. Here the suggestion is that *knowledge synthesis* in practice basically involves the knowledge of the private domain at the situation of practice (see Figure 14.2). The exceptions would be cases where the nurse becomes involved in retrieving and accessing knowledge from the public domain in order to address the issues of the situation, such as in looking something up in the *Physician's Desk Reference* or consulting the Internet. Hence, the synthesis between the knowledge of the public and private domains needs to be assumed to occur on an ongoing basis for practitioners.

Synthesis From Other Perspectives

Knowledge synthesis carried out in nursing practice, of course, is much more complicated than just coordinating knowledge distributed in the four spheres. It involves a synthesis and use not only of nursing knowledge but also of knowledge from many sources and disciplines. Knowledge synthesis is carried out by nurses in practice by eliciting nurses'

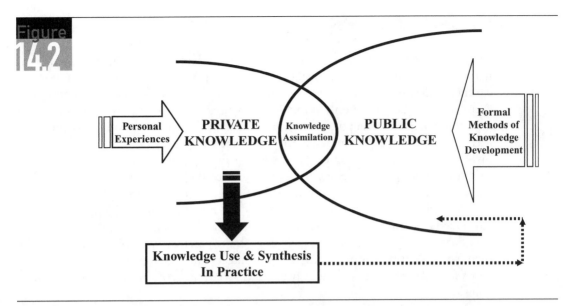

Figure 14.2

Knowledge Use and Synthesis in Practice.

---

personal knowledge, drawing situation-specific knowing, and sometimes accessing public knowledge of all sorts. The work of Benner and her colleagues (Benner & Tanner, 1987) has suggested that nurses at various levels of expertise are engaged in this synthesis using different types of processing. From a different perspective, Gadow (1995) suggests a "clinical epistemology" to describe practitioners' synthesis in nursing assessment in which both general and particular knowledge are brought together to another level at which "knowledge is co-authored by client and nurse together in their relational narrative" (p. 26). This focuses on synthesis in terms of process.

As described by these two approaches, synthesis involves a set of rather complex processes that cognitive psychologists, neuroscientists, and philosophers have tried to specify during the past 3 decades. I am not going to address this aspect of synthesis—that is, the mental, existential, or experiential processes involved. My focus with the proposed nursing epistemology is not with the nature of this processing but with the product of such processing as knowledge. Because we are interested in the development of nursing knowledge, the focus is on what is produced through such synthesis in practice and how we might be able to identify such products as valuable knowledge in nursing.

Methods to Accumulate Synthesized Knowledge

Viewed from the knowledge development perspective, we need to have access to exemplary knowledge syntheses that are produced by nurses in practice. Hence, I propose that in addition to the need to develop knowledge in the four spheres from a formal perspective, we need to develop methods and approaches appropriate for an accumulation of synthesized knowledge in nursing. Synthesized knowledge is only evident as the product of nursing practice. Thus, it can be revealed only through an in-depth, post hoc analysis of practice within the perspective of critical narrative epistemology.

Exemplary Practice Scripts

Critical narrative epistemology, then, can be understood as knowledge that is based on narrativity of human activity. Further, it includes critique that is required to compare, contrast, and reinterpret narratives of practice in order to discover "good" practice. Such knowledge can be gained only through accessing actual practice, exposed to a specific analytic method. The analytic method, then, must involve scripting, analysis, critique, and identification of exemplary practice scripts. Hence, this phase of knowledge development involves nurses actively practicing in the knowledge of generation activities.

Practice scripts must come from nurses about their practice in clinical situations and may deal with a case or a specific nursing event. An in-depth, critical analysis of a practice script may be done by the nurse or a researcher in order to identify knowledge embedded in the practice with respect to its content and to examine the nature of selection, coordination, and synthesis that is apparent in the practice. Exemplary practice scripts then can be identified through such analyses and critique. Exemplary practice scripts are new knowledge of synthesis, which becomes a part of that ever-evolving stock of nursing knowledge.

Process of Critical Reflective Inquiry

For this process, then, I propose an application of critical reflective inquiry (Kim, 1999) as a method to develop knowledge embedded in nursing practice. This method of inquiry is understood to be couched within the critical narrative epistemology. Further, it is founded on the ideas in (a) action science (Argyris, Putman, & Smith, 1985; Argyris & Schön, 1974) and Schön's reflective practice (1991) and (b) critical philosophy (Habermas, 1986) and the critical reflection of Freire (1972). However, this method is not necessarily only interested in discovering new, synthesized knowledge of good practice. It also aims to understand the nature and meaning of practice to practitioners and how to correct and improve the practice through self-reflection and critique (see Table 14.3).

The method includes (a) narratives or scripting, (b) reflection and analysis, and (c) critique and emancipation as three phases through which a researcher or a practitioner can gain critical knowledge of synthesis in practice. The *descriptive phase* involves a narrative description by the practitioner of a specific instance, situation, or case of practice. Descriptive narratives of actual practice in specific clinical situations are written by nurses, including the description of nurses' actions, thoughts and feelings, as well as the circumstances and features of the situations.

The *reflective phase* involves a careful analysis of narratives in a reflective mode with three different foci: (a) reflecting against standards or the espoused theories in the action science perspective, (b) reflecting on the situation, and (c) reflecting on intentions. From the knowledge development perspective, the reflective phase is involved in identifying how the synthesis of knowledge, both the public and personal, is done in practice. From this phase, models of good practice, theories of application, and knowledge regarding the process of practice can be identified and constructed. It is also possible to discover systematic inconsistencies, poor practice, or ineffectual routinizations that exist in practice.

Table 14.3	Phases in Critical Reflective Inquiry		
Phases	**Descriptive Phase**	**Reflective Phase**	**Critical/Emancipatory Phase**
Processes	• Description of practice events (actions, thoughts, and feelings) • Examination of descriptions for genuineness and comprehensiveness	• Reflective analysis against espoused theories (scientific, ethical and aesthetic) • Reflective analysis of situation • Reflective analysis of intentions	• Critique of practice regarding conflicts, distortions, and inconsistencies • Engagement in emancipatory and change process • Description of practice models
Products	• Descriptive narratives (scripts)	• Knowledge about practice processes and applications • Self-awareness	• Learning and change in practice • Self-critique and emancipation • Synthesized models of practice

The third phase in this method is the *critical/emancipatory phase* that is oriented toward correcting and changing less-than-good or ineffective practice, or ineffectual routinizations that exist in practice. It aims to move forward to future assimilation of new innovations emerging in practice. This phase involves critical discourses that are aimed at discovering the nature and sources of distortions, inconsistencies, and incongruence between the actual practice and the expected or desired practice. The process uses self-dialogue, critique, and argumentation and can lead to self-emancipation regarding practice and a change in practice.

Conclusion

My experiences in the application of the method of critical narrative theory in actual practice settings indicate that the method is useful both to novices and experts in discovering the knowledge embedded in practice in synthesized forms. In addition, the nurse can understand the nature of one's practice through reflection and critique. Certainly the synthesizing that exists in practice does not necessarily involve knowledge drawn from the four spheres I have identified in nursing epistemology. Often the practice reveals that the knowledge in situ is not inclusive, well organized, or consistent with the systematized knowledge of the discipline, especially on the surface. However, through critical reflection, analysis, and critique it is possible to identify what sorts of knowledge

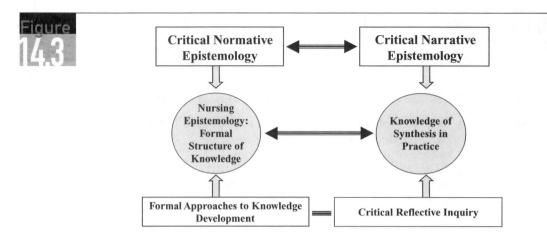

Knowledge Development in Nursing.

are synthesized and coordinated to bring about specific practice in situations. Thus, critical narrative epistemology applying the method of critical reflective inquiry is an approach to develop knowledge for the discipline, linking the formal structure of nursing epistemology to synthesis in practice (see Figure 14.3).

REFERENCES

Argyris, C., Putnam, R., & Smith, D. M. (1985). *Action science.* San Francisco: Jossey-Bass.

Argyris, C., & Schön, D. (1974). *Theory in practice.* San Francisco: Jossey-Bass.

Benner, P., & Tanner, C. (1987). How expert nurses use intuition. *American Journal of Nursing, 87*(1), 23–31.

Bhaskar, R. (1986). *Scientific realism and human emancipation.* London: Verso.

Freire, P. (1972). *Pedagogy of the oppressed.* New York: Continuum.

Gadow, S. (1995). Clinical epistemology: A dialectic of nursing assessment. *Canadian Journal of Nursing Research, 27,* 25–34.

Good, B. J. (1994). *Medicine, rationality, and experience: An anthropological perspective.* Cambridge, UK: Cambridge University Press.

Habermas, J. (1971). *Knowledge and human interests.* (J. J. Shapiro, Trans.). Boston: Beacon Press.

Habermas, J. (1986). *Knowledge and human interests.* Cambridge, UK: Polity Press.

Kim, H. S. (1994). Practice theories in nursing and a science of nursing practice. *Scholarly Inquiry for Nursing Practice: An International Journal, 8,* 145–158.

Kim, H. S. (1996a). Pluralism: viable options for applying theory to knowledge. Paper presented at the 1997 Nursing Knowledge Impact Conference II. University of Rhode Island, Kingston, Rhode Island.

Kim, H. S. (1996b). Nursing epistemology as a human practice science. In T. Bjerkreim, J. Mathisen, & R. Nord (Eds.), *Vision, viten og virke* [Vision, knowledge and impact], (pp. 36–45). Oslo, Norway: Universitetsforlager AS.

Kim, H. S. (1997). Terminology in structuring and developing nursing knowledge. In I. M. King & J. Fawcett (Eds.), *The language of nursing theory and metatheory* (pp. 27–36). Indianapolis, IN: Sigma Theta Tau International Center Nursing Press.

Kim, H. S. (2000a). *The nature of theoretical thinking in nursing* (Rev. ed). New York: Springer.

Kim, H. S. (2000b). Directions for theory development—For an increased coherence in the new century. In N. Chaska (Ed.), *The nursing profession: Tomorrow and beyond* (pp. 271–286). Thousand Oaks, CA: Sage.

Schön, D. (1991). *The reflective practitioner* (2nd ed). San Francisco: Jossey-Bass.

Unifying Nursing Language: Communicating Nursing Practice*

15

Joanne McClosky Dochterman
Dorothy A. Jones

I n 1973 Kristine Gebbie and Mary Ann Lavin held the First Conference on the Classification of Nursing Diagnoses, a conference designed to classify health problems within the domain of nursing (Gebbie & Lavin, 1975). This group later became known as the North American Nursing Diagnosis Association (NANDA). Over the years, other classifications, including the Nursing Interventions Classification (NIC) and the Nursing Outcomes Classification (NOC), were developed. As NANDA, NIC, and NOC have grown, each group has worked independently to classify, name, and define diagnoses, interventions, and outcomes in three separate structures. In an effort to promote the consistent use of a unified disciplinary language by all nurses, NANDA and the Center for Nursing Classification and Clinical Effectiveness at the University of Iowa (home to NIC and NOC) created a virtual NANDA, NIC, and NOC (NNN) Alliance to facilitate movement toward the

*This chapter is an edited version of parts of *The Unifying of Nursing Language: The Hormonization of NANDA, NIC, and NOC*, by J. M. Dochterman and D. Jones, 2003, Silver Spring, MD: American Nurses Association. Used with permission. Project funded by a grant from the National Library of Medicine (R13 LM07243).

development of a unified nursing classification. This chapter presents the process, content, and outcomes of a project funded by the National Library of Medicine (Dochterman & Jones, 2001). The invitational conference addressed the issues of the importance of language for nursing and the need to harmonize the work of the three organizations. The collaborative process used to achieve the goal of creating a common unifying structure for nursing language is presented along with the proposed structure.

The Groundwork for Unification

For more than 25 years, nurses have struggled unsuccessfully to consistently communicate nursing practice to others. The extensive narrative about patient care in the literature includes descriptions about patient behaviors and reactions, along with specific actions taken by nurses to respond to patients' experiences. In recent years, increased attention has been paid to successful outcomes and changes in plans of care. Methods of documentation have varied over the years with multiple differences observed in terms of both the language and format used to document patient care. Streamlined checklists, critical pathways, and problem-oriented charting have been put in place to reduce documentation and respond to changing regulations related to reimbursement.

In the midst of these changes, nurses have created a variety of documentation forms but have been hindered by a lack of a common disciplinary language that effectively communicated patient problems, supporting data, related nursing actions, and outcomes. As a result, nursing practice is poorly communicated to patients/clients, to other nurses, to other health care providers, and to policy makers. The essence of professional nursing lies within the dynamic nurse–patient relationship. It is important that nursing language captures a portion of this experience directly related to patient behaviors and experiences. Nurses worldwide need to be able to use and expand the language they use so that nursing practice can be articulated, evaluated, and included in discussions of cost-effective, quality patient care.

Issues and Challenges in Using Nursing Language Classifications

As noted, Kristine Gebbie and Mary Ann Lavin held the first National Conference in 1973 on the Classification of Nursing Diagnoses to present "a clear articulation of those health problems that comprise the domain of nursing and the classification of the problems into a taxonomic system" (Gebbie & Lavin, 1975, p. v). Since that time, other classification systems (e.g., Nursing Intervention Classification, Nursing Outcomes Classifications) and language data sets (e.g., Nursing Management Minimum Data Set) have been developed to organize and describe nursing diagnoses, interventions, nursing sensitive patient outcomes, and other components of the care episode (e.g., staffing, cost). By 2001 the American Nurses Association had recognized eight nursing classification systems, two nursing data sets, and two nomenclatures (Coenen, McNeil, Bakken, Bickford, & Warren, 2001).

This proliferation of nursing language classification systems has resulted in a lack of unified disciplinary language, leading to confusion among nurses in practice across specialties and settings. Although mapping efforts associated with the development and use of terminology models (e.g., The Systemized Nomenclature of Medicine, or SNOMED) are under way, these efforts are designed to relate different languages "behind the scene" and are untested to date. Even when the reference terminology models are successful for the collection and comparison of nursing data, they do not assist the clinician or student to learn or to use the language at the bedside. The inconsistent use of nursing languages in documenting patient problems and responses has minimized nursing's visibility and compromised the contributions of nurses to quality and cost-effective patient outcomes. Lack of consistent language to describe nursing practice has significantly reduced the integration of nursing language and clinical reasoning approaches to academic curricula across programs. This has led to a growing number of new graduates with limited knowledge of nursing language, culminating in inconsistent documentation of patient problems. Failure to communicate nursing practice effectively has limited reimbursement and nursing's ability to provide policy makers with data needed to change and inform health policies.

In addition, the development of substantial content for the domain of nursing has been compromised, and the growth of the science has been restricted. The problems nurses solve each day when they respond to patients with multiple problems are poorly articulated. As a result, knowledge development and clinical investigation are negatively impacted. The multiplicity of language classification systems has also decreased the inclusion of nursing language within information systems, further impeding nursing's ability to communicate its disciplinary contributions to patient outcomes. Although nursing has gained the attention of policy makers (Testimony, 1999), and there is a willingness to include nursing language in health care information systems, system developers also want to harmonize nursing language and move toward a more unified language that is responsive to nurses globally.

Contributions of a Common Unified Structure for Nursing Language

The time has come for development of a common unified structure for nursing language. Within existing terminologies, certain points of consensus have been reached, particularly within the NANDA, NIC, and NOC Classification. Although these three classifications have been linked with each other (Johnson, Bulechek, Dochterman, Maas, & Moorhead, 2001), the lack of a common organizing structure fails to provide a visual indication that the three classifications are related. Developers of these structures share common thinking around nursing language and professional nursing. The development of a common unifying structure for these nursing languages will provide significant contributions for nursing knowledge development, clinical practice, education policy, and information systems development. These contributions were culled from the literature and from our collective experience and are acknowledged as follows:

For *Knowledge Development*, a unified structure will

■ Enable scientists to focus on concept development and isolate the essential content of the discipline.

■ Contribute to the definition of nursing science and professional nursing practice.
■ Support the contributions of language to knowledge development and the development and use of mid-range and practice theory.
■ Articulate the phenomena of concern to the discipline and lead to the development of a new knowledge.

For *Clinical Practice*, a unified structure will

■ Improve the articulation of diagnoses, interventions, and outcomes.
■ Reduce the complexity of integrating these three elements of nursing care.
■ Differentiate more clearly the contributions of the discipline to cost-effective quality care.
■ Reflect the complexity of clinical nursing practice.
■ Contribute to nursing's visibility in evidence-based practice.
■ Help to standardize documentation across settings and improve communication among nurses and other care providers.
■ Create movement toward a standardized nursing assessment.

For *Education*, a common unified structure will

■ Guide faculty in curriculum development and evaluation.
■ Foster the integration of language into nursing curricula at all program levels.
■ Organize the language of the content of the discipline for teaching clinical decision making.
■ Help to provide graduates with knowledge and experience for communication of nursing judgments, interventions, and measurement of outcomes.

For *Research*, a common unified structure will

■ Guide researchers in development, testing, accuracy, and refinement of nursing diagnoses, interventions, and outcomes.
■ Promote the development and testing of predictive models that will link patient outcomes to practice contributions across clinical specialties.
■ Facilitate research to identify high-incidence problems that are critical for all nurses to know and resolve.
■ Facilitate the integration of nursing knowledge into clinical databases that are used for effectiveness research.

For *Health Policy*, a common unified structure will

■ Help to integrate nursing information within the electronic patient record and national nursing database used for health policy decision making.
■ Provide a structured, unified framework for capturing clinical nursing information.
■ Help to create an accurate model for administrators and insurers to determine the cost of nursing care.
■ Facilitate reimbursement for specific dimensions of nursing practice related to patient problem identification, interventions, and outcomes.
■ Help to accurately define provider mix and complexity of patient care used to make patient assignments and to allocate resources.

For *Information Systems*, a common unified structure will

- Create an improved structure for inclusion of nursing language into new and existing information system models.
- Aid in the development of a database that fosters the mapping/linking of diagnoses, interventions, and outcomes across terminology models.
- Improve data access, storage, and retrieval needed by researchers, clinicians, policy makers, and administrators.
- Enable systematic evaluation of existing terminologies and their relevance and use in clinical practice.
- Increase the overall use of nursing languages and long-term viability of NANDA, NIC, and NOC internationally.

Background for a Framework for Unifying Language

The developers of the proposed common structure for the language of nursing used the clinical reasoning process and problem solving along with the work of Donaldson and Crowley (1978) and the American Nurses Association's *Social Policy Statement* (1995) to guide the creation of a unifying structure. This knowledge provided a framework that fostered the linkages among NANDA, NIC, and NOC classifications.

Nursing language developers have historically dealt with classifying phenomena of concern to nursing. Changes that result from nursing interventions are measured and described by the achievement of outcomes. Problem solving and clinical reasoning have been used to process information about the patient experience. Problem solving is structured with a model that relies on data (cues) obtained through assessment, resulting in a judgment or the identification of a patient problem (diagnosis). Nursing's goal is to relieve the problem by linking the judgment and related data to interventions "that restore function, promote comfort and foster optimal health" (Jones, 1997, p. 80). Outcomes are then measured and responses to interventions are observed. Within nursing the clinical reasoning process is guided by the *Standards of Clinical Nursing Practice* (1998) published by the American Nurses Association.

Donaldson and Crowley (1978) cited three core nursing principles that also informed the developers of the proposed common unifying structure. These principles include (a) concern with principles and laws that influence life principles, well-being, and optimum functioning of humans, sick and well; (b) concern with the patterning of human behavior in interaction with environment in critical life situations; and (c) concern with processes that effect positive changes in health status.

The American Nurses Association's *Social Policy Statement* (1995) provided additional focus for developers. In particular, the *Social Policy Statement* states that "the phenomena of concern to nurses are human experiences and responses to birth, health, illness and death" (p. 8). The *Statement* goes on to define concepts that are central to the creation of a common structure, including (a) diagnoses, "the identification of responses to actual or potential health problems"; (b) interventions, "actions nurses take on behalf of patients and families or communities . . . to improve, correct, or adjust physical, psychological, spiritual, cultural and emotional conditions"; and (c) outcomes that evaluate "the effectiveness of interventions in relation to identified outcome" (pp. 1, 9).

The Invitational NNN Conference: Drafting a Common Structure

The invitational conference was held at the Starved Rock Conference Center in Utica, Illinois, August 12–14, 2001. The grant project objectives are listed in Table 15.1. The purpose of the conference was to develop a first draft of a common unified taxonomic structure for three of the classifications of NANDA, the NIC, and NOC. Twenty-five participants, knowledgeable in the development, testing, and refinement of classification systems, were invited to participate in the conference. Representatives from Omaha and Home Health Care systems were among those who were invited but declined the request to participate. The meeting convened with 24 participants, including 22 nurse experts, a keynote speaker, and a staff person.

Methods Used to Develop a Common Unified Structure

The conference began with a keynote presentation on the science of classification presented by Geoffrey Bowker, professor in the Department of Communication at the University of California at San Diego. Dr. Bowker has spent his academic career studying the structure of knowledge in various disciplines. His presentation reinforced the need for nursing classifications and placed the current nursing work in the context of development, articulation, and growth of knowledge. Dr. Margaret Lunney spoke on the need for a common structure, and sessions were focused on the structures of NANDA, NIC, and NOC, as well as other nursing classification systems and data sets currently in use.

Although all participants were familiar with some of the systems, this review helped to ensure a common starting place for each conference participant. Discussions related to each presentation helped to uncover issues and to offer solutions in areas of concern. The time spent examining existing nursing terminologies helped each member establish some common expectations, enthusiasm for the current project, and the importance

Table 15.1

Conference Objectives Structure

1 Articulate the assumptions underlying each language (diagnoses, interventions, outcomes).
2 Identify issues that will need to be addressed to achieve a common taxonomic structure.
3 Examine existing taxonomic structures currently in use clinically.
4 Prepare a first draft of a "White Paper" on the common taxonomic structure linking NANDA, NIC, and NOC.
5 Plan strategies for dissemination and feedback of the White Paper at venues, including an open forum at the April 2002 NANDA, NIC, and NOC conference.
   Following the dissemination and feedback of the document:
6 Develop a position paper detailing the need for the common structure and the methodology used to develop the proposed structure.
7 Create mechanisms to integrate feedback and to disseminate the final structure to nurses globally.

Table 15.2	Guidelines for Constructing a Common Organizing Structure: The Desiderata

The users of the proposed structure will include:
1 Developers of NANDA, NIC, and NOC, and other classifications.
2 Practicing nurses, students, and other clinicians who wish to locate a particular diagnosis, intervention, or outcome.
3 Developers of information systems who will use the structure to organize screens.
4 A host of others, including faculty, for use in courses and curriculum design, researchers, and policy makers.

Ten Desiderata for Developers
1 *Simplicity of Structure:* Keep the structure simple—two levels above the concept level seems to work, naming them domains and classes.
2 *Parsimony of Groups:* The second level (classes) should have about 25 to 30 groups; the first level (domain) less than 10. More than this is hard to handle mentally and is beyond what can be easily put onto a computer screen.
3 *Clear Language:* The names of groups (domains and classes) should be clear, short (three words or fewer), and descriptive enough to know what kind of diagnoses, interventions, and outcomes are included.
4 *Formal Definitions:* Each domain and class should have a definition.
5 *Distinct Groups:* The structure should minimize need/desire to cross-reference; classes/domains should be distinct so that diagnoses, interventions, and outcomes can preferably be placed in only one location.
6 *Graceful Evolution:* The structure should resonate with users and be similar to what is now familiar so that the move to a new structure is relatively easy.
7 *Domain Completeness:* An "other" category (not elsewhere classified) should not be included.
8 *Theory Neutral:* The structure should be useful in any institute, nursing specialty, or care delivery model regardless of philosophical orientation.
9 *Other Discipline Friendly:* Headings (domains and particularly classes) should preferably be recognizable and useful for all disciplines (e.g., process and body system).
10 *Scientific Common Sense:* The structure should look and feel scientific but also reflect common sense.

of the work at hand. Much of the work was accomplished in four work groups that met following the overview sessions. Guidelines for constructing a common organizing structure were provided (see Table 15.2) for the groups by identifying the expected users and articulating 10 desiderata for developers.

Review of Organizing Structures

The six organizing structures that were sent to every participant in advance and that were reviewed at the conference were NANDA's Taxonomy 2, NIC's Taxonomy, NOC's Taxonomy, Gordon's Functional Health Patterns, Home Health Care Classification's 20 components, and the Omaha System's Structure. The six structures were selected because they are used frequently in clinical practice. They are commonly acknowledged as front-end clinical terminologies useful in helping practicing nurses to plan and document care. Each of the structures selected has an organizing structure thought to be helpful to the purpose at hand.

North American Nursing Diagnosis Association (NANDA) Taxonomy 2

The NANDA Taxonomy 2 (NANDA, 2001) was approved for adoption by the NANDA members at their conference in April 2000. At the time it consisted of 12 domains (e.g., health promotion, nutrition) and 46 classes (e.g., health awareness, ingestion). Each domain and class has a definition, and a total of 155 diagnoses were included at the third level of taxonomy.

Nursing Interventions Classification (NIC; 3rd ed.)

The NIC taxonomy (McCloskey & Bulechek, 2000) consists of 7 domains (e.g., physio-logical: basic, behavioral) and 30 classes (e.g., activity and exercise management, coping assistance). Each domain and class has a definition. The 486 interventions available at the time of the project were placed in the classes at the third level of taxonomy.

Nursing Outcomes Classification (NOC; 2nd ed.)

The NOC taxonomy (Johnson, Maas, & Moorhead, 2000) consists of 7 domains (e.g., functional health, physiologic health) and 29 classes (e.g., energy maintenance, growth & development). Each domain and class has a definition. The 260 outcomes then available were placed in the classes at the third level of taxonomy.

Gordon's 11 Functional Health Patterns

The Functional Health Patterns (Gordon, 1994) contain 11 pattern areas (e.g., nutrition-metabolic, health perception-health management, elimination) and are used by numerous educators, students, and clinicians to organize the nursing assessment data and informa-tion from physical examination to arrive at nursing diagnoses. Gordon has organized the NANDA diagnoses into 11 patterns, and the new NANDA Taxonomy 2 domains reflect a modification of the Functional Health Patterns.

Home Health Care Classification (HHCC)

The 145 diagnoses and the 160 interventions in this system (Saba, 1992) were developed for home healthcare nurses to use in practice and are classified in 20 categories (e.g., activity, bowel elimination, cardiac, cognitive). The classification reflects diagnoses, in-terventions and outcomes. The 20 components are at a class level of some of the other classifications and may be helpful in the design of a common structure.

Omaha System

The Omaha System, developed in the mid-1970s for use in community health (Martin & Scheet, 1992), contains three schemes for problems, interventions, and outcomes. Forty problems are organized in four domains: environmental, psychological, psychosocial, and health-related behaviors. The intervention scheme consists of four broad categories (e.g., the first category is health teaching, guidance, and counseling) and 62 targets for intervention. The outcome ratings are measured by ratings using three 5-point scales for concepts of knowledge, behavior, and status.

Major Outcomes of Group Work

Although using the same guidelines, the outcomes of group work took several forms. Some developed assumptions, others raised issues, some worked on new classes and domains, and others drafted integrated language within one framework.

Assumptions

Two of the four work groups spent part of their time identifying the assumptions on which a combined taxonomic structure for NANDA, NIC, and NOC would be based. One of the groups identified four assumptions, whereas the other group identified nine assumptions. The following list combines the ideas of both groups.

1 Nursing classification (NANDA, NIC, and NOC) describe the phenomena of nursing practice and represent the clinical judgments nurses need to make.
2 Nursing classifications represent the knowledge base of nursing and relate to all settings and specialties.
3 Nursing classifications are useful for clinical practice, education, research, and administration.
4 The nursing classifications are advanced enough to identify key concepts that can be harmonized.
5 The classifications need to address individual, family, community, and health system dimensions.
6 Classifications evolve and change as nursing changes, and a structure can evolve to handle these changes.
7 Classifications can capture the holistic nature of nursing's perspective.

Issues

Several issues were obvious at the beginning of the discussion in the work groups. Two principal issues were:

1 Dealing with their own sense of territoriality regarding the various languages represented. Participants had to agree up front in the dialogue that each person would keep an open mind and would try to think in terms of what the best overreaching structure would be regardless of personal or professional inclinations. This proved to be surprisingly easy once the small group work began. The various language

developers were pretty evenly divided in each group allowing everyone to have a say in the product of the group with no language dominating.

2 Concern about composing a framework that encompassed patient-focused concepts with nurse-focused concepts. Some of the participants voiced a concern that it was not appropriate to combine patient-focused diagnoses and outcomes with nurse-focused interventions. Others felt that because all three (diagnoses, interventions, outcomes) are in the domain of nursing, an overreaching framework could encompass all three. After some discussion they agreed that if they didn't try they would never know. By the time all of the groups had completed their work, there was general consensus that a unifying structure was possible and that, although the approaches by each group were different, the initial drafts of structures had many similarities.

Results

One group produced a list of new classes for all three structures, another identified new classes and domains, whereas a third group placed the current classes of NANDA, NIC, and NOC in a modified version of the Gordon Functional Health Pattern structure. A fourth group identified new domains and placed the current classes in these domains according to type of recipient (i.e., individual, family, community). Each of these drafts was discussed in terms of the issues and challenges it presented.

The final session of the 3rd day was spent identifying the common challenges and the direction the group desired to take on each challenge. For example, the group was unanimous in its desire that the new structure include both new classes and new domains in which the labels of all three classifications could be placed. Although the importance of family and community was acknowledged, the majority of participants did not want to see these as domains. There was total agreement that the terms used should clearly communicate the type of concepts included and that the words used should be familiar to clinicians. On the 3rd day of the conference, the group adjourned midday in high spirits, expressing the feeling that they had accomplished a lot and that they believed that, though a perfect document was not possible, a final draft of one common structure could be achieved.

Post Conference Activity: Synthesizing a Common Structure

Immediately following the conference a small group consisting of Johanne Dochterman (NIC), Dorothy Jones (NANDA), Sue Moorhead (NOC), and Kay Avant (NANDA) met to prepare a first draft of the proposed structure based on the work of the four groups and the general discussion of the 3 days. Owing to the structure of NANDA, it was desirable to have both the current president (Kay Avant) and the past president and co-organizer of this conference (Dorothy Jones) participate in the postconference activities.

Following a brief discussion of the four proposed structures from the conference work groups, the postconference task force decided that a first step would be to compare the two drafts of new classes with each other as well as with the modified Gordon classes prepared by the third group. When this was done, a number of similarities were noted—although named differently, the same classes were identified. The task force discussed each of the alternative names and selected the one that communicated the best or chose a new name. The end result of this exercise was 28 potential classes.

The next step was to organize these classes into domains. One group at the conference had produced four new domains that were well received by the participants. The task force used four domains plus one other suggested in the discussion as the initial starting point for the domains of the common structure. Each of the 28 classes was then placed in one of the five domains. At this point the five domains were labeled health/life style, physiological function, psychosocial function, life principles, and environment/health protection.

As the process evolved, some of the classes were thought to be relevant to two of the domains, with the greatest amount of redundancy seen between health/life style and psychosocial function. For example, the classes of activity/exercise and sleep/rest were initially placed in both health/life style and psychosocial function. After discussion of these and other classes placed in two locations, each class was placed in only one location where it was thought to fit best. The placement was helped by the definitions of each domain that the postconference group generated. As work progressed, it became apparent that the proposed domain of life principles was overlapping with the domain of health/life style and because the life principles domain had only one class in it (values/beliefs, which includes spirituality), it was decided to combine these domains, calling them, at this time, health/life style.

After some editing, a new proposed structure, consisting of four domains— health/life style, physiological, psychological, and environmental/health protection—as well as 27 classes were all created. The task force reviewed each of the issues that were raised by the four groups against the proposed structure and determined that the proposed structure had addressed each of the concerns. For example, various participants strongly indicated that the new structure must be able to accommodate growth and development, medications, and the care in the community.

A few months after the conference, this draft of the proposed unified common structure was sent to each conference participant for review and feedback, along with a set of questions that addressed particular aspects of the proposed structure (e.g., should the comfort class be divided into two classes—physical comfort and physiological comfort, and then be placed in different domains?). Based on the comments, changes were made in the proposed structure. For example, the word "health" was taken out of the titles of two of the domains and two of the classes, with the rationale that all of this pertained to health. Definitions of two of the domains and some of the classes were changed and titles of some of the classes were changed. All changes were made in the interest of keeping the practicing nurse in mind and focusing on what the practitioner would find most helpful and easiest understood to understand.

The 2002 NNN Conference: Presenting the Proposed Structure

At the April 2002 NNN Conference in Chicago, the proposed unifying structure was disseminated and was further discussed by a larger community. During this conference, attended by over 300 individuals from the United States and nearly a dozen other countries, a plenary session was held with 90 minutes devoted to presentation of the process used, the proposed structure and discussion. All participants had copies of the draft and proposed structure. A lively discussion ensued. One suggestion was to post the draft and structure on the Web and allow more time for feedback. One week after the conference the paper and structure were posted on the Web sites of both NANDA and the Center for Nursing Classification and Clinical Effectiveness. Feedback was requested through the list serve. Based on the feedback during the discussion period at the conference and the responses received from the Web postings, the paper and structure were again revised. Among the major revisions were (a) a change in the name of the first domain from lifestyle to functional, (b) a change in the definition of three of the domains and several of the classes, (c) the addition of emotional class, and (d) a name change from safety promotion class to risk management. Several other minor changes were made to reduce wordiness and to improve consistency in format.

Although several of the issues raised have been resolved by changes in names and definitions, some differences of opinion remain that cannot be reconciled in one structure. The revised structure will not be entirely to everyone's liking. This is the nature of consensus. It is also the nature of nursing—nurses work in a variety of settings with different philosophical orientations and levels of skill. The effort was to achieve a common structure. To account for all of nursing practice is a tall order. Nonetheless, we believe that the result is a very good beginning—a harmonization of all views has been accomplished.

Proposed Taxonomy of Nursing Practice

The proposed structure—consisting of 4 domains and 28 classes—integrates the work of all participants and working groups at the conference and takes into account the reflection and feedback of participants following the conference. This new structure is different from the existing structures of NANDA, NIC, and NOC, but it is not a radical departure from any of them. This is considered favorable inasmuch as it favors none and at the same time forms an effective transition to the use of a common structure. The structure is also in the public domain, available for use by any group or individual (see Table 15.3). The proposed structure meets the desired guidelines for a common structure. The two-level structure is simple, consistent with existing structures and will be easy for clinicians to use. The number of classes (parsimony of groups) is not overwhelming. The names of the domains and classes are clear and each has a formal definition. The names will also be familiar to members of other disciplines allowing for use across disciplines if desired. All classes are listed in only one domain. The classification is theory neutral and may be used with any philosophical orientation as well as any specialty or care delivery model.

The unifying structure was developed so that the NANDA, NIC, and NOC developers (as well as others, if desired) could place their diagnoses, interventions, and outcomes in these same classes and domains. Initially, these are likely to be separate publications each using the same structure, but over time and perhaps with some modifications, the languages can be placed together and published together in the one structure. Information systems can use the one structure to help students and practicing nurses locate and select the appropriate diagnosis, intervention, or outcome. The use of one common

Table 15.3	Taxonomy of Nursing Practice

Domains

I. **Functional Domain:** Includes diagnoses, outcomes, and interventions to promote basic needs.	II. **Physiological Domain:** Includes diagnoses, outcomes, and interventions to promote optimal biophysical health.	III. **Psychosocial Domain:** Includes diagnoses, outcomes, and interventions to promote optimal mental and emotional health and social functioning.	IV. **Environmental Domain:** Includes diagnoses, outcomes, and interventions to promote and protect the environmental health and safety of individuals, systems, and communities.

Classes

Activity/Exercise—Physical activity, including energy conversation and expenditure.	**Cardiac Function**—Cardiac mechanisms used to maintain tissue profusion.	**Behavior**—Actions that promote, maintain, and restore health.	**Health Care System**—Social, political, and economic structures and processes for the delivery of health care services.
Comfort—A sense of emotional, physical, and spiritual well-being and relative freedom from distress.	**Elimination**—Processes related to elimination and excretion of body wastes.	**Communication**—Receiving, interpreting, and expressing spoken, written, and nonverbal messages.	**Populations**—Aggregates of individuals or communities having characteristics in common.
Growth and Development—Physical, emotional, and social growth and development milestones.	**Fluid and Electrolyte**—Regulation of fluids and electrolytes and acid base balance.	**Coping**—Adjusting and adapting to stressful events.	**Risk Management**—Avoidance or control of identified health threats.
Nutrition—Processes related to taking in, assimilating, and using nutrients.	**Neurocognition**—Mechanisms related to the nervous system and neurocognitive functioning, including memory, thinking, and judgment.	**Emotional**—A mental state of feeling that may influence perceptions of the world.	
Self-Care—Ability to accomplish basic and instrumental activities of daily living.	**Pharmacological Function**—Effects (therapeutic and adverse) of medications or drugs and other pharmacologically active products.	**Knowledge**—Understanding and skill in applying information to promote, maintain, and restore health.	

Table 15.3	Taxonomy of Nursing Practice (Continued)

Sexuality—Maintenance or modification of sexual identity and patterns.

Physical Regulation—Body temperature, endocrine and immune system responses to regulate cellular processes.

Roles/Relationships—Maintenance and/or modification of expected social behaviors and emotional connectedness with others.

Sleep/Rest—The quantity and quality of sleep, rest, and relaxation functions.

Reproduction—Processes related to human reproduction and birth.

Self-Perception—Awareness of one's body and personal identity.

Values/Beliefs—Ideas, goals, perceptions, spiritual and other beliefs that influence choices or decisions.

Respiratory Function—Ventilation adequate to maintain arterial blood gasses within normal limits.

Sensation/Perception—Intake and interpretation of information through the senses, including seeing, hearing, touching, tasting, and smelling.

Tissue Integrity—Skin and mucous membranes to support secretion, excretion, and healing.

structure should facilitate the identification of linkages among diagnoses, interventions, and outcomes and, thus, encourage research that examines the relationship. Nursing curricula can be designed using the structure as a framework. It is also possible that in time the structure's 28 classes will evolve into a common assessment tool usable by all nurses to collect and communicate patient data.

Conclusion

Having a nursing language facilitates communication among nurses and with other providers. Using nursing language can promote the following:

■ Describing the substantive content of the discipline.

- Defining the elements of care and assigning a cost based on the parameters such as complexity and acuity.
- Developing a database that can be analyzed and used to predict staffing mix and care requirements.
- Articulating the focus of nursing practice and nursing's unique contribution to patient care outcomes to other disciplines.

When nursing care is documented with standardized language, the resulting data can be aggregated and studied. The results of nursing care are known. Changes in practice can be made based on the results of research that used real clinical data. New avenues of research using clinical databases based on the documentation, actual care delivered, and outcomes achieved are opened. Nurses can study the cost and effectiveness of care.

The proposed Taxonomy of Nursing Practice is a structure specifically designed for the integration of NANDA, NIC, and NOC and can also be used by other language developers and others who desire to organize or index nursing content. Within this proposed framework, gaps in language about the human experience and the nurse–patient relationship can be identified and studied. The presentation of diagnoses, interventions, and outcomes in one unifying structure will facilitate teaching and use of the languages and will further the goals of the profession as they relate to delivering and assuring quality patient care. We believe that this effort in collaboration and harmonization is one more step toward a preferred future.

Epilogue: Continued Developments and Unifying Nursing Language

The recommendations put forth in the document *Unifying Nursing Languages: The Harmonization of NANDA, NIC, and NOC* (Dochterman & Jones, 2003) were subsequently addressed by NANDA and the Center for Nursing Classification at the University of Iowa, respectively. The results of this work were presented at the 2004 NNN Alliance meeting in Chicago held on June 29, 2004. In addition, each language classification group has continued to address the implementation of the proposed unified language structure in publications and presentations (Dochterman & Bulecheck, 2004; Moorhead, Johnson, & Maas, 2004; NANDA, 2005). Each group has also worked to place their existing languages into the unified structure and publish this work in an appendix to their current publications. This work will continue to be addressed in subsequent national meetings.

Placement Issues and Recommendations

For NANDA, all but 2 (deficit diversional activity and delayed surgical recovery) of the 167 nursing diagnoses approved in 2004 could be placed into the new structure. Reviewers found that the NNN taxonomy pointed to the need for more environmental nursing diagnoses, whereas the placement of risk diagnosis required further discussion and clarification.

Table 15.4	Comparison of the Number and Percent of Nursing Diagnoses (NANDA), Interventions (NIC), and Outcomes (NOC) by Domain		
Domain	NANDA	NIC	NOC
Functional	41 (25)	105 (20)	123 (37)
Psychological	54 (32)	220 (43)	69 (22)
Psychosocial	64 (38)	97 (18)	96 (29)
Environmental	6 (1)	90 (18)	35 (11)

NIC was able to place 514 interventions (2004) in the proposed domains. There was some concern that although all interventions may fit better in other classes (e.g., the knowledge class of interventions) they only placed one intervention in a class and decided that the issue may need further discussion. In addition, the placement of interventions in pharmacological function and health system were considered essential for inclusion in this harmonization structure. The group found placing the language into only four classes was less complex; not necessarily as effective as the current NIC structure but workable. This approach stressed the importance and need to continue working toward one structure that would reflect nursing diagnoses, interventions, and outcomes.

The group working on outcomes—NOC—placed all of their 330 (2004) nursing outcomes within the new structure. The use of one structure allowed for gaps to be more easily identified and could lead to the development of new nursing diagnoses, interventions, or outcomes.

The proposed unifying structure was considered by all three groups to be workable. In general, there was support to continue discussion and refinement of the structure and to make revisions as needed. The groups did agree that the proposed structure provided a visual picture of all three languages that may increase the use of nursing languages in teaching, practice, and documentation systems. In addition, it was thought by some that the standardization of nursing language could also be complemented by a standardized nursing assessment that would support evidence-based practice. Table 15.4 reflects the distribution of each language within the new structure.

Future Directions

The need for standardized nursing language is essential to the communication and documentation of nursing practice. The growth of nursing language and the implementation of nursing classifications into information systems within clinical practice settings continually grows. The American Nurses Association's (ANA) *Nursing Practice Information Infrastructure* (2006) has recently developed a Web site (http://www.nursingworld.org/npii/about.htm) to discuss standardized nursing languages and update nurses on national developments and standardized documentation. The ANA believes that standardizing nursing documentation will help reduce errors, promote patient safety, complement the electronic record of the future, and communicate quality and continuity of patient care by nurses.

As the development of nursing language grows internationally, it will create new opportunities for international nursing research and knowledge development. Work on the development of a standardized nursing language began nearly 35 years ago. It has experienced a continuous evolution over the years. There are currently 13 data sets, nomenclatures, and classification systems approved by the ANA. However, the need for unity in advancing standardized nursing language is critical. Although nursing language does not describe all of nursing practice, it does reflect the problems nurses solve, the judgments nurses make within their scope of practice, and the interventions used to achieve quality outcomes of care. For nursing to be visible, language developers will need to move toward a unified classification structure or a reference terminology that embraces the accomplishments of all language developers to enhance the impact of the nursing profession on patient care.

REFERENCES

American Nurses Association (ANA). (1995). *Nursing's Social Policy Statement.* Washington, DC: American Nurses Publishing American Nurses Association.

American Nurses Association (ANA). (1998). *Standards of Clinical Nursing Practice* (2nd ed.) Washington, D.C.: American Nurses Publishing, American Nurses Association.

American Nurses Association (ANA). (2006). *Nursing Practice Information Infrastructure* (http://www.nursingworld.org/npii/about.htm). Silver Spring, MD: American Nurses Association.

Coenen, A., McNeil, B., Bakken, S., Bickford, C., & Warren, J. J. (2001). Toward comparable nursing data: American Nurses Association criteria for data sets, classification systems and nomenclatures. *Computers in Nursing, 19*(6), 240–246.

Dochterman, J. M., & Jones, D. (2001). *Collaboration in nursing classification: A conference* (National Library of Medicine Conference Grant Proposal, R13 LM07243). Washington, DC: ANA.

Dochterman, J. M., & Jones, D. (Eds.). (2003). *Unifying nursing languages: The harmonization of NANDA, NIC, and NOC.* Silver Spring, MD: American Nurses Association.

Dochterman, J. M., & Bulechek, G. (Eds.). (2004). *Nursing interventions classification* (4th ed.). St. Louis, MO: Elsevier.

Donaldson, S. K., & Crowley, D. M. (1978). The discipline of nursing. *Nursing Outlook, 26,* 113–120.

Gebbie, K., & Lavin, M. (1975). *Proceedings of first national conference on classification of nursing diagnoses.* St. Louis, MO: Mosby.

Gordon, M. (1994). *Nursing diagnosis: Process and application.* New York: McGraw-Hill.

Johnson, M., Bulechek, G., Dochterman, J. M., Maas, M., & Moorhead, S. (2001). *Nursing diagnoses: outcomes, interventions: NANDA, NOC and NIC linkages.* St. Louis, MO: Mosby.

Johnson, M., Maas, M., & Moorhead, S. (Eds.). (2000). *Nursing outcomes classification* (2nd ed.). St. Louis, MO: Mosby.

Jones, D. (1997). "Nursing knowledge and outcomes: An integrative perspective." Linking nursing knowledge to practice outcomes: Knowledge impact conference

II proceedings. Ed. Roy, C. & Jones, D. Chestnut Hill, MA: Boston College Press. (p. 77).

Martin, K. S., & Scheet, N. J. (1992). *The Omaha System: Application for community health nursing.* Philadelphia: Saunders.

McCloskey, J. C., & Bulechek, G. M. (Eds.). (2000). *Nursing interventions classification* (3rd ed.). St. Louis, MO: Mosby.

Moorhead, S., Johnson, M., & Maas, M. (Eds.). (2004). *Nursing outcomes classification* (3rd ed.). St. Louis, MO: Mosby.

North American Nursing Diagnosis Association (NANDA). (2001). *Nursing diagnoses: Definitions and classification 2000–2001.* Philadelphia: NANDA

North American Nursing Diagnosis Association (NANDA). (2005). *Nursing diagnoses: Definitions and classification 2005–2006.* Philadelphia: NANDA

Saba, V. K. (1992). The classification of home health care nursing: Diagnoses and interventions. *Caring Magazine, 11*(3), 50–57.

Testimony presented at the National Committee on Vital and Health Statistics (NCVHS), Subcommittee. (1999) (testimony "Updates on Nursing Diagnoses Classification, by President, Dr. Dorothy Jones").

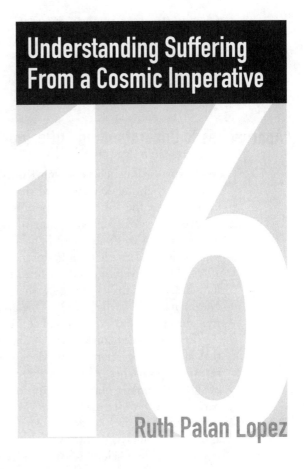

Understanding Suffering From a Cosmic Imperative

Ruth Palan Lopez

uffering has been a topic of concern for humanity from the beginning of time. Many disciplines, from theologians and philosophers to social scientists and international politicians, have struggled to understand the concept of suffering. Nurses also struggle with the suffering of humankind. Anyone who has supported a woman in childbirth, cared for a sick child, or attended to a dying elder has experienced suffering. Nurses have seen suffering on patients' faces, heard it in their cries, and felt it in their hearts. Despite the integral part suffering plays in nurses' work, knowledge development about this human response remains obscure and abstract. Can one examine, measure, or develop knowledge about a concept that may only be observed in patient responses to the experience but not the concept itself? Is it possible to make generalizations about suffering or is it so subjective that only the sufferer can have knowledge of it?

One answer to this paradox may be is found in Sister Callista Roy's paradigm of knowledge as a universal cosmic imperative. The philosophical underpinnings of this perspective provide the necessary support to examine the concept of suffering. Knowledge as a universal cosmic imperative provides not only a middle ground in the quantitative and qualitative debate, but most important, it provides a philosophical foundation that supports multiple theories and research methodologies. In this way knowledge is integrative. Knowledge as a universal imperative provides nurse scholars with vast possibilities for exploration of the complex concept of suffering. This chapter highlights Roy's philosophical assumptions and shows how they illuminate this author's theoretical model of suffering.

Approaches to Understanding Suffering

Many nurse scholars have acknowledged the central role that suffering plays in nursing. Florence Nightingale recognized that good nursing care could prevent suffering, "the symptoms or the sufferings generally considered to be inevitable and incident to the disease are very often not symptoms of the disease at all, but of something quite different— of the want of fresh air, or of light, or of warmth, or of quiet, or of cleanliness, or of punctuality and care in the administration of diet, or each or of all of these" (Nightingale, 1946, p. 6). Travelbee (1966) defined the task of the professional nurse as assisting the individual and families to cope with and find meaning in their illness and suffering. For Newman (1994), suffering offers the opportunity to transcend a situation and allows for transformation and expansion of consciousness.

In order to develop knowledge about suffering, nursing must work from a paradigm that allows integration of knowledge from many disciplines as well as from various research approaches. Although there is agreement on the significance of the concept of suffering among nurses, the approach to the phenomenon differs depending on the paradigm from which one operates. For nurse scholars, a paradigm provides a perspective from which research questions are asked, research is designed, methods are selected, and data are analyzed, interpreted, and applied (Monti & Tingen, 1999). A paradigm is important in a scientific community because it provides a framework for resolving problems, conducting research, and deriving theories and laws.

The concept of paradigm was popularized by Thomas Kuhn (1996) who primarily used the term to refer to a disciplinary matrix, shared beliefs, and values. Paradigms referred to exemplars or shared examples that students of a discipline learn and from this perspective they are able to solve similar disciplinary problems when they arise. Kuhn's work has been influential in nursing. For nearly 20 years, the notion of paradigm shifts has been accepted as a way of referring to a set of beliefs and assumptions about how knowledge develops within a discipline and explaining how and why ideas are formulated as they are (Thorne, Kirkham, & Henderson, 1999).

The Debate About Approaches to Knowledge

In the nursing literature, discourse about paradigms has primarily taken the form of a debate between those who use quantitative and qualitative methods (Stajduhar, Balneaves, & Thorne, 2001; Thorne et al., 1999). There is much discussion regarding the role of subjective and objective truths and for singular and multiple realities (Stajduhar et al., 2001). Although a gross generalization, for the purpose of pedagogy, the quantitative approach is exemplified by the paradigm of positivism and the qualitative approach is exemplified by the paradigm of interpretivism.

The ontology of positivism is a causal determinist view of reality. The world is predictable, knowable, and measurable. Reality is single, tangible, and can be understood as separate parts. In contrast, the interpretivism paradigm views reality as multiple, constructed, and holistic. Events can be explained and their meaning for people uncovered, but behavior cannot be predicted or controlled. Parts can only be understood in context.

From the perspective of positivism, the researcher and subject are considered independent. Knowledge arises from experimentation and observation. This is distinguished from the epistemology of interpretivism that holds that knowledge is grounded in empathic communication with the subjects of research. The investigator and subject of investigation are interactive and inseparable. Values are inseparable from the research process. In contrast, the positivist attempts to remove values and spirituality from the process of knowledge development.

When taken to their logical extremes, neither paradigm is not without its critique. Critics of the positivist paradigm complain that it is methodologically inadequate to study concepts and issues important to nursing. It has been called reductionistic, outmoded, and restrictive. It cannot be used to develop personal, ethical, or aesthetic knowledge (Chinn & Kramer, 2004). The positivist perspective provides an inadequate perspective to fully understand suffering because the concept is so abstract and immeasurable.

Alternatively, interpretivism has been criticized as relativistic and unable to establish guidelines for practice or make ethical or moral claims. The acceptance of multiple realities means that there cannot be generalizable knowledge. Further, the philosophy of rejection and destruction does not allow for reconstruction (Stevenson, 2001). Although helpful for developing knowledge related to personal and aesthetic knowing, it is inadequate for developing ethical knowledge. From this perspective, suffering is viewed as unique for each individual and generalizations about the phenomenon cannot be drawn.

Within a philosophical perspective, these two views of reality are incommensurate and mutually exclusive. This paradigm dispute is similar to a political debate in which neither side is willing to listen or hear one another. Rather than consider the other's complete argument in relation to its objective, the criticizer tends to attack a particular point out of context. The debaters tend to dismiss an entire theory if parts are considered inadequate. Furthermore, each side uses its own philosophical assumptions to frame the debate thereby playing the game using different rules. What is more, both sides personalize and exaggerate the opposition by using extreme positions such as logical positivism and relativism to propel their criticism (Peile, 1994).

Integration as an Alternative

The debate between singular and multiple realities detracts from the discipline's collective thrust toward knowledge that makes meaning and can be credibly applied within a practice discipline (Stajduhar et al., 2001). Knowledge that is useful for nurses requires integration. Fortunately, nurses are not bound to this all-or-nothing thinking. A resolution of the debate involves a synthesis of both sides. Not a mixture or compromise between the two, but the development of an entirely new paradigm that in a holistic way is more than the sum of its parts (Peile, 1994). This concept of synthesis is not unfamiliar to nurses. In clinical practice, nurses regularly demonstrate synthesis. For example, when identifying a patient problem from assessment data or understanding the pattern of the whole. Nurses recognize universals and commonalities but highly value uniqueness and individuality of person.

Stajduhar and colleagues described this synthesis as the "middle ground" position (Stajduhar et al., 2001). It is not sloppy or theoretically weak but supported by a rigorous and scholarly appreciation for the complexities inherent in a practice science. The result of synthesis can be the emergence of a worthy paradigm to guide the nursing discipline and promote a framework by which nurses can attend to general truths and the relational and contextual factors in any clinical situation. It must support research questions and methodological approaches that create knowledge applicable both to the general and to the particular, variation and common themes.

The Universal Cosmic Imperative

One such paradigm is presented by Sister Callista Roy (2001; chapter 10, this volume), in which knowledge is viewed as a universal cosmic imperative. Although the paradigm and its philosophical assumptions are based on the life and work of the theorist, Roy points to a sententious moment, at the 1983 Rogerian Conference in New York City. She was pondering the relativistic philosophical underpinnings of Rogers' work and contrasting these ideas to her own. As there was not a word in existence to capture the essence of her idea, she coined the term *veritivity* from the Latin word *veritas*, meaning truth. She marked the insight by drawing a light bulb on a piece of paper (C. Roy, personal communication, April 23, 2002). Roy has continued to refine and clarify the core premise of veritivity—that there is an absolute truth and a convergence of the universe into a unity of oneness with the truth, the creator (Roy, 2000).

Roy has contrasted three worldviews—rationalism, relativism, along with her new concept, vertitivity to discuss knowledge integration. The rationalist knows truth through empirical fact, and the relativist knows truth only in relation to the thinking person. For Roy, veritivity is knowing in its highest form and is the integration of the unity of truth. Veritivity is the absolute truth that leads to the values of conviction, commitment, and caring (Roy, 1988).

In 1995, Roy set the stage for the idea of the unity of knowledge by exploring the practice issues raised by the philosophical perspectives of realism, relativism, interpretivism, and humanism. She cautioned nurse scholars that truth does not lie unequivocally on one side or the other and foreshadowed the emergence of knowledge as a cosmic imperative as she described the "oneness of the rainbow" that one sees when looking at knowledge (p. 82).

At one of the nursing knowledge conferences described in the appendix, Roy expanded the philosophical assumptions of veritivity to explore the ontological and epistemological perspective of knowledge as universal imperative. The cosmic perspective includes unity, purposefulness, and promise. The perspective on knowledge is systematically supported on philosophical and scientific grounds and equally well supported by mysticism. Although seemingly unrelated, mystics, scientists, and philosophers all share an interest in the nature of reality, the struggle to attain a clear vision of reality, and the transformation of consciousness that accompanies such vision.

Unity

Knowledge viewed as a cosmic imperative provides the middle ground between the positivist who searches for the one true reality and the interpretivist who searches for multiple realities. Roy's philosophical assumption of unity demonstrates how one can find unity in diversity and is supported by noted philosophers and scientists. As an example, Roy cited Aristotle, who believed that all knowledge is of the universal. She also supported her assumptions with works by Pantheists that claim that a creator includes Himself in everything that is.

Kabbalah, Jewish mysticism, adds additional insights into the perspective of the cosmic imperative. The first characteristic of knowledge as cosmic imperative is unity. According to Kabbalah, creation is made up of spheres of consciousness. From the Creator's perspective, one would see that everything in creation is connected to a center, the source of creation (Cooper, 1997). As one raises the level of awareness, two things happen—one's perception of multiplicity dissolves, while at the same time, each level is reflecting all others. Similarly, if one examines a human being from a microscopic level, one sees a multitude of cells. But if one raises the level of awareness to the whole person, one sees just one person. One also could examine the family, the town, the Earth, the universe, and as the investigator raises the level of awareness, the boundaries dissolve and things become more and more unified. Yet, despite the fact that the boundaries disappear, each level is a reflection of all levels. If one chooses to see a town, it includes all the individuals and all their individual biological cells. Consequently, one can possess both unity and plurality at the same time. In the process, one can choose to focus on separateness or unity.

Purposefulness

Roy's second characteristic of purposefulness refers to the notion that both the universe and knowledge have meaning and purpose. She noted that a mechanistic view of immutable laws that control the motion and interaction of material objects was supported by Galileo and Newton's principles of classical dynamics. But, as a deeper understanding of the universe is gained, it becomes more and more evident that the universe did not happen by chance. When faced with the apparent randomness of relativity, Einstein said that he could not believe that God plays dice with the universe (White & Gribbin, 1994).

Kabbalah also provides a beautiful analogy that illustrates the essence of purposefulness. According to one of the central figures of Kabbalah, Rabbi Isaac Luria (1534–1572) held that during creation, the vessels containing the light of creation shattered, and the light became concealed as holy sparks. Every particle and being in our physical universe contains sparks of holiness. Our task, according to Luria, is to release each spark from the shell and raise it up to return to its original state. The sparks are raised through acts of loving kindness, of being in harmony with the universe, and through higher awareness (Cooper, 1997).

Promise

The promise for the future that is the characteristic of the cosmic imperative and is based on the conviction that together people will decide what kind of a universe we will inhabit and that creation will converge toward an omega point. Roy (chapter 10, this volume) supported the philosophical assumption of a future convergence in an omega point with work from a Christian paleontologist, de Chardin, and an atheist physicist, Tipler. Both wrote about a coming together in a final end point of singularity. The promise for the future lies in human participation in transformation (Roy, 1996). Roy used the work of Swimme and Berry (1992) to support the notion that we are now entering a period of creativity in which the entire earth community will participate, and together people will decide what kind of universe we will inhabit.

This sentiment is echoed by one of the major tenets of Kabbalah, the world is an integrated whole, not a collection of parts. We are not just individuals, but are integral members of a global community. Support is also garnered by the teaching that The Holy One found it necessary to create all the things in the world so that there should be a central light of awareness with many vessels encircling it (Cooper, 1997). Rabbi Zalman Schachter-Shalomi, World Wisdom Chair at Naropa Institute and a pioneer in efforts to foster interfaith dialogue, was quoted as saying, "The flag does not wave in the wind; the wind does not wave the flag. The flag and the wind are interweaving" (p. 14). Similarly, human beings are an integral part of creation and creating. The actions of women and men are significant. One word, one thought, one gesture, can change the direction of the creative process.

Roy summarized her philosophical assumptions for the 21st century as: Persons have mutual relationships with the world and with a God figure; human meaning is rooted in an omega point convergence of the universe; God is intimately revealed in the diversity of creation and is the common destiny of creation; persons use human creative abilities of awareness, enlightenment, and faith; and persons are accountable for the processes of driving, sustaining, and transforming the universe (Roy, 1997; Roy & Andrews, 1999, chapter 10, this volume).

A Theoretical Model of Suffering

Theory is a set of statements that tentatively describe, explain, or predict relationships between concepts that have been selected and organized as an abstract representation of some phenomenon. It is a plan showing "where you are, what you may try to do, and where you may choose to go" (Morse, 1996, p. 75). Similarly, the theoretical model of suffering presented here is a tentative representation of the current thinking of this author. It is the current state of a work in progress (see Figure 16.1).

Suffering involves an experience or sensation that is perceived by the individual and interpreted as painful or harmful and causes the individual to experience in his

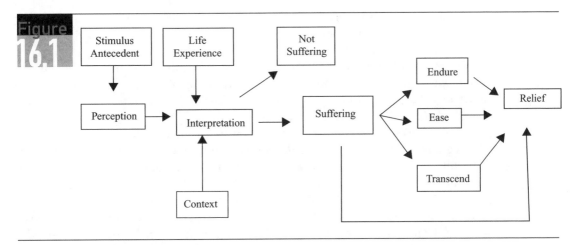

Proposed theoretical model of suffering (Lopez, 2006).

or her whole being in a sense of distress. Proposed components of the model include stimuli, perception, and interpretation. Interpretation is influenced by life experience and context. The consequence of suffering is endurance, ease, or transcendence. The final concept in the model is relief.

Stimuli—Antecedents to Suffering

There are many potential antecedents to suffering. Although suffering and pain are often used interchangeably, it is clear from the literature that although suffering may be associated with pain, one can suffer from offenses other than pain, and experience pain without suffering. Copp (1974) found that the patients' response to pain, which she called suffering, began even before the pain and included many anticipatory fears that sometimes were even more acute than the eventual pain. Chapman and Gavrin (1993) examined the relationship between pain and suffering in cancer. They suggested that pain and suffering are related concepts that share the common ground of negative emotion, but the relationship was seen as imperfect. The suffering of patients with cancer was discussed not merely as physical but as having multiple causes, including psychological and social origins. Starck (1992) examined the extent to which the management of suffering was a feature of the nursing home organization and found that elderly people in nursing homes suffered from multiple losses, including physiologic, psychosocial, and economic, as well as losses of the human spirit. Simply using a biomedical model and equating suffering with pain runs the risk of overlooking all the other contributing factors to suffering such as the existential, emotional, and spiritual.

Perception—Characteristics of the Person Who Suffers

In order to progress to suffering, the stimulus must be perceived by the individual. A person who does not have perception of a painful stimulus or recognize a distressing event will not proceed to suffer. One's perception of a stimulus can be altered by such things as anesthesia, neurological impairments, or pharmacologic agents. In addition, altered cognition as in dementia can effect how one perceives a stimulus.

Cassell (1982, 1991) maintained that in order to suffer, one must be a knowing person with a sense of past, future, aims, and purpose. The defining characteristic of suffering included the presence of perceptual capacity (sentience), factors undermining quality of life, and an aversive experience. According to this definition, suffering is a phenomenon of conscious human existence that appears to require high-level cognition. This requirement for high-level cognition appears to exclude people with dementia from being vulnerable to suffering. However, clinical experience and common sense finds that this is not the case. Persons with dementia are at profound risk for suffering. Although people with dementia may loose their public and social selves as a result of how they are perceived by others, research indicates that the private sense of self persists into the late stages of the illness (Downs, 1997; Small, Geldart, Gutman, & Scott, 1998). Everyday living can produce profound suffering in people who may perceive family members as strangers and become lost in their own homes.

Life Experience and Context

Suffering is an intensely subjective, holistic experience that has been expressed in the biography and lived world experiences of patients (Gregory, 1994). Kahn and Steeves (1986) described suffering as a private lived experience of a whole person, unique to each individual. Although a person may experience pain or discomfort in one particular body part, only the entire person experiences suffering. In addition, it is the person's evaluation of the experience that may cause suffering and not the experience itself.

What one person may find intolerable another may not find as offensive. In addition, what may cause suffering for an individual in one setting or time, may in another place and time not be as distressing. The context of the experience also seems to play a role in whether a perceived stimulus will be interpreted as suffering. If a tragedy is considered needless or senseless, for example, in some way that adds to the burden of misery. Similarly, if suffering is the consequence of a futile treatment or intervention, suffering is enhanced.

Interpretation

An individual may suffer or not suffer based on his or her interpretation of the stimulus or event. For example, a person who is a piano virtuoso may suffer from a hand injury, whereas another individual may find the injury inconvenient and painful, but it may not produce suffering. Suffering originates in the meaning or lack of meaning that one finds in the experience. According to Frankl (1984), the founder of logotherapy, man's search for meaning is the primary motivation in his life (p. 105). This meaning is specific and unique in that it can and must be fulfilled by the individual. Thus, people find or create meaning for themselves.

The human propensity to interpret all events and experiences has encouraged many thinkers to conclude that a fundamental need or drive for meaning is an innate part of the human mind. People seek meaning in ordinary events just as they seek meaning in life generally. The same factors that guide the effort to make sense out of life in general shape the daily efforts to make sense out of individual experiences. According to Sommer and Baumeister (1998), people have four basic needs for meaning. People need a sense of purpose in life and want to perceive their current activities as relating to future outcomes. People desire a feeling of efficacy or control and seek to interpret events in ways that support the belief that they have control over their outcomes. In addition, people want to view their actions as having value and being morally justified. Finally, people want a sense of positive self-worth. They seek ways to establish that they are good, admirable, and worthy individuals with desirable traits. Threats to a person's ability to find meaning in an experience may cause a person to suffer.

Consequences of Suffering—Endure, Ease, Transcend, Relief

Suffering has meaning in itself. Although one would not advocate causing suffering, people can grow, mature, and find meaning through suffering. There are four consequences of suffering: endure, ease, transcendence, and relief. Patients can endure suffering. While enduring, the person is living the experience of suffering. Suffering is eased when the experience, although still present, is less intense.

Suffering can be also be transcended. A person who transcends suffering is able to find meaning despite the misery of the circumstance. Although at times man is helpless to change a situation, he is capable of changing himself (Frankl, 1984). Nurses cannot change their patients or find meaning for them. But nurses' holistic model of care, which incorporates community and emphasizes the uniqueness of the individual, supports people as they struggle to find meaning.

Ultimately, nurses want to relieve the suffering of their patients. There are times when nurses can remove the antecedent to suffering and assist the patient to find relief. However, there are times when patients face suffering that nurses are powerless to ameliorate. Not all suffering can be prevented, relieved, eased, or transcended. During such times of suffering, the nurse can be present, to assist the patient to endure and find meaning in the experience. Suffering is a human experience in which nurses take part.

Application of the Paradigm to the Model

The paradigm of knowledge as a cosmic imperative illuminates the theoretical model of suffering and provides direction and energy to investigate the concepts and draw propositions. The core of the perspective is the assumption of verivitity with the three characteristics of unity, purposefulness, and promise related to the suffering model.

Individuals and Universals

The highly individualistic, subjective nature of suffering would make it nearly impossible to study using a positivistic paradigm. In contrast, the interpretivistic paradigm's focus on multiple realities would allow for an investigation of one person's experience of suffering, but it does not allow for generalization about the experience. Roy's assumption of diversity within unity supports the study of individual's experiences of suffering, while at the same time, sustains the notion of a universal truth within the experience. One can study the individual and one's uniqueness or raise the level of awareness to find unity or commonality in the phenomenon. Roy's assumption of unity supports a phenomenological methodology whereby one examines many persons' lived experiences to find the essences of the phenomenon, that is, the commonalities or universals.

Common Purposefulness

The philosophical assumption of purposefulness and meaning provides energy at many levels. For the nurse providing care to suffering people, purposefulness is the energy that fuels his or her motivation and caring actions. Purposefulness and the search for meaning also help move suffering people through the experience as shown in the proposed model of suffering (Fig. 16.1). The search for meaning can ultimately be at the root of the suffering experience, whereas finding purpose and meaning is the end to suffering. Likewise, purposefulness drives the nurse researcher who searches for answers to questions on how to ease and relieve suffering.

Just as the flag and wind can be seen as "interweaving," the nurse, patient, and the family can be seen as "intersuffering." As a witness to human suffering, one may ask, "Who is suffering?" Is it the patient, the patient's family, or those providing care? The suffering of these groups are inextricably interrelated such that the perceived distress of any one may amplify the distress of the others (Cherny, Coyle, & Foley, 1994). Empathic distress results from the perception by the patient of the distress his or her condition is having on family, friends, and caregivers. This can contribute to a perception that his or her ongoing existence is causing the distress of others. In addition, family members and caregivers can experience empathic distress from the suffering of the patient.

Rogers (1994) uses the term *pandimensionality* to express a nonlinear domain whereby human beings are connected in such a way that another's suffering can become incorporated into one's own life. Empathic suffering can occur when a patient, the family, and/or the caregivers suffer as a result of empathizing with the suffering of another. From a unitary perspective, the suffering of humankind everywhere is the suffering of all (Nelson, 2001). Likewise, as Roy has noted, all persons share a common purposefulness.

Promise in Suffering

Similarly, the promise for the future lies in human participation in the search for meaning and in transcending suffering. Roy's philosophical assumption of promise supports the view that creation is not completed but is constantly becoming, evolving, and ascending. Yet all human beings share a common destiny. According to Kabbalah, a person can be transported from a place where there is nothing new to a place where there is nothing old, where everything renews itself (Matt, 1995, p. 99). From the perspective of the universal cosmic imperative, nurses have the capability and potential for healing the world.

Future Knowledge Development

A rich understanding of the concept of suffering is made possible by using Roy's paradigm to frame our understanding of suffering. Many propositions can be drawn from the model of suffering as illuminated by the cosmic imperative. The concepts in this theoretical model are abstract and, in their current state, immeasurable. However, propositional statements lend themselves to research questions and verification. Examples of propositional statements include:

- Certain stimuli are more likely to cause suffering.
- Altering the level of perception will alter the potential for suffering.
- Certain life experiences make people more resilient or more prone to suffering.
- Nurses are able to identify suffering in patients.
- Working with patients who are suffering may cause suffering in the nurse.
- Purposefulness and meaning have a protective effect on suffering.

Conclusion

The major advantage of knowledge as a universal cosmic imperative is that it provides the middle ground position as described by Stajduhar et al. (2001). It supports an ontology whereby there can be one reality with diverse perspectives. Accordingly, epistemologically, knowledge can be developed for both individualizations and generalizations. The paradigm is capable of guiding the nursing discipline to appreciate general truths and contextual factors in any clinical situation. It supports both qualitative and quantitative methods. The assumptions are rigorous and supported with scholarship.

Knowledge as a universal cosmic imperative is a relatively new paradigm, developed by a nurse theorist for the discipline of nursing. It is rigorously supported by the work of scholars ranging from Aristotle and de Chardin, to Issac Luria and Rabbi Zalman Schachter-Shalomi. As suggested by Peile (1994), it is not a compromise in the quantitative versus qualitative debate, but an entirely new paradigm that in a holistic way is more than the sum of its parts. It brightly illuminates the concepts and linkages in this author's theoretical model of suffering and will support the investigation of this concept using both qualitative and quantitative methods.

REFERENCES

Cassell, E. J. (1982). The nature of suffering and the goals of medicine. *The New England Journal of Medicine*, *306*(11), 639–645.

Cassell, E. J. (1991). Recognizing suffering. *Hastings Center Report*, *21*(3), 24–31.

Cherny, N. I., Coyle, N., & Foley, K. M. (1994). Suffering in the advanced cancer patient: A definition and taxonomy. *Journal of Palliative Care*, *10*(2), 57–70.

Chapman, C. R., & Gavrin, J., (1993). Suffering and its relationship to pain. *Journal of Palliative Care Medicine*, 9(1), pp. 5–13.

Chinn, P. L., & Kramer, M. K. (2004). *Integrated knowledge development in nursing*. St. Louis: Mosby.

Cooper, D. A. (1997). *God is a verb*. New York: Riverhead Books.

Copp, L. A. (1974). The spectrum of suffering. *American Journal of Nursing, 74*, 491–495.

Downs, M. (1997). The emergence of the person in dementia research. *Aging and Society, 17*, 597–607.

Frankl, V. E. (1984). *Man's search for meaning* (3rd ed.). New York: Simon and Schuster.

Gregory, D. (1994). The myth of control: Suffering in palliative care. *Journal of Palliative Care, 10*(2), 18–22.

Kahn, D. L., & Steeves, R. H. (1986). The experience of suffering: Conceptual clarification and theoretical definition. *Journal of Advanced Nursing, 11*, 623–631.

Kuhn, T. S. (1996). *The structure of scientific revolutions* (3rd ed.). Chicago: The University of Chicago Press.

Matt, D. C. (1995). *The essential Kabbalah: The heart of Jewish mysticism*. New York: HarperCollins.

Monti, E. J., & Tingen, M. S. (1999). Multiple paradigms of nursing science. *Advance of Nursing Science, 21*(4), 64–80.

Morse, J. M. (1996). Nursing scholarship: Sense and sensibility. *Nursing Inquiry, 3*, 74–82.

Nelson, M. L. (2001). Helping students to know and respond to human suffering. *Nursing Science Quarterly, 14*(3), 202–204.

Newman, M. A. (1994). *Health as expanding consciousness* (2nd ed.). New York: NLN.

Nightingale, F. (1946). *Notes on nursing: What it is, and what it is not*. Philadelphia: Lippincott.

Peile, C. (1994). *The creative paradigm*. Aldershot, UK: Avebury.

Rogers, M. E. (1994). The science of unitary human beings: Current perspectives. *Nursing Science Quarterly, 5*, 27–34.

Roy, C. (1995). Developing nursing knowledge: Practice issues raised from four philosophical perspectives. *Nursing Science Quarterly, 8*(2), 79–85.

Roy, C. (1988). An explication of the philosophical assumptions of the Roy adaptation model. *Nursing Science Quarterly, 1*, 26–34.

Roy, C. (1997). Future of the Roy model: Challenge to redefine adaptation. *Nursing Science Quarterly, 10*(1), 42–48.

Roy, C. (2000). The visible and invisible fields that shape the future of the nursing care system. *Nursing Administration Quarterly, 25*(1), 119–131.

Roy, C. (2001, October 25–27). *Knowledge as cosmic imperative and impact on the health care system*. Paper presented at the Knowledge Impact Conference, Newton, MA.

Roy, C., & Andrews, H. A. (1999). *The Roy adaptation model* (2nd ed.). Stamford, CT: Appleton & Lange.

Small, J. A., Geldart, K., Gutman, G., & Scott, M. A. C. (1998). The discourse of self in dementia. *Ageing and Society, 18*, 291–316.

Sommer, K. L., & Baumeister, R. F. (1998). The construction of meaning from life events: Empirical studies of personal narratives. In P. T. P. Wong & P. S. Fry (Eds.), *The human quest for meaning* (pp. 143–161). Mahwah, NJ: Lawrence Erlbaum Associates.

Stajduhar, K. I., Balneaves, L., & Thorne, S. E. (2001). A case for the "middle ground": Exploring the tensions of postmodern thought in nursing. *Nursing Philosophy, 2*(1), 72–82.

Starck, P. L. (1992). The management of suffering in a nursing home: An ethnographic study. In P. L. Starck (Ed.), *The hidden dimension of illness: Human suffering* (NLN Publication No. 15-2461; pp. 127–153). New York: National League for Nursing (NLN).

Stevenson, C. (2001). Paradigms lost, paradigms regained: Defending nursing against a single reading of postmodernism. *Nursing Philosophy*, *2*, 143–150.

Swimme, B., & Berry, T. (1992). *The universe story*. San Francisco: Harper.

Thorne, S., Kirkham, S. R., & Henderson, A. (1999). Ideological implications of paradigm discourse. *Nursing Inquiry*, *6*, 123–131.

Travelbee, J. (1966). *Interpersonal aspects of nursing*. Philadelphia: Davis.

White, M., & Gribbin, J. (1994). *Einstein: A life in science*. New York: Penguin.

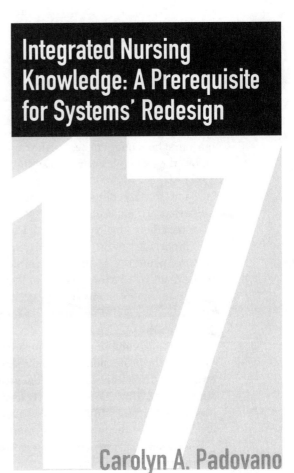

Integrated Nursing Knowledge: A Prerequisite for Systems' Redesign

Carolyn A. Padovano

A s nurses in the new millennium, we are challenged to transform the health care system and advance nursing's preferred future. Using integrated nursing knowledge for practice has been cited as paramount throughout the years by nurse scholars. "If we can not name it, we can not control it, finance it, teach it, research it, or put it into public policy" (Clark & Lange, 1992, p. 109). More than a decade since the authors made this statement nurses lack unity around knowledge needed for practice and useful strategies to communicate that knowledge to others. The development of nursing knowledge for practice has proliferated. Programs of research that name, describe, and relate phenomena of practice and its outcomes have increased. However, the ongoing challenge continues to be nursing's inability to speak with one voice as the profession strives to be a leader in the health care industry by facilitating systems' redesign.

This chapter examines the elements required to successfully transform the health care environment in this new millennium. Responding to the challenge articulated by Clark and Lange, the key formula we will explore, is as follows: Integrated Nursing Knowledge + Integrated Nursing Systems + Integrated Public Policies = INTEGRATED HEALTH CARE.

Premises and Approach

The first component of the formula, integrated nursing knowledge, contains three characteristics or guiding principles described by Roy (chapter 10, this volume). The principles that serve as the framework for this discussion of an integrated nursing knowledge perspective include unity, purposefulness, and promise. I propose that unity of knowledge must first be brought to bear as the fundamental requisite for redesigning nursing systems before the principles of purposefulness and promise can be realized (Padovano Corliss, 1997).

The second component of the formula, integrated nursing systems, contains four areas that are most crucial to redesigning systems in nursing. These include ethical systems, educational systems, practice systems, and technological systems. To highlight the importance of an integrated nursing knowledge perspective in redesigning these systems in nursing, I will give examples where nursing has limited success in responding to the challenge "name it, control it, finance it, teach it, and research it." Bridging the gaps in nursing systems will give nurses the ability to take a stand on exactly what the profession represents to itself and to society; hence, succeeding in the challenge to name it and thereby to have an impact.

The third component of the formula, integrated public policies, considers three levels on which the profession must understand issues affecting the patient and the health care environment. Within this component, are levels in which the profession must actively participate within the health care arena to evoke change. The three levels include the professional, the institutional, and the societal. Nursing action to integrate these three levels can make the nursing profession a force in public policy.

The final premise is that by transforming nursing systems and public policies based on integrated nursing knowledge, nursing is capable of ultimately integrating our health care system. When this is accomplished our profession will have evolved into our preferred future of redesigned health care systems where nurses are leaders in making the systems effective in meeting health needs. This is the outcome term of the formula.

The Need for Integrated Nursing Knowledge

Nurse scholars have articulated their concern that the profession has few consistent definitions of terms used by nurses and little consensus on standards, for some time. They have recommended that agreements on these foundational issues are necessary to avoid professional exclusion and/or extinction within the health care arena. As exhibited in the nursing literature and in an international study, *Universals of Nursing: Consensus and Action* (Padovano Corliss, 1994), nursing has continued to deliberate on the body of knowledge that represents the profession. A landmark study conducted by the International Council of Nursing (ICN) Board of Directors served as the catalyst for revisiting this discussion (Styles, 1995) on a global level. The ICN examined the legal and political positions of the nursing profession by analyzing the uniformity in the profession's regulatory systems worldwide. The study purported that the concept of nursing had no singular, universal meaning across countries. Additionally, there were no consistent standards for education or practice across countries, internationally. As a result, several nursing groups began to reexamine whether or not commonalties in nursing language and standards were actually available (Clark & Lange, 1992).

A common understanding of what nursing means and a common language used to describe nursing practice are basic to integrated nursing knowledge (see chapter 15, this volume). This is an initial step in reaching the desired goal of integrated health care. Support for integrated nursing knowledge has been discussed not only in historical debates, but it has also been met with acceptance in current scientific literature and conferences. An example is the series of conferences held in the northeastern part of the United States between the 1980s and 2001 (Appendix, this volume). During this era, nurse scholars from around the world convened to discuss emerging nursing knowledge. The highlight of these conferences occurred in 1998 when a consensus statement (see chapter 1, this volume) was developed on the nature of the person, the nature of nursing, the role of nursing theory, and the linkages between understanding of person, nursing, and theory related to nursing practice.

Redesign of the Four Nursing Systems

The significance of integrated knowledge can be seen by examining the four nursing systems on which the profession needs to focus to affect practice. Knowledge integration underlies change in ethical, educational, practice, and technological systems, thus supporting health care redesign.

The Ethical System: The "Name It" Challenge

Nursing, like other service professions, has a social mandate to develop knowledge and practice for the good of society and its individual members. Nursing practice takes place largely within the health care delivery system. However, the goals and commitments of the profession necessitate ongoing scrutiny both of the immediate practice environment and of the wider context in which health care occurs. In a time of health care crisis, nurses are the major moral voices on health care issues. We focus on the moral implications of and professional responsibilities related to promoting the health and flourishing of individuals within society. Although it is widely recognized that the current United States health care system is disorganized and chaotic, there remains less agreement about the best way to reorganize the system to provide quality and equitable care. The moral challenges of contemporary health care provision are multiple and complex, requiring the highest level of ethical knowledge. Grace (1998) identifies that professional advocacy includes the challenge to accurately conceptualize the source and implications of problems in order to address them on behalf of the social good. Given that the primary focus of health care delivery has shifted from the good of the person to the economic bottom line, a strong articulation of values related to the social good and nurses' concomitant moral commitment are crucial.

The level of integrated knowledge related to ethical and moral accountabilities is best understood by examining the basic documents in which the profession addresses these issues. *Nursing's Social Policy Statement* and *The Code of Ethics for Nurses with Interpretive Statements* developed by the American Nurses' Association (ANA) as well as federal, state, and international statutory regulations, are the existing records of this undertaking. *Nursing's Social Policy Statement* is the U.S. document that explains to society what nursing is and describes the profession's mission. The first draft of the policy statement was circulated by the ANA Congress for Nursing Practice in 1980. The purpose of this policy statement was to define the scope of nursing practice, including specialization. In it, the precise definition stated is that nursing is "the diagnosis and treatment of human responses to actual or potential health problems" (American Nurses Association, 1980). In addition, theory application, nursing action, and evaluation were described. A task force of the ANA Congress for Nursing Practice developed the 1995 revision with significant input from the various units of the professional organization. The effort of this task force was to present clinical nursing practice within the evolving health needs of society and to set a direction for the future. Rather than a specific definition of nursing, this revision focused on essential features of nursing practice and dealt more specifically with advanced nursing practice (American Nurses Association, 1995).

Incongruities in earlier statements evoked action among nursing specialty groups that led to the revision of the document (American Nurses Association, 2003). The three major components of the current statement concern the definition of nursing, the knowledge base for nursing practice, and regulation of nursing practice. This version clearly builds on the earlier statements. Specifically, the policy statement names underlying values and assumptions in statements such as "humans manifest an essential unity of mind, body, and spirit"; "humans' experience is contextually and culturally defined"; and "the interaction between nurse and patient occurs within the context of the values and beliefs of the patient and the nurse" (p. 3). The document provides both a statement of nursing's professional stewardship and to express nursing's continuing commitment to the society to whom it is accountable.

The Code of Ethics for Nurses has also been revised. The initial version was published in 1985 and later an extended process led to major changes. Nurses believed that although core nursing values were identified in the early version, the document did not provide timely guidance for practice. The ANA established a task force in 1996 (Michigan Nurses Association, 1997), which summoned input from all ANA members at the national and state levels throughout 1997. In 1998 a revised version of the initial code was sent to the Ethics Committee and with their input a draft was presented for adoption at the ANA Convention in 1998. However, the House of Delegates recommended that the final version expand and clarify the Code of Ethics as it related to ethical decisions and nursing actions (Thompson, 1998). Thus, additional work was done to complete the document. The revised code (American Nurses Association, 2001) includes nine provisions and interpretive statements that emphasize the nurse's role as a patient advocate and the obligation to protect the health of the public. The language of the revision takes into account the vast challenges in the nurse's work environment in the 21st century.

Both of these documents represent nursing as articulated by the major professional organization. They are far reaching and broad in their application, with some amount of consensus. For example, domestic and international codes of ethics for nurses (International Council of Nurses, 2000) are in agreement in their tenet to safeguard society from illegal, incompetent, and unethical parties. However, they encompass many, but not all, of the concerns related to defining the nursing profession. Further, as Sawyer (1989) noted, the mere existence of several, independent codes of ethics evidences a yet nonunified knowledge base. This fragmentation is further noted with the increasing numbers of specialty organizations that address similar issues from the perspective of their particular memberships. It is, therefore, paramount for nursing to refine these documents on an ongoing basis to reflect professional unity and collaboration.

Further, the pervasive import of federal, state, and international statutory regulations provide additional exemplars concerning the necessity for unity of knowledge. Statutory schemes expressly, although often ambiguously, delineate the boundaries and restrictions within which nurses are allowed to practice. In *The Nursing Regulation: Moving Ahead* project, initiated by the International Council of Nursing with the support of the W. K. Kellogg Foundation and other development agencies, a worldwide study was conducted involving 77 countries (Affara & Styles, 1990). The findings exhibited (a) inadequate and restrictive definitions of nursing, (b) expressions of scopes of practice that precluded nurses from practicing according to their education and experience, (c) inconsistent use of terminology, (d) varying degrees of government control in nursing practice, (e) lack of consensus on categories of nursing personnel, (f) a spectrum of role responsibility and accountability, (g) multiple standards for competency, and (h) a multitude of credentialing procedures.

In the United States, the National Council of State Boards of Nursing took a major step toward consistency in standards in 1999 by adopting uniform licensure requirements for Registered Nurses (RNs) and Licensed Practical Nurses (LPNs)/Licensed Vocational Nurses (LVNs). This unity was achieved by "willingness to place emphasis on the public good; willingness to compromise; and willingness to trust other boards" (National Council of State Boards of Nursing, 1999). Although increased consistency in licensure requirements is recognized as appropriate in a world in which nurses and patients cross state lines, this same consistency has not been extended to the advanced practice level. Uniform Advanced Practice Registered Nurse Licensure/Authority to Practice Requirements have been proposed, but not yet acted on.

The worldwide and U.S. regulatory situation provides a challenge for the profession to move toward unity of nursing knowledge needed to redesign its ethical system. The redesigned system is derived from and further affects the principles of purposefulness and the promise of integrated knowledge. The construction of uniform nursing and statutory documents will include legal definitions of practice, licensing laws, and employment, health care, and reimbursement policies. In this way, the goal of unity of nursing knowledge is reinitiated and the cycle continues. Nurses will inevitably attain the common purposefulness of accountability through an improved understanding of what is practiced, how one practices, where one can practice, and what benefits one will derive from this practice. With these changes nurses can be thus in a position to identify, assert, and certify their status to the public, to employers, and among the health care professions.

In addition, the purposefulness of this knowledge is recognized by society when people can feel with conviction that they are better protected from fraud, abuse, and incompetence. It is axiomatic that the promise of nursing knowledge and the future of nursing will become less an elusive idea and more a reality when the ethical system is redesigned. The refocused vision will use professional nurses as effective advocates, proposing and creating legislation that will affect future generations. The continuity of the cycle is ensured when nurses strive to achieve, refine, and maintain unity of knowledge through collaboration within the redesigned ethical system.

The Educational System: The "Teach It" Challenge

The key area that derives from and shows the impact of the unity of nursing knowledge on the nursing profession is its educational system. The ramifications are identified in three substantive categories: the entry level into practice debate, the development and design of nursing curricula, and the accreditation of academic institutions. These topics of frequent contention are representative of significant issues affecting the nursing profession. The issue of a clear knowledge base is even more crucial in education as the faculty shortage deepens and, as a result, potential students are denied admission to nursing programs. Ultimately, this worsens the shortage of nurses to provide care for an aging population.

The discussion concerning entry level for professional nursing and related requirements has been documented since the late 1940s (Brown, 1948). This lack of unity around entry levels was noted as late as 1990 when one survey identified that of 61 responding state boards of nursing only 23 had a formal position on entry (Styles, Allen, Armstrong, Matsuura, Stannard, & Ordway, 1991). In fact, the uniform core licensure requirements (National Council of State Boards of Nursing, 1999) clearly state that "state-approved registered nursing programs are all types of programs designed to prepare individuals for entry into practice and RN licensure, including diploma, associate degree, baccalaureate, generic master's and nursing doctoral programs" (p. 3). Incredibly, having one preparation for entry into the nursing profession remains as enigmatic and unattainable as it was nearly 65 years ago. The lack of clarity about essential knowledge and educational requirements for professional nursing practice is the prima facie evidence of the need for unity of nursing knowledge.

The literature continues to report that the most widely recognized legal mechanism for ensuring basic competence for entry into practice remains licensure. However, in an attempt to respond to the rapidly changing health care environment and to ensure accountability to patients, the American Nurses Credentialing Center (ANCC) also recognizes certification as an indicator of competence. The Open Door 2000 program has expanded this function. This 21st-century model of credentialing allows nurses to demonstrate competence over the lifetime of their career. For example, the program offers differing levels of certification for associate degree and diploma prepared registered nurses, and offers higher levels or board certifications for nurses with baccalaureate and higher preparation (Maryland Nurses Association, 2000). This is one step toward the desired systems redesign.

Curricula development and design is a second area where fragmentation is pervasive. Several authors support reconstructing nursing's educational curricula altogether. For example, the role of nursing history and the inclusion of liberal arts education have been cited as imperative, not elective, content for nursing students (Keeling & Ramos, 1995). A related review of the literature by van Maanen (1990) noted that American nursing theories evolved from knowledge of the sciences, whereas European nursing models appeared to have evolved from knowledge of the humanities. The diverse beginning points and the lack of blending of multiple realities both derive from and contribute to the lack of collaboration in knowledge development. The inability to converge on universal knowledge, compromises nursing's ability to effect change and promote the common, national or global good.

Education Systems and Accreditation

The absence of uniform, mandatory mechanisms for the accreditation of academic institutions is a further instance where having unity of nursing knowledge would be beneficial to the profession, its students, and society. Fragmentation not only exists in the structure of nursing curricula as noted, but it also exists when choosing an accreditation agency for nursing schools. In one study of nursing schools,

> findings revealed that nearly a quarter of respondents intend to continue with the National League of Nursing Accrediting Commission (NLNAC), whereas thirty percent indicated they have already switched to the Commission on Collegiate Nursing Education (CCNE) or intend to do so. (Bellack, Gelmon, O'Neil, & Thomsen, 1999, p. 53)

However, half of the remaining respondent schools stated that they intend to be accredited by both agencies, whereas the other half stated that they were undecided. The authors concluded that this is an end to single-source school accreditation and a beginning of a new market-oriented approach. Although no further studies of this kind have been reported, in the fifth year of its program, the CCNE reported that more than 60% of existing baccalaureate and master's degree programs had affiliated with the American Association of Colleges of Nursing (AACN)–sponsored process (American Association of Colleges of Nursing, 2002). The inherent fragmentary process of *choose your own standard* has the potential to further nursing liabilities and create detrimental health outcomes for patients.

The challenge for the profession to focus on unity of nursing knowledge in redesigning its educational system will further affect the principle of purposefulness. Accomplishing closure with respect to entry-level requirements acts as the springboard for starting the cycle of unity of knowledge.

Purposefulness of Knowledge

Purposefulness of knowledge is reflected as standards of curricula development and design, when they are envisioned and become tangible. As new curricula models emerge, they will hopefully enable convergence of theory and clinical teachings yet at the same time promote multiple realities and theoretical diversity. In turn, commonalities in education can trigger effective and uniform regulations for accreditation from governmental entities and protect the public from harm caused by lack of knowledge. Consistent with the cyclical premise, is the promise of knowledge activated as future students and faculty receive assistance and warranties for identifying accredited institutions. Unity of knowledge can be the common basis for modifying and improving standards.

The Practice System: The "Control It, Finance It" Challenge

Unity of knowledge within the nursing profession is particularly significant in the practice arena. The ramifications associated with unity of nursing knowledge for practice becomes apparent when scrutinizing *The Nursing Standards of Practice* and the accreditation process of health care institutions. These guidelines for nursing practice, despite differences in their values, tenets, and ideologies of an originating group, are inevitably incorporated in some manner by all nursing individuals, groups, factions, and associations.

The Standards of Nursing Practice as defined in the United States by the ANA describe a standard of care or performance at a level that can be judged and serve as an indicator of quality nursing practice. The ANA has been developing nursing standards since 1966. They published the first "official" *Standards of Practice* in 1973. In 1988 the ANA's Congress of Nursing Practice created a task force to conduct a national consensus for definitions of standards in order to revise the national clinical practice standards. The ANA (1991) cited that "organized nursing must reach consensus and speak with a unified voice on the matter of standard setting for professional practice" (p. 2). The results of the national consensus project were so significant that the ANA's Congress of Nursing Practice had to establish a standing committee entitled the Nursing Practice Standards and Guidelines Committee to continue the standards work on an ongoing basis (Minar Baugh, 1999).

In 1998, the ANA, with the assistance of 35 national specialty organizations, published the work.

The revised standards later were reviwed and revised by the ANA Congress on Nursing Practice & Economics (CNPE) resulting in *Nursing: Scope and Standards of Practice* (ANA, 2004). The stated goal within the standards is "to improve the health and well-being of all individuals, communities, and populations through the significant and visible contributions of registered nurses utilizing standards-based practice" (*Nursing: Scope and Standards Practice*, ANA, 2004, p. viii). The time and energy put into this project illustrates the relevance of unity of knowledge in practice. Such unity could greatly facilitate agreement by large governing organizations and their members.

Practice Systems and Accreditation

Various accreditation bodies for health care institutions, such as the Joint Commission on Accreditation of Healthcare Organizations (JCAHO) and the National Commission for Quality Assurance (NCQA), prescribe that if an institutional entity reaches "deemed status," it has attained the minimum health and safety standards for patients. In response to this perpetuating definition that reflects institutional accreditation needs rather than the needs of people, the American Academy of Nursing (AAN) conducted a study that examined characteristics of hospitals that retained highly qualified nurses and that exhibited best practices and outcomes (Kramer, 1990). As a result of this study, the ANA—through the ANCC—has established a formal accreditation program for hospitals that acknowledges excellence in nursing services. This program is entitled the Magnet Nursing Services Recognition Program (Aiken, Havens, & Sloane, 2000). The "magnet status" for hospitals identifies high-quality nursing care, that is, maximum care, unlike the previously mentioned deemed status that is minimum care. In the past, the absence of unity of nursing knowledge prevented accrediting bodies (like JCAHO and

NCQA) from ensuring that professional nursing personnel were employed, and, therefore, nurses were replaced by less experienced, less educated technicians. More recently, data are accumulating that this change endangered patients with mortality being linked to the ratio and education of nurses caring for patients (Aiken, Clarke, Cheung, Sloane, & Silber, 2003; Aiken, Clarke, Sloane, Sochalski, & Silber, 2002).

Practice Redesign and Unity

The implications for the profession in redesigning its practice system and moving toward unity of nursing knowledge would be actualizing of the purposefulness and promise of knowledge. Developing standards for practice that expressly and uniquely identify nursing's clinical goals and objectives is the genesis for the cycle of achieving further unity. When uniform accreditation systems are ascribed to and institutions mobilize toward achieving and maintaining accreditation, the purposefulness of nursing knowledge will lead to positive outcomes for patients. Regulatory, educational, and health care systems will respond by adapting their objectives to ensure conformity with the accreditation process. The nexus is then made to the promise of knowledge by providing future nurses, nursing professionals, and patients with aspirations of maximum, not minimum, standards. As these maxims are modified and revamped, they once again complete the cycle back to attaining unity of knowledge.

The Technological System: The "Research It" Challenge

The technology sector is also invested in seeking unity of nursing knowledge. As noted earlier, a common language is basic to integrated nursing knowledge. The impact of this requirement is best noted by investigating the struggles to attain a unified nursing language system and the continued existence of a multiplicity of classification systems.

Nursing language is described as

> the universe of written terms and their definitions comprising nomenclature of thesauri that are used for purposes such as indexing, sorting, retrieving, and classifying varied nursing data in clinical records, in information systems. . .and in literature and research reports. (National Institute of Nursing Research Priority Expert Panel on Nursing Informatics, 1993, p. 31)

The development of nursing language has been closely tied to the development of technology. For example, the first national conference on nursing diagnosis was called in response to the need to develop language for use in a computer system in the outpatient clinics at St. Louis University Medical Center (Gebbie & Lavin, 1975). As early as 1984, the definition of nursing informatics referred to applying computer science to nursing processes (Chastain, 2003). By 1994 nursing informatics was recognized as a nursing specialty by the ANA with its own scope and standards of practice. Technology is viewed as a tool for nurses to bring data to the level of knowledge where it can manage and improve communication. Simpson (2003) discussed the relationship of nursing informatics to assessment of quality of care. Such assessments can identify the value and true contributions of nursing to the process of patient care. However, the author noted that without nursing-specific taxonomies, there are not specific measures to make assessments against.

For a number of years, parallel classification systems for nursing language were developed, but these systems varied in purpose, scope, structure, and level of abstraction (Henry, 1995). Examples of such systems include (a) The NANDA Taxonomy (NANDA, 1992), (b) The Nursing Interventions Classification (McCloskey & Bulechek, 1992), (c) The Home Healthcare Classification System (Saba & Zuckerman, 1992), (d) The Omaha Community Health System (Martin, Scheet, & Stegman, 1993), (e) The Nursing Intervention Lexicon and Taxonomy study (Grobe, 1992), and (f) Outcome Classification Systems (Iowa Outcomes Project, 2000). Lang and Jacox (1993) warned the profession that if consensus is not reached on these data elements within the nursing arena, the risk of exclusion of nursing from large databases, such as governmental agencies, private health care organizations, and proprietary data dictionaries would be realized.

Significant efforts have been made to deal with the lack of unity of nursing language needed to redesign nursing's technological system. Nurses working to develop The North American Nursing Diagnosis Association (NANDA), Nursing Intervention Classification (NIC), and Nursing Outcomes Classification (NOC) have worked to develop an integrated taxonomy of nursing practice as a common unified structure for nursing language (Dochterman & Jones; chapter 15, this volume). Nursing language (nursing diagnosis, interventions and outcomes) are organized into four domains named: functional, physiological, psychosocial, and environmental. The classes within the domains are listed to include classes of diagnoses, interventions, and outcomes. Further, on the international level, the ICN has led an effort for about a decade to generate a common language with the stated aim of increasing nurses visibility in describing and documenting care internationally (De Back, 2002). The most recent version—consisting of a multiaxial structure—addresses nursing phenomena, nursing action, and nursing outcomes and continues to be validated through international clinical testing. These developments are encouraging, but they provide evidence of a consistently nonunified nursing language system.

Multiple projects in the public and private area recognize the need for a universally accepted standardized clinical language as fundamental to dealing with the issues facing the health care community worldwide. For example, one project noted that it draws from the more than 30 researched standardized health languages that have been developed (Ergo Partners, 2004). Unity of nursing knowledge is needed to maintain the discipline's inclusion in the important ongoing work related to creating standardized electronic health care records.

Nurses can be leaders in this movement by drawing on the principles of unity, purposefulness, and promise of the knowledge of the discipline. Unity of knowledge will be realized with the maturation of a unified nursing language and its parallel data banks. This would prompt a reaction within the purposefulness of nursing knowledge, as it would enable collaboration and mutual transfer of information within the nursing profession. A practicing nurse in Nepal would have immediate access and comprehensive understanding of data from a nursing professional in the United States. Purposefulness of the nursing knowledge would become equally self-evident as health care agencies achieve collaboration through implementation of mutual information exchanges. The incorporation of a unified nursing language into an existing database would therefore abate Lang and Jacox's fears of professional alienation and increase nursing's visibility in and contributions to practice outcomes. The inevitable promise of nursing knowledge will take seed in the hopes for improved patient care facilitated by destruction of geographical boundaries and the formation of regional alliances promoting and ensuring technological advances.

The "Putting It Into Public Policy" Challenge

Redesigning nursing systems, as described by incorporating the key elements (unity, purposefulness, promise) of an integrated nursing knowledge perspective, is necessary and required in the "Name It, Control It, Finance It, Teach It, Research It" challenge. The next essential movement of putting it into public policy will be advanced when nursing understands and prioritizes the most pressing health care issues facing the profession, health care institutions, and society and actively participates in effecting these problems on all these levels. Today, understanding this complex health care environment in which we live is indeed overwhelming. We are bombarded by the facts of ongoing inflation in health care costs, the increasing numbers of Americans with inadequate or no health care coverage, and the increasing numbers of lawsuits served by patients/consumer groups pertaining to abuses in managed care. In addition to this chaotic environment, we also live in a world where shorter hospital stays, restricted provider panels and services, denials of care/coverage, and inflated deductibles and co-payments are acceptable norms.

The context in which nurses work, as previously sketched in brief, is the context that nursing as a prominent health care profession must understand when faced with prioritizing and solving health care issues. One of the most pressing, contemporary issues facing the nursing profession, health care institutions, and society is the actual lack of nursing personnel. The shortage of nurses is well documented, and future projections are alarming. In reporting the supply and demand projections of registered nurses for 2000 to 2020, the National Center for Health Workforce Analysis (2002) reported a shortage of 6%, or 110,000 nurses, in 2000. Using trend analysis, the Center identified that the shortage is expected to quadruple to 29%, or close to 1 million nurses, by 2020. The shortage is affected by the driving forces and trends related to both projected supply and demand. The needed supply of registered nurses to care for patients is affected by the declining number of nursing school graduates, the increasing age of working nurses, declines in relative earnings, and the availability of alternative job opportunities.

There was a decline in numbers of students taking the RN licensing examination from 96,438 in 1995 to 76,618 in 2003 (American Association of Colleges of Nursing, 2004). At the same time, there is an increase in the number of nurses departing the workforce in search of less stressful and higher-paying careers. Buerhaus (2002) noted that given the decreased number of young RNs over 2 decades, "enrollments of young people in nursing programs would have to increase at least 40 percent annually to replace those expected to leave the workforce through retirement" (p. 5). Even as the AACN reported some increases in enrollments in entry-level baccalaureate programs, they also noted that qualified applicants are being turned away by schools because of insufficient numbers of faculty, clinical sites, classroom space, clinical preceptors, and budget constraints (American Association of Colleges of Nursing, 2004). Today faculty shortages have emerged as a major factor affecting the supply of nurses, with 614 faculty vacancies identified at 300 nursing schools in 2003 with the number growing annually.

While the supply forces are discouraging, the factors affecting the demand simultaneously add to the overall projection of nursing shortages. Major factors driving the trend toward an increasing demand for nurses include the increasing population numbers, the aging of the population, and the greater demand per capita for health care (National Center for Health Workforce Analysis, 2002). The nursing profession understands such issues as the nursing shortage. Nursings challange is to participate actively in analyzing trends and to deriving solutions that can be put into public policy. The nursing shortage issue is representative of issues to be resolved using an integrated nursing knowledge framework. The integrated knowledge that is embedded in ethical, educational, practice, and technological systems is essential for effecting public policy at the professional, institutional, and societal levels.

For public policy to deal with the nursing shortage at the professional level it would have to utilize integrated nursing knowledge from ethical, educational, and practice systems to promote recruitment and retention efforts, as well as increase opportunities/resources for funding. Subsequently, to deal with the nursing shortage at the institutional level, public policy would have to use integrated nursing knowledge from ethical and practice systems to increase staffing ratios and eliminate mandatory overtime. Last, to deal with the nursing shortage at the societal level, public policy would have to use integrated nursing knowledge from practice and technology systems to promote patient and institutional safety standards and to transform reimbursement/financing structures to accurately reflect the care that is provided.

Conclusion

In conclusion, the key formula for transforming the health care environment and evolving the nursing profession into a preferred future is: Integrated Nursing Knowledge (Unity, Purposefulness, Promise) + Integrated Nursing Systems (Ethical, Educational, Practice, Technological) + Integrated Public Policies (Professional, Institutional, Societal) = INTEGRATED HEALTH CARE.

REFERENCES

Affara, F., & Styles, M. (1990). Nursing regulation moves ahead. *International Nursing Review, 37*(4), 307–310.

Aiken, L. H., Clarke, S. P., Cheung, R. B., Sloane, D. M., & Silber, J. H. (2003). Education levels of hospital nurses and patient mortality. *Journal of the American Medical Association, 290*(12), 1617–1623.

Aiken, L. H., Clarke, S. P., Sloane, D. M., Sochalski, J., & Silber, J. H. (2002). Hospital nurse staffing and patient mortality, nurse burnout, and job dissatisfaction. *Journal of the American Medical Association, 288*(16), 1987–1993.

Aiken, L. H., Havens, D. S., & Sloane, D. M. (2000). The magnet nursing services recognition program: A comparison of two groups of magnet hospitals. *American Journal of Nursing, 100*(3), 26–36.

American Association of Colleges of Nursing (2002). *Commission on Collegiate Nursing Education retains its status as a nationally recognized accrediting agency by the U.S. Department of Education.* Press release retrieved on April 4, 2004, from http://www.aacn.nche.edu/acceditation/July02release.htm.

American Association of Colleges of Nursing (2004). Nursing shortage fact sheet. Retrieved April 17, 2004, from http://www.aacn.nche.edu/Media/Backgrounders/shortagefacts.htm.

American Nurses' Association. (1980). *Nursing: A social policy statement.* Kansas City, MO: Author.

American Nurses' Association. (1991). Task force on nursing practice and guidelines: Working paper. *Journal of Nursing Quality Assurance, 3*, 1–17.

American Nurses' Association. (1995). *Nursing's social policy statement.* Washington, DC: Author.

American Nurses' Association. (2001). *The code of ethics for nurses with interpretive statements.* Washington, DC: Author.

American Nurses' Association. (2003). *Nursing's social policy statement.* Washington, DC: ANA.

American Nurses' Association. (2004). *Nursing: Scope and standards of practice* (p. viii). Washington, DC: ANA.

Bellack, J. P., Gelmon, S. B., O'Neil, E. H., & Thomsen, C. L. (1999). Responses of baccalaureate and graduate programs to the emergence of choice in nursing accreditation. *Journal of Nursing Education, 38*(2), 53–61.

Brown, E. L. (1948). *Nursing for the future.* New York: Russell Sage Foundation.

Buerhaus, P. (2002). Guest editorial: Shortages of hospital registered nurses: Causes and perspective on public and private sector actions. *Nursing Outlook, 50*(1), 4–6.

Buerhaus, P. I., Staiger, D. O., & Auerbach, D. I. (2003). Is the current shortage of hospital nurses ending? *Health Affairs, 22*(6), 191–198.

Chastain, A. R. (2003). Nursing informatics past, present, and future. *Tennessee Nurse, 66*(1), 8–10.

Clark, J., & Lange, N. (1992). Nursing's next advance: An international classification for nursing practice. *International Nursing Review, 39*(4), 109–112.

DeBack, V. (2002). The ICNP: Achieving the goal of an international language. *International Nursing Review, 49*(2), 68.

Dochterman, J. M., & Jones, D. A. (2003). *Unifying nursing languages: The harmonization of NANDA, NIC, and NOC.* Washington, DC: American Nurses Association.

Ergo Partners–Electronic Medical Record Solutions. (2004). *Standardized languages.* Retrieved April 17, 2004, from http://www.ergopartners.com/key-standardized.asp.

Gebbie, K., & Lavin, M. (1975). *Proceedings of first national conference an classification of nursing diagnoses.* St. Louis, MO: Mosby.

Grace, P. J. (1998). *A philosophical analysis of the concept of "advocacy": Implications for professional–patient relationships* (Hodges Library Thesis 986.G73). Knoxville: University of Tennessee.

Grobe, S. J. (1992). Nursing intervention lexicon and taxonomy: Preliminary categorization. In K. C. Lun, P. Degoulet, T. E. Piemme, & O. Rienhoff (Eds.), *MedInfo92* (pp. 981–986). Geneva, Switzerland: North-Holland.

Henry, S. B. (1995). Nursing informatics: State of the science. *Journal of Advanced Nursing, 22*(6), 1182–1192.

260   Nursing Knowledge Development and Clinical Practice

International Council of Nurses. (2000). *The ICN code of ethics for nurses*. Retrieved November 13, 2004, from http://www.icn.ch/icncode.pdf.

Iowa Outcomes Project. (2000). In M. Johnson, M. Maas & S. Moorhead (Eds.). Nursing Outcomes Classification (NOC) (2nd ed.). St. Louis: Mosby.

Keeling, A. W., & Ramos, M. C. (1995). The role of nursing history in preparing nursing for the future. *Nursing & Healthcare: Perspectives on Community*, *16*(1), 30–34.

Kramer, M. (1990). The magnet hospitals: Excellence revisited. *Journal of Nursing Administration*, *20*(9), 35–44.

Lang, L. L., & Jacox, A. (1993). Using large data bases in nursing and health policy research. *Journal of Professional Nursing*, *9*(4), 204–211.

Martin, K. S., Scheet, N. J., & Stegman, M. R. (1993). Home health clients: Characteristics, outcomes of care, and nursing interventions. *American Journal of Public Health*, *83*(12), 1730–1734.

Maryland Nurses Association. (2000). ANCC to make certification available to all registered nurses through Open Door 2000 program: Reflects growing recognition of certification as an indicator of competence. *Maryland Nurse*, *2*(2), 19.

McCloskey, J. C., & Bulechek, G. M. (1992). *Nursing intervention classification*. St. Louis: Mosby.

Michigan Nurses Association. (1997). Members have opportunity to help revise ethics code, standards of clinical nursing practice. *Michigan Nurse*, *70*(6), 8–9.

Minar Baugh, V. (1999). Standards and guidelines, the cornerstone of professional nursing practice. *Georgia Nursing*, *59*(1), 35.

NANDA. (1992). *NANDA nursing diagnoses: Definitions and classifications 1992–1993*. Philadelphia: Author.

National Center for Health Workforce Analysis. (2002). *Projected supply, demand, and shortages of registered nurses: 2000–2020*. Washington, DC: U.S. Department of Health and Human Services.

National Council of State Boards of Nursing. (1999). *Uniform core licensure requirements: A supporting paper*. Retrieved April 17, 2004, from http://www.ncsbn.org/resources/complimentary_ncsbn_uclr.asp.

National Institute of Nursing Research Priority Expert Panel on Nursing Informatics. (1993). *Nursing informatics: Enhancing patient care*. Bethesda, MD: U.S. Department of Health and Human Services, U.S. Public Health Service, National Institutes of Health.

Padovano Corliss, C. (1994). *Universals of nursing: Consensus and action*. Ann Arbor, MI: University Microfilms International.

Padovano Corliss, C. (1997). Implications for health and social policy. In C. Roy & D. Jones (Eds.), *Knowledge conference proceedings 1996: Developing knowledge for nursing practice: Three philosophical modes for linking theory and practice* (pp. 127–137). Chestnut Hill, MA: BC Press.

Phippen, M. L. (1990). The search for common standards and guidelines is a collaborative effort. *The Association of Peri-Operative Registered Nurses Journal*, *52*(2), 212–214.

Roy, C. (2000). A theorist envisions the future and speaks to nursing administrators. *Nursing Administration Quarterly*, *24*(2), 1–12.

Saba, V. K., & Zuckerman, A. E. (1992). A new home health classification method. *Caring Magazine*, *11*(9), 27–34.

Sawyer, L. M. (1989). Nursing code of ethics: An international comparison. *International Nursing Review*, *36*(5), 145–148.

Simpson, R. L. (2003). The role of IT in health care quality assessment. *Nursing Administration Quarterly*, *27*(4), 355–359.

Styles, M. M. (1995). *Project on the regulation of nursing.* Geneva, Switzerland: International Council of Nurses.

Styles, M. M., Allen, S., Armstrong, S., Matsuura, M., Stannard, D., & Ordway, J. S. (1991). Entry: A new approach. *Nursing Outlook*, *39*(5), 200–203.

Thompson, L. W. (1998). Nursing ethics: The ANA code for nurses. *Tennessee Nurse*, *61*(6), 23, 25–29.

van Maanen, H. M. T. (1990). Nursing in transition: An analysis of the state of the art in relation to the conditions of practice and society's expectations. *Journal of Advanced Nursing*, *15*, 914–924.

Impact on Health and Patient Care—Exemplars for the Future

Introduction

In a rapidly changing world, the health and well-being of society remains a central focus of concern to nurses worldwide. It is critical that the nursing knowledge, guided by multiple philosophical and theoretical perspectives, be used to shape and inform health care for the human community, globally. The ability to clearly translate and articulate nursing knowledge can occur as the substance of the discipline continues to be identified and refined and its link to clinical practice exemplified.

Part IV contains exemplars that depict the application of nursing knowledge emerging from the perspectives of knowledge as process and an emerging integrated knowledge view. Each exemplar reflects core disciplinary values and beliefs about person and environment, health, and nursing. In addition, knowledge from various philosophical and theoretical perspectives is used to shape, interpret, and link theory and research with clinical practice.

In chapter 18, Anne-Marie Barron provides compelling information about the experience of living with cancer from newman's process perspective. Using Newman's *research as praxis* methodology, Barron illuminates the experience of living with cancer, particularly during the terminal phases of the illness. Knowledge revealed using this process adds to our understanding of how individuals continue to live, change, and heal while experiencing a long-term illness.

Jane Flanagan, in chapter 19, intentionally uses knowledge from within a transformative paradigm to shape a practice environment that actualizes a process perspective within a medically informed problem-solving clinical setting. The discussion focuses on the preparation of an environment of care and the nursing staff for change, along with an evaluation of the experience from the perspective of the patient and the nurses. Findings reveal the dynamic and changing impact that patients and nurses experience when there is congruence between the nursing knowledge and the delivery of patient care.

The challenges of sustaining health behavior changes are explored by Diane Berry in chapter 20 within the context of Newman's process perspective. The approach illuminates the human struggle around obesity and sustaining weight loss. The patient exemplar highlights the ability of nurses to move beyond fixing a problem, such as excess weight, to uncovering the meaning of life issues surrounding the person's ability to make life choices—in this case often unrelated to excessive eating. The discovery of this knowledge is useful in developing and shaping new modes of nursing care that affect costs, health issues, and the human experience.

Valuing different integrated strategies that embody multiple epistemological approaches to knowledge development is explored and extended by Nancy Dluhy in chapter 21. In mapping existing knowledge of chronic illness and symptom distress, the author describes what is known about the experience and explores the barriers that compromise translating this knowledge into practice. The mapping process and use of knowledge in practice is influenced by a number of issues, including the volume of information available, the multiple assumptions that underlie the dominant disciplinary perspective informing the knowledge available around chronic illness, and multiple worldviews and language used to communicate the phenomena. The author uses Hesook Suzie Kim's *Critical Narrative Epistemology*, described in chapters 12 and 14, as a framework to guide the development of a proposed *model of negotiated symptom management* as an approach to knowledge assimilation in chronic illness and its use and impact on clinical practice.

Roy's epistemological perspective on *knowledge as the cosmic imperative* is applied to clinical practice in chapter 22 by Debra Hanna. The author further relates the concepts of this perspective to unity, diversity, conformism, and chaos. Using exemplars from clinical practice, the author poses new strategies for nursing knowledge development, including exploration of the concept of unity and human existence. This work suggests that a focus on the ontological purpose of nursing "makes room for the mystery" of nursing's presence and patients' responses and celebrates a connectivity to a higher power.

Donna Perry and Katherine Gregory's discussion in chapter 23 offers an application of philosophical and theoretical knowledge to clinical practice on a global level. The exploration links nursing's contract with society and the promise to contribute to the common good (American Nurses Association, 2003) with the role nurses can play in promoting global understanding and human rights. The concept of tolerance is expanded to one of understanding. Transcendent pluralism is a new concept introduced by the authors to acknowledge the human potential for good; the authors also expand the concept of environment. When nursing knowledge is developed in a transformative mode, it can explicate nursing as focusing on values of common purpose, unity, diversity, and subjectivity with the ultimate goal of justice and global understanding.

Presentations included in part IV challenge nursing knowledge development and provide guides for the advancement of clinical practice, research, and the theoretical and conceptual approaches to knowledge development during this new century. The presentations offer applications of several philosophical perspectives and offer the reader strategies to impact world health and recognize the multiple opportunities nurse have to affect the social order of the world.

References

American Nurses Association (Ed.). (2003). *Nursing's social policy statement*. Silver Spring, MD: ANA.

Margaret Newman's Theory and Research Method: A Case Illustration

Anne-Marie Barron

ewman's theory of health as expanding consciousness (HEC) and research method provided the theoretical framework and primary research method for the study, *Life Meanings and the Experience of Cancer* (Barron, 2001). The problem that motivated the study was the suffering of cancer patients. It was hoped that further understanding of pattern, meaning, expansion of consciousness, and spirituality in the experience of individuals with cancer would yield important insights into the experience and suggest nursing strategies that would ultimately relieve suffering and promote comfort. Three research questions were used to guide this study. Namely, How do the life patterns described by persons with cancer express meaning and expansion of consciousness over time? What facilitates or hinders expansion of consciousness? How is spirituality manifested in the narratives of persons with cancer?

Newman's (1994) research method was the primary one used in the study. Her theory was used to guide understanding of the participants' experiences using interviews that focused on a discussion of meaningful people and events, identification of patterns, and recognition of consciousness expansion. Phenomenology was also used as a secondary methodology to analyze questions that address experiences across the participants.

The final phase of the research design was the analysis of the participants' narratives in relation to spiritual perspectives revealed during the interviews.

There were 22 participants in the study; most had advanced forms of cancer. This chapter presents a case description of an individual participant to illustrate how Newman's theory and method both guided understanding of the experience being studied and offered the possibility of meaningful nursing encounter—research as praxis. Identifying information has been changed to preserve confidentiality.

Newman's research methodology that calls for a two-interview protocol was developed and implemented. The first interview focused on a discussion of the important people and events in the participant's life as well as their current circumstances. Following the first interview, a narrative was developed, identifying key issues, people, and events of the participant's life. The participant's story was then summarized and chronologically ordered and the person's life pattern was identified and depicted diagrammatically. The second interview focused on sharing the summary and pattern and reflecting with the participant on the narrative summary, personal reflections and meaning, and pattern as displayed until the participant felt that all of the components described were accurate. The following is Derek's story as revealed using the process noted above.

Derek's Story

Derek was a 22-year-old college student when he participated in the study. He had a very aggressive form of lymphoma and was hospitalized to participate in an experimental bone marrow transplant research protocol during the time of the study interviews. He articulately described his life and current situation and offered rich examples of the power of Newman's method and theory. Grappling with life-threatening illness shifted Derek's perspective in profound ways, expanding his understanding of himself, those around him, and his sense of universal wholeness. His struggle had led to a new personal awareness and consciousness expansion. He was confronting the biggest obstacle of his life—as he would say, "my highest mountain"—with grace and courage. His reflection and engagement during the interviews deepened his sense of understanding and connection—research as praxis. He spoke very movingly about his appreciation for the opportunity to reflect and share some of the most important concerns and understandings of his life through participation in the research.

Derek had grown up while living with his brother, sister, and parents in a small community. His family was close, and they were deeply connected to this community. His father owned a small business in town, and from an early age, Derek helped out at the store. He had lots of contact with people in the community through that work. Derek had always known that he was surrounded by love, but his cancer diagnosis led to a deeper realization of the meaning of that love. Prior to his diagnosis, Derek described himself as an introvert, largely keeping to himself and enjoying solitary activities.

Derek was a junior in college when he was diagnosed with lymphoma. This was followed by several rounds of chemotherapy. Each treatment had helped for a period of time, but the lymphoma kept recurring. He and his family had investigated research protocols throughout the country and around the world and had traveled a great distance to participate in the experimental bone marrow transplant protocol.

Because the particular transplant protocol Derek was preparing for was still considered experimental, his insurance company refused to pay for it. Derek and his parents had already flown across the country and checked into the hospital when they received word from the insurance company that neither the hospitalization nor the procedure would be covered. They were devastated, believing that this was their final option for treatment. People back home became aware of their plight and were outraged. They wrote letters and raised money. Derek was deeply moved:

> it's a small town and so the mayor set up a bank account, I mean people just started donating everything. They donated money, and friends donated like airline tickets for back and forth, and I just couldn't believe the outpouring. I didn't think like I affected that many people, just everyone. I guess they ran a newspaper article, even a little TV ad, a news segment, and strangers and people we knew and friends of friends that kind of knew us [responded] and I just couldn't believe it. I was overwhelmed. I'm still overwhelmed...and it's one of those things I'll always remember for the rest of my life, of course...that friends did help and stuff. And hopefully [in the future] I'll become at least rich, I don't know about famous, but a little well off. I'll be able to donate to like hospitals and charities to further research and things like that...And it's one of those things I'll remember forever and never forget...It was a morale—a huge morale booster.

Later the insurance company reconsidered and agreed to pay for at least a portion of the expenses.

Derek had been diagnosed with cancer just as he felt that the plans for his life were becoming clear. He was working on career goals he was excited about and was beginning to plan for graduate school. Traveling down the highway was the metaphor Derek used to describe his experience with cancer and with life.

> It was just like I was getting my life going. I got on the freeway, and I was going, and everything was going as planned. The traffic was clear and I could pretty much go where I wanted to, wherever I could take myself and all of a sudden it was just like the road's clear, but I can't go any further. It was like everyone was just going by and I just sat there.

Derek and his family had spent a grueling 15 months since the initial diagnosis. There were enthusiastic starts to new treatments followed too quickly by bitter disappointments. They had literally searched the world with the hope of identifying an option that held the possibility of a cure. Derek kept hoping to be able to return to school. He related each failed treatment to his plans to return to school. The goal of returning to school fueled his hope and sustained his coping, but the quest for treatment was exhausting. He described the failure of option number six:

> they were saying "all you have left is a bone marrow transplant. You have to have one" and then they were saying, "well we can give it to you but it's going to be 50–50." So 50% chance I'll make it and 50% chance I won't. So we were like, oh my gosh, last choice and it's a 50–50 choice, and we didn't like that. I didn't, my parents didn't, no one liked

that. So it's like just a really huge depression. Yeah, and we were like, okay, now since I've branched off on another road, and now there's kind of the ultimate detour that I'm not going to make it and. . .just really depressing for everyone. So that's the last option, and it might work and it might not. No one's sure. So we're like going to have to go with it, there's nothing else. We have to do this. So we're like, well we're going to try it. . .We were like okay, well screw this, we're going to do this, and I'm going to make it whether—we're going to make it through now and we're going to do this final option because there's nothing else left.

And all of a sudden methotrexate pops up, and the doctor in Chicago says "Try this," and all of a sudden there's this magic bullet...This has to work. Everyone's like, "It's going to work. We're going to make this work". . .So beginning of the summer, we tried the high dose methotrexate. . .And so the summer passes and I'm doing fine, and then the fall passes and I'm doing fine. The methotrexate kind of stopped working, and it's like, okay, well we still have the bone marrow transplant to do. . .Seems like my detours were kind of shattered, and I had just learned to go—and basically I'd go through [the bone marrow transplant] and see what would happen. I had to do it.

At that point Derek was very sick. He and his parents approached the treatment center where they had expected the bone marrow transplant. They were told that Derek was no longer eligible for the transplant because he was too sick, but they kept seeking possibilities. Summing up their sense of urgency at that time, Derek said, "In this whole damn world, there's got to be one more option." Derek would have gone to the ends of the earth:

[The center on the West Coast] had basically refused, so we're like, "We'll go anywhere. We'll go to China for acupuncture." I've never had acupuncture. I was like, I'll take herbs and do whatever I have to because I'm going to beat this. I've been through so much there's no way it's going to kill me. . .I'm going to just get well, and all these chemos didn't work, and now we have this road, and I seem to fit beautifully, and so we're going to do that. We have this new road.

The next option offered respite from suffering and anguish.

so we got our flashing light [on the East Coast], and I kind of go back to the spring where everything was like it's going to end. So like my grandparents, my grandparents bought me the Harley-Davidson, and it was just like I couldn't believe how much everyone loved me, and like it was great, but I felt so sad—like I'll be able to get it and learn to ride it and then I'm just going to stop. Then up pops the light to [the East Coast] and everyone was like—cheer, party!

I was sick and I was just sick as a dog. I couldn't move, I was sleeping, I was tired. I'd throw up all the time. Basically it was like everything was rolling to an end kind of of—there was this hope [on the East Coast].

Derek was feeling very hopeful about the treatment.

They gave me the chemo, and I felt bad; then right after the chemo, they gave me the bone marrow transplant, and it's like they sat me down and hooked me up to the bone marrow and I watched it drip in, and it was just like I got a new lease on life. And it was like I can feel me soaking up, I feel my bones sponging up the bone marrow. They're going, "Oh this is what we need." Thank you, thank you, thank you.

Derek had grown a great deal since his diagnosis with cancer. He appreciated his inner strength and the power of love in new and deeper ways.

Just to realize, I don't know—I guess it's a huge just gigantic mountain, an obstacle, and I was able to climb it. . .Yeah, it's just like, "Wow I'm tough!" Basically, soon as I get over this mountain, nothing's ever going to stop me ever again. But it's just [that] I never realized just how much love and support everyone had around me. So I have this huge appreciation now, just being able to live life and going on with life; and just that there are always people around me, when something does happen, that I can turn to—and that I will help if someone needs to be helped. I will help to the best of my ability.

Derek was not religious per se, but his experiences following his diagnosis had deepened his personal life philosophy and spirituality.

And going through this has made me think about that [religion, spirituality, and personal philosophy]. . .What you believe is right for you, but what I believe is, and I mean ever since grade school, that's one of the—it seems like one of the questions you always get asked eventually, is, "What church do you go to?" I always say I don't go to church. They think I'm screwy, but now, as I—it seems like we start off in our small, little. . .sphere, and we're just a little tiny speck. But as we grow and mature, I mean our sphere gets bigger and kind of encompasses more of the whole. . .As we grow and learn and just develop, our sphere encompasses more of the whole thing, but we're all just a little section and we believe what we want to. We believe what we believe is right and basically it's like— don't hate anyone. I mean we're all part of the same thing. So. . .it's pointless to hate people because, I think it's like protons, and everything—the whole universe—are made out of all the same things, just protons; this is like science. . .But it's just like everyone's different, but everyone's made of the same protons, and neutrons, and electrons. So it's pointless—I know you have people you don't get along with or you just don't like—but it's pointless [to hate], because we're all part of the same thing.

And I was worried that it was kind of weird that I had no religion. This is kind of my own personal religion for myself, my own personal thoughts, and I'd like to learn about everything in the whole universe. And I know I'm not going to be able to comprehend it, but I'd like to learn as much as I can to expand my own personal universe to encompass as much as I can get out of life. Basically, go to school, live with people, travel, read, watch the Learning Channel. I love the History Channel and Discovery [Channel]; [I] just absorb as much of this universe as I can while I'm here. And I think it starts all over again on the other side of the universe, again. There's something else. . .like reincarnation. Like I'll be me but. . .just because I'm somewhere else, it will be just completely different. It won't be anything like this over here, like a whole new spot on the other side of the universe, and I'll try to extend and learn everything I possibly can. Hopefully, I'll still have the same philosophy, and I won't get locked into a specific place.

Derek described what he believed to be his parents' philosophy of choice of religion and spirituality:

I think my parents are saying, "It's like here's the piano, and you just press whatever key you want to press. And you go and press all the keys over here and see what they sound like. Press all the keys over here and see what they sound like and whatever key you like the best...Like do whatever you want and play the whole thing; just go with one." So, I'm just trying to play the whole piano, seeing what I can do while I'm here. Now that I've got this new lease on life, I've got to go out and make the most of what I can.

As the first interview ended, Derek reflected on his participation in the research. He expressed appreciation for the opportunity that the research had offered and related his openness to participating in the study to the new perspective he had developed since becoming sick. His earlier pattern of introversion had shifted dramatically. The openness and expansiveness he had experienced were life altering. The study participation had reinforced his growth and facilitated deeper levels of awareness.

I'm surprised at myself. I want to thank you for coming to talk with me today. I didn't realize how much it helped...I'll be happy to go through it [the summary and pattern] over and over...So don't go through life in your little ball, experience the whole thing. It's just like, I grew up with my parents and I always knew they loved me and I loved them, but it just didn't, the realization didn't take place until all this happened. I mean I knew they loved me and I loved them, but I just didn't express it really...But now I've learned to be open to people—and make sure you tell your mom you love her every day and give your dad a hug and all that sort of stuff. Take every opportunity to do everything.

The pattern identified for Derek was: introversion, terror, transformation to deep realization of universal wholeness, interconnection, and profound love. Learning, loving, and living in a bubble early in life and later heroic journey, seeking health and slaying the monster. When the pattern was shared, Derek's response was, "That's perfect!" The diagrammatic depiction of pattern was an ascending line of loops across the description of his life's story. It was an attempt to represent his expanding awareness and understandings. He suggested that the ascending line contain sine curves rather than loops. He described climbing sine curves as representative of the peaks and troughs of his life. Cancer represented the biggest dip. He also suggested that double arrows, intending to represent connection with important others in his life be changed to intersecting circles.

At the conclusion of his participation in the study, Derek said, "I felt so good after we talked. To talk about it, to talk to another person. I realize how good it felt to talk about things like that. It really felt great afterwards...I've thoroughly enjoyed it." Derek made remarkable movement in his development as a result of his struggle with lymphoma. The chaos of the crisis had led to experiences of profound love, deep self-awareness, and transformation.

Supporting and Extending Newman's Theory

Derek, like other participants in the study, was on a journey of seeking meaning in his experience with cancer. The chaos and challenges of the diagnosis were major disruptive factors in the lives of all of the participants. When understanding and meaning were gained, as with Derek, there was integration at a higher level of development. The process of the research was valuable for the participants, as Derek articulately described.

This research process used underscores the importance of the intentional, compassionate presence of the nurse as patients suffer and struggle to move beyond their suffering. Newman's research methodology is also her model for nursing care (research as praxis). The research itself offered therapeutic engagement and self-discovery in the immediate situation, which led to pattern recognition and expansion of consciousness. This study, as others utilizing Newman's method, demonstrates the power of Newman's clarity about research as praxis.

Findings from this study support earlier research with Newman's method and the experience of cancer. Moch (1991) utilized Newman's method in combination with phenomenology and phenomenological nursology in her study of women with breast cancer. In her research three themes were identified: changing relatedness, identifying meaning in the experience, and adding new perspectives about life. Newman (1995) studied the experience of cancer and identified themes across the participants' patterns: deprived childhood, lack of connectedness, and reaching a turning point.

Although this study was not explicitly an intervention study as Endo's (1998) study of women with ovarian cancer was, her key finding of pattern recognition as a significant nursing intervention was certainly supported. Participants in both studies found that pattern recognition led to further self-awareness and insight, which facilitated consciousness expansion. Studies utilizing Newman's method are inherently intervention studies.

The findings related to spirituality in this study support important aspects of earlier studies using Newman's method and underscore the significance of spirituality as described by Newman (1989). Although spirituality as a term had limited meaning to a number of participants, Newman's method, with its distinct focus on meaning, invited moving reflections on spiritual perspectives. The spiritual perspectives revealed by participants offer further clarification of the human experience of struggle and transformation within the context of life-threatening illness. The study contributes to further understanding of how chaos can lead to a transformational process that creates movement toward increasing complexity, expansion of consciousness, and wholeness. The focus on meaning and pattern shifted the experience of suffering to a broader perspective that, in itself, brought meaning and alleviated suffering. Participants in this study actively sought meaning in their struggle with suffering. Although initially immobilizing for some, the struggle led to a process of inner reflection, reaching out, and taking action that resulted in greater understanding of self, others, and the environment. The research interviews invited the participants to share and deepen their understanding and appreciation of what was most important and cherished. From that larger perspective, suffering was lessened.

The alleviation of suffering is a central focus for nursing practice. Newman's theory and method for research and caring offer powerful insights for nurses as they engage with patients who are suffering. In both research and practice, nurses using Newman's framework facilitate movement from anguish to self-awareness, insight, and transformation. Newman's work and the research and practice that have been generated from her conceptualization of health as expanding consciousness illuminate the deepest aspects of nursing practice—suffering, meaning, spirituality, possibility, and transformation.

REFERENCES

Barron, A. M. (2001). Life meanings and the experience of cancer. *Dissertation Abstracts International, 54*, 3. (UMI No. 30-08589)

Endo, E. (1998). Pattern recognition as a nursing intervention with Japanese women with ovarian cancer. *Advances in Nursing Science, 20*(4), 49–61.

Moch, S. (1991). Health within illness. *Journal of Advanced Nursing, 15*, 1426–1435.

Newman, M. (1989). The spirit of nursing. *Holistic Nursing Practice, 3*(3), 1–6.

Newman, M. (1994). *Health as expanding consciousness* (2nd ed.). New York: National League for Nursing.

Newman, M. (1995). Recognizing a pattern of expanding consciousness in persons with cancer. In M. Newman (Ed.), *A developing discipline* (pp. 159–172). New York: National League for Nursing.

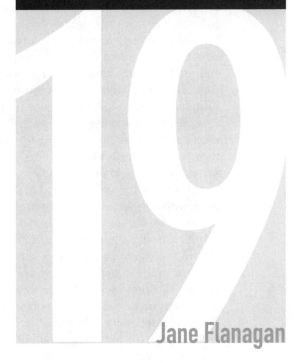

The Nursing Theory and Practice Link: Creating a Healing Environment Within the Preadmission Nursing Practice

Jane Flanagan

This chapter presents an exemplar of care from a study that was conducted in the preadmission clinic (PAC) of a surgical unit (Flanagan, 2002) using knowledge generated from nursing theory to guide the research. The basis for this study was a model of care known as the preadmission nursing practice model (PNPM). The PNPM has incorporated concepts from several nurse theorists and linked them with the clinical practice setting. Knowledge from Rogers' (1990) science of unitary humans, Newman's (1997) theory of health as expanding consciousness, Watson's (1996) theory of transpersonal caring, and Roy's (Roy & Andrews, 1999) adaptation model, in particular the perspective on the cosmic imperative (see chapter 10, this volume) was drawn upon to form an integrated framework for the study. The planned changes in clinical practice were intended to be guided by integrated nursing knowledge to design a patient care delivery model that would change the clinical experience for the nurse and patient. As a result, the purpose of the study was to understand the experience of the nurses and patients who were exposed to this new practice model. Findings from one of the nurses experiences are reported below.

Background

There were several prompts within the practice environment that instigated a need for change in the nursing care delivery model. Two were most influential: (a) a developing body of research that was being generated around the same day surgery population and (b) the reflections of the nurses in team meetings related to clinical encounters with patients and their responses to the impending surgical experience.

First, findings from several studies being conducted with the ambulatory surgery population suggested that having surgery was a stressful time in people's lives. In these studies, people described being overwhelmed by the experience, anxious about the outcome and unprepared for recovery at home (Jones, Coakley, & Flanagan, 1999; Jones, Dauphinee, Coakley, & Fernsebner, 1998).

Secondly, the nurses working in this surgical setting consistently reported in team meetings that patients preparing for surgery often shared much about themselves and their life experiences with their nurse. It seemed to the nurses that patients were expressing a desire to be known by their health care providers and a need to reflect on many issues both related and unrelated to the surgical encounter. The result of these findings along with other emerging issues prompted the nurses under the leadership of the nurse researcher to change the practice delivery model and examine its impact on nurses.

As a result, the nurse researcher met with the staff weekly to review exemplars of care and explore and identify the problems in the practice setting. Several nursing theorists were explored and their work shared and discussed with the nursing staff. The nursing theorists included were Rogers, Newman, Roy, and Watson. The staff found the convergence of ideas about person, health, and environment useful to their practice. These concepts were reflected in each of these nurse theorist's philosophies. They were as follows: (a) the person is an unfolding being and open energy system, (b) the nurse as one who is open to the exchange of energy, and (c) together, the nurse and patient have an ability to increase their awareness of experiences and transcend to a higher level of consciousness.

Several steps were then taken to create an environment of caring. The redesign of the patient care setting included: (a) decorating of individual office spaces as suggested by Watson (1996); (b) inviting patients to share their story, as suggested by Newman (1994); (c) performing therapeutic touch, relaxation exercises, guided imagery, or prayer with patients to enhance relaxation and promote comfort; and (d) incorporating follow-up visits into the PAC program.

Methods

To understand the nurse–patient experience of participating in this model of care, a study using a phenomenological approach was conducted. Questions were generated to explore the experience from the perspective of both the nurse and the patient. The focus of this discussion is on the nurses' responses. Within this context, the following questions were asked of the nurses participating in this study:

1 What was the overall experience of being with this patient like for you?
2 What is the experience of being a nurse working in the PAC where this revised care delivery model (PNPM) is practiced?

Within this study, 3 nurses cared for 10 patients using the revised care delivery model. Following exposure to PAC, patients usually had surgery and were admitted to recover in the hospital for a short stay. They were then discharged to home. Data was also obtained from patients but this discussion will focus on the nurses. There were four specific data collection points for the nurse during the study: (a) prior to the initial PAC visit, (b) after the initial PAC visit, (c) before and after the follow-up visits (at least two) on the inpatient unit, and (d) the first postoperative visit or phone call (usually 2–4 weeks post discharge). The nurses recorded their thoughts and reflections at each of the time points. See Table 19.1 for questions that guided the nurse's reflections at all data points.

The nurses were asked to be contemplative, intentional, open to the interaction, and able to pursue the potential of a healing relationship as they engaged in each point of data collection. To be contemplative, the nurse took sufficient and deliberate time to become centered prior to the patient encounter. Intentionality was established by being present and open to the experience with each individual, encouraging the patient to tell his or her story in such a way as to uncover its meaning and purpose to the person. To establish presence, the nurse interacted with the patient in a way to promote mutuality, sharing, trust, and commitment. To pursue the healing relationship, the nurse established a partnership with the patient and remained connected with him or her by continually contacting the patient, following up on the healing journey at mutually agreed intervals throughout the hospitalization and recovery at home.

The nurse researcher interviewed the three nurses after they had the post discharge call or visit with the patient and asked, "What was the overall experience of being with this

Table 19.1

Questions Used to Guide Nurse's Reflections at all Data Collection Points During the Study

1 What have you done to prepare yourself for seeing patients today?
2 How does it feel for you to practice within this new model of care?
3 Did you ask the patient about significant people and events?
4 If yes, what was that like? If not, why not?
5 Did you offer to pray, do therapeutic touch or relaxation exercises with the patient? If yes, what did you do?
6 Why did you choose to do what you did?
7 What was it like for you to visit the patient on the inpatient unit?
8 What do you do to care for yourself before or after seeing the patient on the hospital unit?
9 What was it like to call the patient at home?
10 Were they recovering from surgery in a way that met your expectations?

patient like for you?" This interview was taped, and all of the tapes were then transcribed and analyzed by the nurse researcher. Data analysis was completed in two steps—first, by reviewing the nursing data following each nurse–patient interaction and second, by examining the data across all of the nurse interactions.

The Exemplar

The following is one exemplar from the study. Like many of the nurses in the practice, ST had more than 20 years of varied nursing experiences. Being encouraged to create a practice environment was a new experience, but she actively participated by decorating her office in a way she felt made people feel welcome. This nurse described her office in this way:

> I mean, I have all kinds of things in the room that they (patients) can relate to. I have peaceful and pretty artwork, but I also have pictures of me, and things that are important to me. You know, subtle pictures about me that maybe they can relate to as well. I have the chairs arranged to welcome them, so they can feel comfortable. I have books out that may spark their interest, and, of course, I softened the lighting. I guess I want them to connect to me in whatever way is comfortable. When you have a little of you out there, it allows them to not feel like they are the only ones sharing everything that is so personal. You know all about them—this changes that, makes it more us. This way I say, I tell you something, if you tell me something.

During the pre-reflection, the nurse described things she did to prepare herself for seeing the patient. During this time period, it was expected that the nurses would take time to meditate and center so that they could be better prepared to be fully present with the patients. Often, however, nurses described meeting their own basic physical needs such as getting something to eat or drink. These same needs were also reflected as the primary concerns nurses had when caring for patients such as nutrition, hydration, toileting, and safety. ST reflected on the experience this way:

> You know, I don't normally ask myself how I feel before a I see a patient or what do I need before I see a patient—I just go see the patient. It's been funny because I need to go the bathroom and will need to get water, but I normally don't ask myself or allow myself to do those things. I just take the next patient and in the middle of it think I have to go to the bathroom or I have to get a drink. So now I've been taking better care of myself because I've been thinking I need a drink and then I get one. So I just had lunch, and I feel pretty good about taking another patient. I did notice when I took the last patient there was quite a pile of blue slips [indicates there are patients to see]. I had that funny reaction to the Newman question: Tell me about significant people and events in your life. Who knew someone would say no one [is significant], but I'm ready to tackle it again. It does amaze me how much it opens people up.

The patient ST met with was a 69-year-old gentleman coming in with cancer, and he was facing a major procedure. His wife accompanied him to the visit. The nurse reported that the patient appeared healthy, pleasant, and nervous. Within the interaction, the nurse tried to connect with the patient, but this was difficult because his wife answered many of the questions for him. The nurse invited this patient to share his story the way that Newman (1994) suggests (i.e., "Tell me about significant people and events in your life." ST reported:

> So we did some deep breathing, imagery, and TT [therapeutic touch] and I asked the Newman question. And, it really took me by surprise, because he was really quite quiet up until this. The wife is an RN, and he really let the wife answer every question that I had. When we got to the significant people and events, the wife looked at me like, "I'm about to stab you for making my husband cry." I think she anticipated that he would react that way, and he did. I had to sit with a little bit of silence while he was coming up with his answer, and I hate you (researcher) already because it's very hard for me to sit in silence. I would much rather continue talking and put words in patients' mouths because it makes me feel comfortable. Then he said that it had been really, really hard for him, and he was more afraid than he thought he could ever be, [in] that he did not think this could ever really happen to him because his mother's 101 years old, and it made him feel vulnerable, and it also made him truly love his family. He held his wife's hand and said, "my wife has gotten me through." And then the wife stopped giving me the "I'm going to stab you," and she started crying. And I thought, oh, this is just way more crying than I had anticipated happening.

Incorporating this new delivery model of care was a process that took 2 years to completely implement. The nurses felt comfortable with some aspects of the revised practice model almost immediately, such as decorating their office spaces. The medical model, however, was so thoroughly ingrained in all these nurses, all with at least 20 years of experience, that it took time to move toward an integrated, theory guided practice. Although all the nurses recognized the need for a change in the way care was delivered and supported the more process-oriented approach to care, change did not come easily. Nurses stated that they went from knowing all the answers in a prescriptive, medical model to feeling uncomfortable with allowing the story to unfold. ST described her discomfort with this type of practice in this way:

> So it was very uncomfortable for me, but I think it was good for both of them (patient and wife) The experience, it was good, it hurt my abdomen watching them both be sad. I didn't know I was about to open Pandora's box with that question. I never expect that. Obviously, you get deep, and you get deep very quickly when you ask that question. And I think—no, I know that I would have in the past immediately used humor as a coping mechanism, because I couldn't have sat with their sadness like that. I'm not sure what they needed at that point, but it's what I needed at that point. So it's something I need to work on. So I thought that was interesting.

The nurses continued their interaction with the patients on the inpatient units for at least two postoperative visits. This experience provided an opportunity for the nurses to further establish the nurse–patient relationship and also continue with any interventions that may have been agreed on such as the use of therapeutic touch or relaxation exercises.

The nurses recorded their thoughts and reflections before and after each postoperative visit.

It is during these recordings that nurses often described their apprehension about seeing the patient again. The nurses questioned if the patients would remember them. There was also confusion about the role they played with the patient at this point. Were they the meditation nurse, patient advocate, liaison between pre and postsurgery? Sometimes if they had a day off, they felt they abandoned the patient. ST described:

> I was going to come in on Sunday, but I did not feel great and thought he'll be okay until Monday. I saw him today. He's already been through the worst of it and was walking around. I was apprehensive about seeing him today because I had told him I would see him Sunday and then I didn't, and you know they are suffering so much they don't need me to not live up to what I promise. So I kind of felt awful showing up Monday morning saying I know you had a horrible day yesterday, and here I am now. Really didn't get to any meaningful conversation. I told him I would be back. He said thank you very much for the visit and that he was glad to see me. And there was nothing therapeutic going on that I'm aware of. I'll go back, and we'll see what tomorrow brings. You know, I'm sure we need to talk, but I don't know how deep this will get.

ST felt she let this patient down, and these concerns interfered with her ability to be fully present with the patient. Later ST visited the patient again and seemed to be more focused. ST had this to say about this visit:

> Well I refocused, did a little meditation before my visit. He and his wife were glad to see me. I forgot I had taught them both a couple of relaxation exercises. He wanted me to work more on that with him because he was having a hard time focusing on it, so we did that. His wife said they told all of their family and friends about the relaxation I taught them. I thought in some ways our whole purpose, as a human being, is to touch someone positively and have them touch someone positively. It was somewhat quite exciting that this was taking place before my eyes. One of the things I suggested was a visit outside. I said I would take him out if he would like. Interesting[ly], his nurse was like, "Who are you and why are you here?" I just said I wanted to take him outside—and he did also, so we went outside, which he liked even more than I thought he would. The experience with the patient was positive and reaffirming of some of the things I believe, and now I feel quite excited and pleased about it.

Sometimes on the first visit, the nurses were able to have very open dialogues with the patients, exploring meaning and purpose almost immediately. Other times, the dialogue took time to build trust, and a continued relationship. With ST and her patient, it took several visits before he was able to share his thoughts and meanings with her. ST described this sharing after the third patient visit as follows:

> So I went to see him, and really I was not expecting much, but we ended up having this whole conversation about cancer. He said he had been giving those questions I asked him about significant people and events some thought, and he just had to talk about it. He said he was thinking about how he read esophageal cancer is usually found in white-collar workers. He said that when I asked him about significant events, it hit him,

and he started to realize he hated his job when he was 18 and still does to this day. He talked about how he couldn't fall asleep until it was so late, it was time for him to wake up, and he said "I never wanted to wake up." I asked him if he shared that with anybody or did he hold it in? He said he held it in, and he thinks holding in all those feelings for all that time was so unhealthy for him. He had sadness about him but also excitement. He felt it was time to right what was wrong with his life and time to live more fully than he ever did. He knew the changes he had to make and that he had the opportunity was interesting and very refreshing. He said his first priority is to quit work. He said he should have quit a long time ago. He thanked me for all I did, which was really to listen and for once just shut up.

The nurses in the study either contacted the patients by phone after discharge or arranged to visit with them as part of their routine follow-up visit with the surgeon. These visits or phone calls took place 2 to 4 weeks postoperatively. In some situations the 2 to 4 week follow-up call or visit allowed for more dialogue about choices between the patient and nurse. Unfortunately, there were an equal number of disappointing outcomes, and often patients and families reported feelings of anger and frustration, as well as being abandoned and overwhelmed after they left the hospital. Despite this, the follow-up visit or call, by the nurse, was still very much appreciated.

ST attempted to contact her patient at 2 weeks postoperative because he was not returning to see the surgeon for 6 weeks. When ST called his home, she found that he had been readmitted to a local hospital with complications from the surgery. The ambulance took him to the hospital nearest to his home, but both he and his wife tried to contact the surgeon who had completed the original surgery. They were told he would be treated locally now, which left them feeling angry and abandoned. This is how ST described the call she made once he returned home from the local hospital at 4 weeks postdischarge from the surgery.

I called him, and I first spoke with his wife. She was very angry when I called, but happy with me for calling. She talked about how scared she was. I think somehow just talking made her feel better. Then I talked to him. He was so thrilled to hear from me. His voice was so hoarse, so tired sounding. You just wanted to shed tears for him. I was so glad I called him, and I know I made a difference, but I wonder what would be different in this whole thing if our role were to really follow these people. Basically, he felt he was ignored by the hospital, but he saw me differently in all that. He said it was obvious that I cared. Amazingly, he was able to say that somehow for him it was a good experience. He said he felt refreshed. He certainly did not sound that way, so he means that on another whole level. You know when I first met him I thought I'm not getting anywhere with him, but then it just took more time that's all. It really speaks to a whole different role for the nurse.

Study Implications

Findings from this study have many implications for practice. From the nurse's perspective, study results suggested that (a) this revised care delivery model (PNPM) supports interrelationships among practice, theory, and research; (b) reflection is an essential component of nursing practice, for the nurse as well as the patient and family; (c) there is an ongoing need for mentors in the nursing practice setting to help novice and seasoned clinicians approach patient care using disciplinary, as well as other knowledge; (d) practice settings using a model of care such as the PNPM are valued by nurses; (e) nurses practicing within this knowledge driven, theory-based practice framework are advocates for patient healing; and (f) there is an ongoing need for staff development to advance practice and promote the growth of clinicians.

Relationship

Findings from this research also suggested that for truly mutual, sharing relationships to exist, there must be a break from the previously honored self-sacrificing role of the nurse. The tradition of caring *for* patients becomes more inclusive, when the relationship between the nurse and patient is viewed as an interactive one, where nurses care *with* patients in a dynamic partnership.

Use of Disciplinary Knowledge and Patient Care

This preliminary study also suggested that when nurses participated in a model of practice that used disciplinary knowledge and nursing perspective to deliver patient care, there was a renewed commitment to practice and recognition of what nurses gain when they share in the sacred and intimate healing environment of another person. As nurses share in patients' most vulnerable moments, there is a need to create a practice environment that allows for the contributions of nursing knowledge to become visible.

The PNPM

The PNPM clearly linked the clinical environment with nursing values, beliefs, and knowledge. The model acknowledged each individual's potential, recognized the importance of personal growth, support for nursing as process, and viewed the person as a part of a larger, interconnected whole. It also provides significant implications for nursing education, practice, and leadership.

Transformation

Within the study, both nurses and patients were seeking an opportunity within the experience of patient care that was meaningful and purposeful. Freshwater (1998) compared this process of transformation to that of the alchemist and stated that there is a need in the process of change for a fixed ingredient. Freshwater suggested reflection as that essential ingredient to allow for growth and change.

A consistent theme throughout the study was the power of the transformation that each individual experienced during and beyond each nurse patient encounter. Oftentimes this transformation was difficult for the individual participants to articulate in language.

The results of this study support that nurses need to be invited to share the wisdom of their work and that nurses must invite patients to share the deep understandings of their experience. As Picard (1998) and Watson (1999) suggested it would be important to consider this and invite participants to share or express in whatever way they can, in poetry or other art forms, what an experience has been like for them. Such strategies give patients an alternative to tell their story.

Choice Point

Newman (1989) described the importance of critical choice points in people's lives. It is during these times of choice people can come to recognize the need for change in their lives, recognize opportunity for growth and come to a new awareness and expanded consciousness. Newman suggested that the nurse can allow for this transformation through her ability to be open and present with the person. Additionally, Picard (1998), Freshwater (1998), and Johns (1998) recommended that nurses be reflective and allow for reflection of others who are part of the process of transformation. This implies not only that nurses must be reflective in their own practice but invite their patients to be reflective as well.

Mentoring

Mentoring is another essential component of transformation. Mentoring is a process in itself that is often a part educational and practice experiences of a nurse. There is a need for someone to guide the nurse as nurse guides their patients. Each of the nurses in this study described the turmoil they felt in the practice and the sense of urgency driven by lack of time needed to complete tasks. In some cases, it could be argued that the personal transformation was causing conflicts not recognized as such immediately. By reflecting, mentoring, meditating, and journaling, the nurses came to understand this turmoil as part of the process of growth.

Inner Healing and Moving Away

Imposing or enforcing change that can expose a person's vulnerabilities, while not being supportive enough to allow for transformation, can be detrimental. Recognizing that each person has potential, allowing for that potential and encouraging, nurturing, and supporting are essential steps in the process of transformation. Not all the nurses in this study grew at the same pace. At times personal situations held them back, and at other times, it was their ideas about nursing that had been imposed on them that were limiting. They all, however, sought something beyond what they were doing. They wanted to come to know their patients in a more mutually satisfying way. In the end, each had her own pace, and each had her own way.

Nurses, when invited to share their ideas of what could be in practice, often know they are seeking something more. Guidance can be offered by mentors who provide encouragement and, thereby, opportunity for growth. Nurses' stories and patients' stories alike are opportunities to articulate powerful moments of transformation.

Through the experiences of caring, suffering, and joy, mutual growth can occur. Words cannot always express the impact such occurrences have. Artistic expression can allow nurses and patients the vehicle for reflection and, therefore, transformation. The experiences nurses have with their patients are genuine gifts. As people who share their most vulnerable moments, nurses are not only able to assist people to heal, but are able to heal themselves.

Conclusion

In closing, a quote from E. B. White in *Charlotte's Web* captures the transformation that can occur through a mutually caring relationship. Charlotte is reflecting that now Wilbur will be safe from death, and she calls this moment in part her own moment, and it continues with these words:

> A moment later a tear came to Wilbur's eye. "Oh Charlotte," he said. "To think that when I first met you you were cruel and bloodthirsty!" When he recovered from his emotion he spoke again. "Why did you do all this for me?" He asked. "I don't deserve it. I've never done anything for you." "You have been my friend," replied Charlotte. "That in itself is a tremendous thing. I wove my webs for you because I liked you. After all, what's a life, anyway? We're born, we live a little while, we die. A spider's life can't help being something of a mess, with all this trapping and eating flies. By helping you, perhaps I was trying to lift up my life a trifle. Heaven knows anyone's life can stand a little of that." (p. 164)

REFERENCES

Flanagan, J. (2002). Nurse and patient perceptions of the Pre-admission Nursing Practice Model: Linking theory to practice. *Dissertation Abstract International 56* (UMI No. 30-53657)

Freshwater, D. (1998). The philosopher's stone. In C. Johns & D. Freshwater (Eds.), *Transforming nursing through reflective practice* (pp. 177–184). Oxford, UK: Blackwell Science.

Johns, C. (1998). Opening the doors of perception. In C. Johns & D. Freshwater (Eds.), *Transforming nursing through reflective practice* (pp. 1–20). Oxford, UK: Blackwell Science.

Jones, D., Coakley, A., & Flanagan, J. (1999). Nursing diagnosis and defining character-istics at 24 and 72 hours post surgery with general anesthesia: Preliminary results. In M. Rantz & P. LeMone (Eds.), *Classification of nursing diagnoses: Proceedings of the thirteenth conference* (pp. 471–477). Glendale, CA: CINAHL Information Systems.

Jones, D., Dauphinee, J., Coakley, A., & Fernsebner, W. (1998). *Patient response to same day surgery with local anesthesia AORN Final Grant Report,* AORN.

Newman, M. A. (1989). The spirit of nursing. Holistic Nursing Practice, *3*(3), 1–6.

Newman, M. A. (1994). *Health as expanding consciousness* (2nd ed.) New York: National League for Nursing.

Newman, M. A. (1997). Evolution of the theory of health as expanding consciousness. *Nursing Science Quarterly*, *10*(1), p. 22–36.

Picard, C. (1998). *Baccalaureate nursing students and the use of aesthetics in reflective practice.* Unpublished manuscript.

Rogers, M. E. (1990). Nursing: Science of unitary, irreducible, human beings: Update. In E. A. M. Barrett (Ed.), *Visions of Roger's science-based nursing* (pp. 5–11). New York: National League for Nursing.

Roy, C., & Andrews, H. (1999). *The Roy Adaptation Model.* (2nd ed.) Stamford, CT: Appleton & Lange.

Watson, J. (1996). Watson's theory of transpersonal caring. In P. Walker & B. Neuman (Eds.), *Blueprint for use of nursing models: Education, research, practice and administration* (pp. 141–184). New York: National League for Nursing.

Watson, J. (1999). *Postmodern nursing and beyond.* Edinburgh, Scotland, UK: Churchill Livingstone/WB Saunders.

White, E. B. (1952). *Charlotte's web.* New York: HarperCollins.

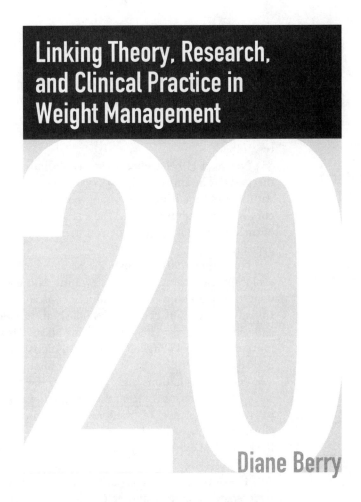

Linking Theory, Research, and Clinical Practice in Weight Management

Diane Berry

Overweight and obesity in the United States have reached epidemic proportions affecting approximately 61% of all adults over the age of 20 (U.S. Department of Health and Human Services [USDHHS], 2001). Obesity is prevalent in both genders, children and adults, and in all major ethnic groups, including African American, Hispanic, and American Indian (Flegal, Carroll, Kuzarski, & Johnson, 1998; Ogden, Flegal, Carroll, & Johnson, 2002; USDHHS, 2001). Overweight and obesity are major contributors to many preventable causes of death including coronary artery disease and Type II diabetes (USDHHS, 2000). Treatment and management of overweight and obesity includes weight management programs using nutrition education, exercise, behavioral modification, medication or bariatric surgery.

Despite short-term weight loss successes, long-term weight reduction has been difficult to maintain. A majority of individuals regain all weight lost within 3 to 5 years (Wadden & Stunkard, 2002). Many clinical interventions designed for weight loss management, have not linked theory and research with clinical practice. The use of Newman's theory of health as expanding consciousness (HEC) to understand changing behavior and sustaining weight loss provides a strong theoretical framework to ground research and access the knowledge needed to understand the human experience (Newman, 1994).

Health as Expanding Consciousness (HEC): A Theory

Health as expanding consciousness (Newman, 1994) is a theoretical framework that provides a useful foundation for understanding the process of weight loss and weight maintenance. Through research, lifestyle pattern recognition occurs in each individual in a reflective process that encourages increased self-awareness for the participant and researcher.

Newman (1994) reflects the whole individual as being greater than the sum of the parts. The individual is a part of an open energy system that is interconnected with and engaged in the evolving pattern of the whole. Unfolding consciousness occurs in partnership between the researcher or nurse and the individual. The pattern of each individual and the environment emerges through dialogue and dynamic energy exchange.

Newman (1990) established a parallel between HEC and Young's (1976) theory of evolution. According to Young, evolution occurs as humans move from potential freedom to real freedom. An individual's consciousness is bound with minimal movement. Initially, the person begins to establish an individual identity with self-consciousness and self-determinism at the centering stage. An intentional turn and the beginning of movement toward a higher level of consciousness are apparent when a conscious choice is made to foster change. It is during this time that new laws are learned and a new awareness of limitations and potential as the beginning of inner growth emerges. The stage of decentering reflects movement toward transcendence of self and movement toward a higher level of freedom. At this moment in time an individual's energy and awareness increases and extends beyond his or her physical boundaries. In addition, the individual experiences expanded time or timelessness as consciousness continues to expand.

The development of narratives using Newman's framework allowed the possibility of understanding pattern and behavior change in women maintaining weight loss through self-awareness, choice, transition, and expansion of consciousness. Studies conducted by Newman and other researchers have found the encounter between participant and nurse allowed both an opportunity for self-expression, integration, and expansion of consciousness (Barron, 2000; Berry, 2004; Endo, 1996, 1998; Lamendola & Newman, 1994; Novaletsky-Rosenthal, 1996; Picard, 1998).

Initial Research

Research conducted using the theory of health as expanding consciousness framework (Berry, 2004) provided the researcher with a firm foundation upon which to develop an intervention for overweight and obese parents of obese children. In the study Berry found that women who were successful at weight loss and maintenance progressed through a process, which oftentimes required several attempts. Initially prior to weight loss, women experienced low self-esteem, low self-awareness, and felt vulnerable. Recognition that weight loss was an issue for the person, there was a new awareness that the weight often came from weighing themselves or a comment made by someone else. Over time, all of the women felt a readiness to make change and came to a point where there was a decision to lose weight. They took control of their lives and actively engaged in the process of weight loss by learning new skills such as portion control, increasing awareness of which trigger foods encouraged overeating, exercising daily, and engaging in self-monitoring by weighing themselves at least weekly. Social support came from family, friends, and women whom they met with weekly at a weight management program. As women learned to maintain their weight loss, they learned personal integration, which they described as increasing self-awareness, self-confidence, and self-esteem. In addition, they felt less vulnerable and more in control of their lives.

Subsequent Research

The initial research grounded in the theory of health as expanding consciousness (Newman, 1994) provided the lifestyle pattern behavioral model of change (Berry, 2004) that was included in the design of a nutrition and exercise education and coping skills training intervention for parents who desired to partner with their children to lose weight and improve their health. The pilot study was a 12-week intervention designed for dyads (parent and child) with a body mass index (BMI) greater than 25. The principal aim was to conduct a randomized pilot study intervention that targeted lifestyle change for overweight or obese parents of obese children. Parents who participated in the intervention were compared to control parents who received the standard nutrition education program at baseline, 3, and 6 months on the following outcome measures: (a) individual physiological indicators (BMI, body fat percentage, daily pedometer steps); (b) health promoting lifestyle behaviors (Health Promoting Lifestyle Profile II [HPLP II]; Walker, Sechrist, & Pender, 1987); (c) eating self-efficacy (Eating Self-Efficacy Scale [ESES]; Glynn & Ruderman, 1986); and (d) family functioning (Family Assessment Device [FAD]; Epstein, Levin, & Bishop, 1976). The related hypothesis was that parents randomly assigned to the experimental intervention would score better on all outcome measures at both time points.

The secondary aim was to compare at 3 and 6 months, the individual physiological (BMI, body fat percentage, daily pedometer steps) as measures of obese children whose parents participated in the experimental intervention that targeted lifestyle change to control parents, who had participated in the standard nutrition program as described below. The related hypothesis was that obese children of the parents who were randomly assigned to the experimental intervention would have lower body mass index, lower body fat percentage, and higher daily pedometer steps when compared at 3 and 6 months to obese children of the control parents who received the standard nutrition education program.

Parents were encouraged to join the research study with their child. During the first 6 weeks of the research study, parents attended nutrition classes taught by a registered dietitian once a week for 45 minutes with their children. Nutrition classes included information on determining portion sizes, better food choices and a nondiet approach, calories, meal planning, food labels, healthy recipe substitutions, and eating out. During the second 6 weeks, the parents and children attended separate classes. The parents were taught by a coping skills trainer and learned about exercise, barriers to weight loss, how to motivate themselves, rebounding from weight loss, and weight loss and maintenance. A registered dietitian taught the children about getting the most out of their metabolism, exercise, self-esteem and self-image, setting goals, and identifying high-risk situations. The groups were small (6 to 10 persons) and discussion was encouraged. Parents also discussed the importance of role modeling for their children and how to encourage positive lifestyle behavior change within their families. Problem solving, conflict resolution, assertiveness training, and behavioral modification were included. In addition, both the children and parents received pedometers and pedometer walking books and were encouraged to work toward a goal of taking 10,000 steps per day. The children and parents exercised twice a week with the exercise physiologists and were encouraged to walk at least 30 minutes on the other 5 days using their pedometers. The pilot study is ongoing, but if findings support that the experimental group improved when compared to the control group, the intervention will be refined and expanded to a family-based intervention designed for the whole family.

In summary, the development and execution of this pilot study would not have been possible without the initial research using Newman's (1994) theory of health as expanding consciousness. Understanding why some individuals were successful at weight loss and maintenance provided the tools necessary to design a theoretically based intervention.

Practice Implications

In clinical practice, a nurse practitioner can use HEC (Newman, 1994) and the lifestyle behavioral model of change (Berry, 2004) to work with families, women, men, and children who are struggling with overweight and obesity. Prevention of Type II diabetes and coronary heart disease are important public health goals. In prescriptive medicine, patients are told to lose weight and many times not given the support and information they need to improve their health. Prescriptive health care has resulted in little improvement in the obesity problem in the United States. However, when reflective practice is used, a relationship develops between the nurse practitioner and patient that empowers the patient to see the possibilities of balancing his or her life in a new way. Behavior change takes time, patience, and a strong commitment. Obesity is a chronic disease like diabetes and hypertension. Patients have to be helped and supported to recognize the importance of the problem to their lives and understand that change, in this case weight loss, is hard work, with no easy solutions. Assisting patients to understand that they must find their own personal balance between nutrition and exercise takes time. This understanding starts with a practice that is theoretically and research based. A nurse practitioner can help the individual work through this process and provide the knowledge and support through the process of adopting new choices and behaviors. The following case study exemplifies the importance of the nurse patient relationship during the period of weight loss and weight maintainance.

Linking Theory and Research to Clinical Practice

Betty was a 46-year-old African American female who presented with a blood pressure of 158/96, taken at her local pharmacy. Her past medical history included obesity since puberty. Family history was positive for obesity, Type II diabetes, hypertension, hyperlipidemia, and coronary heart disease. A dietary history revealed that Betty consumed a diet high in calories, fats, carbohydrates, and few fruits and vegetables. Her physical examination revealed that her height was 66 inches and her weight was 285 pounds. Body mass index was 46.1. Clinically, overweight is defined as a BMI of 25 kg/m^2 or more, up to a BMI of 29.9 kg/m^2; obesity is defined as a BMI of 30.0 kg/m^2 or greater (USDHHS, 1987). Her blood pressure was 156/98, apical pulse 88 bpm, and respirations 20 per minute. The nurse practitioner explained that it would be necessary to start a thiazide diuretic (National High Blood Pressure Education Program, 2003) to control her hypertension and schedule a full physical examination to rule out comorbidities.

The nurse practitioner then asked Betty, "How do you feel about your current weight?" Betty then spoke for 10 minutes about her struggle to lose weight, noting that she had tried many diets and nothing seemed to work. The nurse practitioner queried her further about her diet intake and exercise pattern and asked Betty to keep a food and exercise journal for 3 days and bring it to her physical the following week. In addition, the nurse practitioner asked her to use the next week to reflect on what her future health goals were. Laboratory work was ordered that included a complete blood count, chemistry panel, lipid profile, and thyroid-stimulating hormone, to be drawn before the physical examination.

The following week, Betty returned for her physical examination, and the nurse practitioner met with her in the office before going to the exam room. The nurse practitioner completed a medical history and reviewed her laboratory data with her, which were all within normal limits. Using Newman's HEC framework, the nurse practitioner then queried Betty further asking her to "tell me about the most meaningful persons and events in your life" (Newman, 1994, p. 147). Over the next half hour, Betty shared her life story outlining important events and relationships. The nurse practitioner documented this information and in addition completed the physical examination. The physical findings were within normal limits, except for Betty's obesity and hypertension. As Betty had started taking the thiazide diuretic her blood pressure had decreased to 132/88.

At the completion of the examination, the nurse practitioner shared her results related to the physical examination and asked if she would like to start working toward making healthy behavior change. Betty agreed that this was an important life goal. The nurse practitioner then reviewed some basic dietary changes that she could start making at home such as decreasing portions, becoming aware of her trigger foods, exercising, and weighing herself weekly (Berry, 2004). In addition, the nurse practitioner asked Betty to purchase a pedometer and to start a gentle walking program starting with 10 minutes a day and working up to 30 minutes a day. Betty was asked to record her food and exercise progress in her journal and bring it with her when she returned for her blood pressure check in 1 week.

During the next visit, Betty's blood pressure was evaluated and noted to remained stable at 136/82. In addition her weight had decreased to 281 pounds (4 pound weight loss). Betty also reported walking 20 minutes per day. The nurse practitioner shared the narrative and diagram of Betty's life patterns assessed and developed by the nurse after the last visit. The pattern display was organized chronologically and reflected key phrases, relationships and experiences to Betty by the nurse practitioner. Betty responded positively to the experience, and as she reviewed the pattern display for accuracy she specifically noted that while she had a stable childhood, she began gaining weight as an adolescent and struggled with her weight since that time. After reviewing the entire pattern analysis, Betty's response was, "It is amazing to see it all here. I have always struggled with weight, but to see it in black and white is humbling." Betty gained new insights from the process and decided to join a formal weight loss program at work and continued walking with two of her neighbors. She found the validation and social support from these activities important in moving forward in her goals. Betty met with the nurse practitioner 2 weeks later for a blood pressure and weight check and to discuss her progress.

Betty's blood pressure remained within normal limits (130/80) and her weight had decreased to 277 (8 pound weight loss). During her visit with the nurse practitioner, she felt very positive and committed. She realized that this would take time and that there would be setbacks, but she continued to attend the weight management program each week and was walking 30 minutes a day with her neighbors. She continued to email the nurse practitioner weekly with her weight and followed up with the nurse practitioner every 3 months for a blood pressure and weight check and to talk about her lifestyle behavior change. After 1 year, Betty had lost 52 pounds and continued to work toward her personal goals. She has weaned off her blood pressure medication, continues to attend a weight loss program, and walks 30 minutes almost everyday. Betty realizes that it took her many years to gain the weight, and it will take several years to lose it and then maintain her weight loss. Improved health has brought with it improved self-esteem and improved self-confidence, and she is now working with other family members and friends encouraging them to improve their health as well.

Conclusion

The reflective process that occurs when using the health as expanding consciousness praxis model provided a new way to understand overweight and obesity. The importance of recognizing an individual pattern, provides a strong foundation for the nurse practitioner and researcher to assist those individuals who manifest overweight and obesity as a component of their life pattern. Developing interventions that are reflective and teach individual family members to work toward improved health are important. The praxis methodology allows both the researcher and nurse practitioner an opportunity to come to know the person and understand pattern over time. The researcher or nurse practitioner and participant or patient are able to understand exactly where the individual is in the change process and monitor new expressions of the human experience over time.

Over the past 30 years, the prescriptive behavioral model of change has been limited in that it focused on changing the outward behavior (eating and exercise in this case) but not the whole person. It offered the patient knowledge about what they "should do" and failed to provide long-term support necessary for long-term weight-loss maintenance. The new paradigm of reflective practice, guided by nursing knowledge, offers individuals an opportunity to view health and illness in a new way. In the example above, obesity is seen as a manifestation of the whole, and the nurse and the patient work in partnership to explore pattern and change behavior within the context of the total person experience. The individual is encouraged to make choices in view of personal goals and works with the nurse over time to increase personal awareness and promote actions that will be reflected in improved health. Improving personal health is reflected in understanding one's personal pattern and establishing a balance between food and exercise. Each individual wanting to make change is helped to recognize new opportunities by the nurse and is brought to point where he or she is able to draw from inner energy and strength to make the needed changes. Weight loss and maintenance requires sustained support and takes time. Each individual who embarks on improving health, is ready to change, and makes a decision to lose weight, may go through this process many times before taking control of his or her life and actively engaging in the process (Berry, 2004). He or she may chose to join a weight-loss program and learn new skills such as increasing awareness of food portion control, exercise, and self-monitoring. Social support and validation continue to be an important part of the process and when sustained over time can support the individual during difficult periods in the transition. As noted in earlier work (Berry, 2004), when individuals experience success at one change in lifestyle, others often become easier.

As noted, obesity is a chronic disease like diabetes and hypertension, and each individual who embarks on change will have to be aware of the chronic nature of the disease for the rest of their lives. As one participant shared, "I am like an alcoholic, but I am addicted to food. I lost 50 pounds and have kept it off for 27 years, but each day I have to be aware of what I eat and have to exercise." Those individuals who do lose weight and maintain their weight loss have a new sense of personal integration and balance. Although they continue to improve their health and balance their nutrition and exercise, they have moved to another level of consciousness and feel increased self-awareness, improved self-consciousness, increased self-esteem, and feel in control of their lives (Berry, 2004). Lifestyle behavior change occurs over time and requires deep personal reflection and understanding from the participant or patient working with the researcher or nurse practitioner.

REFERENCES

Barron, A. M. (2000). *Life meanings and the experience of cancer: Application of Newman's method and phenomenological analysis.* Unpublished doctoral dissertation, Boston College, Chestnut Hill, MA.

Berry, D. (2004). An emerging model of behavior change in women maintaining weight loss. *Nursing Science Quarterly, 13*(3), 242–252.

Endo, E. (1996). *Pattern recognition as a nursing intervention with adults with cancer.* Unpublished doctoral dissertation, University of Minnesota, Minneapolis.

Endo, E. (1998). Pattern recognition as a nursing intervention with Japanese women with ovarian cancer. *Advances in Nursing Science, 20*(4), 49–61.

Epstein, N. B., Levin, S., & Bishop, D. S. (1976). The family as a social unit. *Canadian Family Physician, 22,* 1411–1413.

Flegal, M. S., Carroll, M. D., Kuzarski, R. J., & Johnson, C. L. (1998). Overweight and obesity in the United States: Prevalence and trends. *International Journal of Obesity Related Metabolic Disorders, 22,* 39–47.

Glynn, S. M., & Ruderman, J. (1986). The development and validation of an eating self-efficacy scale. *Cognitive Therapy and Research, 10,* 403–420.

Lamendola, F. P., & Newman, M. A. (1994). The paradox of HIV/AIDS as expanding consciousness. *Advances in Nursing Science, 16*(3), 13–21.

National High Blood Pressure Education Program. (2003). *JNC 7 Express: The Seventh Report of the Joint National Committee on Prevention, Detection, Evaluation, and Treatment of High Blood Pressure.* Washington, DC: U.S. Department of Health and Human Services, National Institutes of Health, National Heart, Lung, and Blood Institute.

Newman, M. A. (1990). Newman's theory on health as praxis. *Nursing Science Quarterly, 4,* 161–167.

Newman, M. A. (1994). *Health as expanding consciousness.* New York: National League for Nursing.

Novaletsky-Rosenthal, H. T. (1996). Pattern recognition in older adults with chronic illness. *Dissertation Abstracts International, 57*(10), 6180B. (UMI No. AA69707886)

Ogden, C. L., Flegal, K. M., Carroll, M. D., & Johnson, C. L. (2002). Prevalence and trends in overweight among U.S. children and adolescents, 1999–2000. *Journal of the American Medical Association, 288*(14), 1728–1732.

Picard, C. (1998). *Uncovering pattern of expanding consciousness in mid-life women: Creative movement and the narrative as modes of expression.* Unpublished doctoral dissertation, Boston College, Chestnut Hill, MA.

U.S. Department of Health and Human Services. (1987). *Vital and health statistics: Anthropometric reference data and prevalence of overweight United States, 1976–1980.* Hyattsville, MD: Author.

U.S. Department of Health and Human Services. (2000). *Healthy people 2010: National health promotion and disease prevention objectives.* Washington, DC: Government Printing Office.

U.S. Department of Health and Human Services. (2001). *The Surgeon General's call to action to prevent and decrease overweight and obesity.* Washington, DC: U.S. Government Printing Office.

Wadden, T. A., & Stunkard, A. J. (2002). *Handbook of obesity treatment.* New York: Guilford.

Walker, S. N., Sechrist, K. R., & Pender, N. J. (1987). The Health-promoting lifestyle profile: Development and psychometric characteristics. *Nursing Research, 36,* 76–81.

Young, A. M. (1976). *The reflexive universe: Evolution of consciousness.* San Francisco: Robert Briggs.

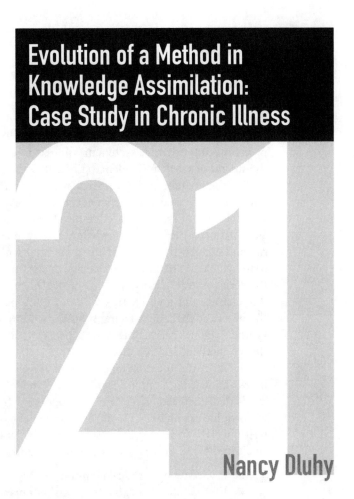

Evolution of a Method in Knowledge Assimilation: Case Study in Chronic Illness

21

Nancy Dluhy

Scientific pluralism emerges as a pervasive theme within contemporary philosophical discourse in nursing (Kim, 1993, 2000; Meleis, 1997; Monti & Tingen, 1999). Equally intense arguments supporting scientific pluralism appear in other disciplines, for example, sociology (Turner, 1989), psychology (Gergen, 2001; Kalmar & Sternberg, 1988; Mikulas, 1995), anthropology (Dressler, 2001), and organizational management (Eulberg, Weekley, & Bhagat, 1988). Within the pluralistic perspective diverse conceptualizations, explanations, and philosophies regarding a given phenomenon are valued. Yet, any one interpretation appears incomplete.

The ensuing discussion focuses on knowledge in a substantive area of nursing. Substantive areas, such as women's health, chronic illness, and gerontology characteristically include diverse interpretations arising across many disciplines. Therefore, a comprehensive understanding of a substantive area requires finding a method to accommodate and assimilate knowledge developed from different perspectives into a systematic whole (Baker, Norton, Young, & Ward, 1998; Dluhy, 1995; Kim, 1989'; Nagle & Mitchell, 1991).

In Search of Method

Valuing diverse forms of knowledge carries an appeal in a discipline that embraces a range of epistemic approaches and theoretical interpretations. Eventually, though, scientific disciplines face the task of systematizing knowledge, a challenge accentuated when dealing with diverse, competing knowledge (Blalock, 1982, 1984). A practice discipline carries a pronounced burden for systematization as interventions defining practice emerge from the weight of scientific evidence (Lang, 1999; Upton, 1999).

Unfortunately, there are no road maps or methods for assimilating diverse, competing knowledge into a coherent system (Dluhy, 1995). This chapter explores the evolution of a method for nursing knowledge development, specifically relating to the synthesis or assimilation of pluralistic knowledge. The author's approach to construct an assimilation method entails strategies initially generated within the philosophy of science and then modified based on knowledge specific to chronic illness. A retrospective meta-analysis of this series of strategies using Kim's critical normative and critical narrative epistemologies (see chapters 12 and 14, this volume) illuminates the philosophical and in particular the practical challenges facing scholars who espouse pluralism. Examining knowledge synthesis efforts raises pragmatic aspects encountered at the intersection of philosophy, theory, method, and practice.

Each of the four distinct methods developed by the author to assimilate chronic illness knowledge is first described in terms of the rationale underlying development and is then analyzed using Kim's epistemology framework. In addition to the underlying philosophical principles, the retrospective analysis also addresses the intellectual hunches, trial and error strategies, and pragmatic considerations inherent in method construction. In chronological order these strategies include:

- 1993: Metatheoretical mapping strategy for knowledge assimilation
- 1998: Model of negotiated symptom management
- 1999: Knowledge synthesis web cluster (practice knowledge)
- 2001: Team strategy—chronic illness consortium model

Metatheoretical Mapping of Substantive Area of Knowledge

In early stages of development, disciplines typically research an array of phenomena, creating a wealth of diverse knowledge. Researchers, even when focusing on similar events, become so specialized that they talk past each other even to the extent of creating unique vocabularies (Blalock, 1982). A maturing scientific discipline faces the task of evaluating and systematizing this disconnected knowledge into a coherent body of knowledge. Scholars in nursing (Hall, 1997; Meleis, 1987) continue to voice a concern that it is time to move beyond philosophical and method debates and begin cumulating knowledge around the substantive aspects of the discipline.

The simple question remains—how do we know all that we know? To address this question, the author (Dluhy, 1995) developed a method to map pluralistic knowledge as a preliminary step in knowledge assimilation. Reasoning that pluralistic knowledge represents different ontological and epistemological positions, a spatial mapping technique was created using the intersection of polarized positions. For example, the person as body or person as soul represent the extreme positions in ontology. Likewise, epistemological positions fall between the extremes of positivism and subjective interpretivism.

In nursing, the four quadrants formed by the intersect of these polarized views tend to be dominated by the physical, cognitive, social, and person-centered, or holistic focus. An extensive review of nursing research and theoretical thinking within chronic illness yielded 20 dominant research programs that could then be located at one point on the spatial map using an analysis of foundational epistemological and ontological positions. This strategy revealed the most extensive scholarly activity in the cognitive quadrant dominated by the work of Lazarus (1966). Though less pervasive, the influence of Selye (1976) and Strauss and Glaser (1974) was evident in two of the remaining quadrants. No dominant foundation was associated with the holistic quadrant (see Fig. 21.1).

The underlying goal driving this mapping effort was to first capture what is known relating to chronic illness and then render it more coherent and useful to practice. Although the mapping strategy illustrates the wealth of knowledge associated with chronic illness, it also raises the potential for discord in trying to bridge the gulf between these knowledge types. Finding a way to accommodate the magnitude of knowledge emerging from disparate epistemological and ontological assumptions presents a nearly paralyzing challenge. Equally evident is the depth of understanding required to effectively uncover the assumptions underlying different perspectives in chronic illness.

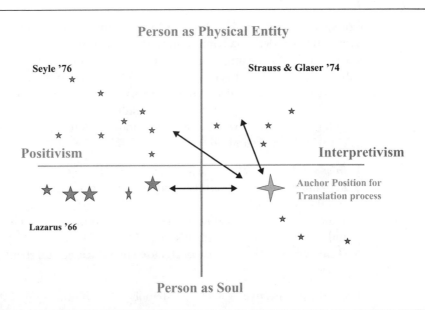

Metatheoretical Map of Knowledge in Chronic Illness.

Uncovering a New Direction

Three barriers became apparent while using this mapping strategy. First, the sheer volume of information and necessary degree of familiarity with the underlying assumptions suggests a need for a group approach for further development. Second, the observed dominance of the cognitive psychology perspective brings into question a potential for scholarly bias. As an example, although holism appears throughout nursing literature, this perspective yielded limited scientific attention in mainstream nursing research on those experiencing chronic illness.

Ultimately, the incommensurability thesis provides the greatest hurdle. This position holds that theoretical worldviews are unique, even creating unique language, and therefore not subject to comparison or integration. Kuhn, the originator of this thesis (1970) refuted this as widespread *mis*interpretation of his writings, asserting that it is in fact feasible to *translate* between frameworks as long as the translator maintains the core or essence of each framework.

After many frustrating trials attempting translation within this mapping strategy, the author came to realize that translation demands a native tongue. Considering the core values of nursing, the anchor position (or native tongue) for translation became quadrant #4, which is most associated with the holistic, person-centered experience (see Fig. 21.1). Whereas there may be many ways to assimilate knowledge within chronic illness, this anchoring position assures that all knowledge is filtered through or reconstructed within a person-centered perspective. This forces the integration of the two primary dichotomies in pluralism within nursing science—body/mind/soul and objective/subjective understanding of the illness experience (Dluhy, 1995).

Epistemic Analysis

On retrospective analysis, there appears to be congruity between the mapping strategy and assumptions underlying Kim's critical normative epistemology for nursing (chapter 12, this volume). One assumption about knowledge indicates that it must be developed partially and selectively but is considered complementary and inclusive versus competitive and exclusive. A second assumption asserts that nursing requires both a science of control and therapy and a science of understanding and care.

Kim (chapter 12, this volume) identifies four epistemic foci for nursing knowledge consistent with these assumptions.

1 *Inferential*—generalized, focused on explaining regularities and patterns.
2 *Referential*—situated hermeneutic, focused on subjective experience, meaning, and the individual.
3 *Transformative*—critical hermeneutic, focused on socially constructed meaning and processes, and the human's social life.
4 *Desiderative*—ethical/aesthetic, focused on values, ethical standards, and aesthetic ideals.

From the perspective of Kim's epistemology, an examination of the chronic illness knowledge plotted on the initial map reveals primarily a referential focus (i.e., dyspnea, fatigue, and uncertainty in illness) or inferential focus (i.e., living with symptoms, meaning in illness, suffering, and redefining life). Synthesizing these aspects, even using an accurate process of translation, still yields an incomplete nursing representation of the world of chronic illness. Kim's model suggests two other domains essential to a comprehensive understanding, the transformative and desiderative focus.

Suggestions of these issues filter through writings in chronic illness, in particular works by Thorne and Patterson (1998, 2001). These authors describe contextual and interactional themes that continue to influence or modify the range of responses and behaviors of those who live with chronic illness. These include the following:

1 Changing societal views of chronic illness, in particular a shift in views on individual responsibility for illness.
2 Continuing impact of mind/body dualism, separating the lived experience from the physical.
3 The silence of other voices as the bulk of qualitative knowledge of the illness experience emerges from advantaged, European-descent, middle-class women not currently in crisis.
4 The abandonment of our moral commitment to those with chronic illness who struggle in a system ill-fitted to their concerns.

This author's interpretation of Kim's epistemology suggests that the desiderative and transformative foci provide context and boundaries to knowledge in the inferential and referential foci. In this way, they serve to redirect, constrain, enlighten, and enliven our substantive knowledge development. A representation (Fig. 21.2) derived from Kim's epistemology depicts knowledge made visible in practice emerging from the traditional research focus (inferential, referential). Understanding developed within the two remaining foci occurs within disciplinary discourse. This representation provides a mode for analysis of the remaining approaches to knowledge assimilation in chronic illness.

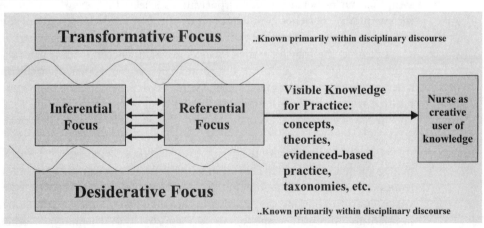

Boundary Function of Transformative and Desiderative Foci.

Model of Negotiated Symptom Management

The next phase in the search for an assimilation method entailed the development of a model of negotiated symptom management (Haworth & Dluhy, 2001). Two notions arising from the mapping strategy provided direction for this work. First, despite the chaos of information in the substantive area of chronic illness, symptom experience emerged as a central concept. Logic suggested that understanding the symptom experience might open an avenue to assimilation. Second, fatigue surfaced as the most frequently encountered symptom across all chronic illnesses. Investigating the nature of fatigue revealed a number of associated characteristics such as vagueness, meaning, the difficulty of giving language to the physical sensation, and the social implications of living with fatigue (Baker & Stern, 1993; Winningham et al., 1994). Hence, the symptom management model developed around this aspect of negotiating this vague, chronic symptom with the nurse who functions in a system historically dominated by an acute illness philosophy.

The model contains five major components—symptom awareness, interpretation, decision making, interaction with nurse, and negotiated management strategies (Haworth & Dluhy, 2001). There is no finite end in this model because the symptom may persist, change, or appear in clusters and require ongoing evaluation. The assimilated model draws on a broad range of symptom discussions within nursing, psychology, sociology, anthropology, and medicine.

Analysis of Symptom Management Model

Using Kim's epistemic foci as a foundation for analysis, perspectives on the symptom experience reflect all four foci, particularly during the phase of the negotiated interaction between the person and the nurse. In the desiderative focus, Haworth and Dluhy (2001) stress the centrality of core nursing values, providing a boundary for the application of this model. The goal of the interaction is not simply finding a quick solution for this symptom but rather using this opportunity to hear the lifeworld of the person, value the symptom experience, and demonstrate the artful, relational work of the nurse. The symptom experience provides for new possibilities.

Likewise, the transformative focus is revealed when the nurse brings an awareness of all the sociopolitical, cultural, and contextual constraints that affect the moment when a person shares a symptom experience with a care provider. The historical evolution of health care alters expectations within this moment of shared knowledge, including which knowledge is valued and even the language given to the symptom (Haworth & Dluhy, 2001).

Notions consistent with the desiderative and transformative foci locate the symptom management model exclusively within nursing. The experiential and referential foci draw from a variety of disciplines, but the two boundary foci serve to reconstruct that knowledge consistent with a nursing worldview. This provides insight into a methodological concern in scientific pluralism, namely, how to reconstruct knowledge from other disciplines congruent with a nursing perspective. Attending to the transformative and desiderative foci may resolve this dilemma (see Fig. 21.3).

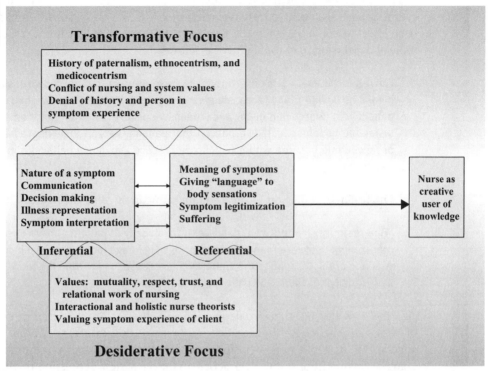

Epistemic analysis of the Model of Negotiated Symptom.

Hearing the Voice of Practice

In 1999, a number of pragmatic, technical, and philosophical events converged resulting in the third strategy. This included recognition that the nurse clinician has little choice but to synthesize what is known for application at least at an individual level, in the management of those with chronic illness. It could prove illuminating to study how nurses actually sort this out to determine an action.

Additionally, computer technology offered a feasible medium to engage in dialogue with practicing clinicians and extract that knowledge. Finally, a growing theme in publications gained impetus and sparked a shift in scholarly thinking toward seeking clinician knowledge, particularly through narratives and reflective practice strategies (Benner, 1984; Litchfield, 1999; Thorne & Hayes, 1997).

In this context, the author created a Web site as a vehicle for assimilating practice knowledge. The *Chronic Illness Knowledge Synthesis* Web site facilitated dialogue among nurse clinicians around key components of chronic illness. Brief paragraphs describing aspects such as depression, living with fatigue, stigma, compliance, meaning in illness, or symptom expression provided the focus for nurse dialogue. Asynchronous (stacked chronologically) comments stored on the Web site permitted ongoing reflection and discussion by the participating clinicians. The real energy (and source for knowledge synthesis analysis) occurred when participants reflected on responses from one another in an effort to challenge, augment, or clarify. As an example, one nurse responded to the topic of depression in chronic illness as follows:

> I have some questions to pose. First of all, have you ever thought of depression in chronic illness as having many faces, stages, or degrees? By that I mean, when we think of a patient with depression in chronic illness, we picture them, or see them as being sad or feeling hopelessness. I've noticed that patients vary in their depression response or face; some become withdrawn, some practice avoidance behaviors in dealing with day-to-day . . .

Other nurses reflect on Diane's comments in an ongoing dialogue.

> [T]he majority of withdrawn, depressed chronically ill patients I have encountered are men. I think there are many reasons for this . . . I have found it more difficult to connect with and break through to the withdrawn, depressed client than the more active angry, sad, or denying client. One patient comes to mind . . .

Analysis provided insights into depression and chronic illness as seen through the eyes of nurses in practice. From extended responses of this nature, the author constructed generalizations about nurses' insights on depression and used these to stimulate on-going discussion. For example, practicing clinicians view depression of chronic illness as markedly different from clinical depression, equating depression to a more global reaction to loss and drawing a connection to finding meaning in the illness experience.

One intriguing addition posed by the nurses was observations of depression emanating not from the illness but rather from interactions with health care providers. Discussions by clinicians emerge in the language of practice and are translated to theoretical language to compare to formal knowledge. Although the narratives among these nurses were intriguing and raised some new insights, limitations seemed inherent in this method. Over the course of 2 years, it was frustrating to sort through the practice language, its lack of unity and in particular the blurring of conceptual meanings in order to analyze the narratives.

Analysis Using Critical Narrative Epistemology

Analysis using Kim's critical narrative epistemology provides shape to the frustrations with this method. In turning her attention to practice knowledge, Kim acknowledges the nurse in practice as "the ultimate synthesizer and knowledge generator" (2001). Further, she states, "since synthesized knowledge is only evident as a product of nursing practice, it can be revealed only through an in-depth, post hoc analysis of practice (2001). Although the Web site strategy attends to these assumptions, serious limitations in methodology surfaced. The first concern, though pragmatic, is significant. Referring again to the representation of Kim's epistemology (see Fig. 21.2) the question can be asked—who is this idealized nurse? Kim, within a critical narrative epistemology, depicts the nurse as the true synthesizer of knowledge in practice. Yet, *nurse* is a term associated with varying levels of education and, therefore, exposed to significantly different breadths and depths of knowledge. Are all nurses reflective knowers of practice and able to give language to practice? What implications does this have for examining the synthesis product we call practice?

Second, postmodern practice discussions tend to portray the nurse in a very favorable manner, posing potential for transformation and artistry (Litchfield, 1999). Are these notions of nursing idealized or pervasive in practice? In other words, is the exemplary practice script coined by Kim (chapter 12, this volume) an accurate reflection of practice behavior? Will the narratives found within practice use knowledge sources similar to those identified by scholars of nursing, or do organizational systems of health care mold and constrain the narratives?

Turning to a different aspect, if knowledge synthesis fundamentally occurs in practice, how does the nurse acquire these synthesizing tools or skills? Does the educational process sow the seeds for this skill? If not, is the experiential process sufficient for assimilation of knowledge into a coherent whole? Additionally, are nurses who are embedded in the context of practice able to distinguish the subtle and not so subtle influences within the organizational and social construction of practice as they reveal their exemplary practice scripts? In other words, how much is all of this synthesis process influenced by the ongoing domination of health care by the medical model and more recently, the consumer, business model? System constraints, the allure of technology, and historical medical dominance are all possible contaminants of the assimilated knowledge that scholars seek to uncover.

Finally, is the notion of good practice tautological? By that I mean, do we identify nurses who we deem (by some external criteria) to be engaged in good practice and ask them to provide exemplars that demonstrate good practice?

Summary

This program of research to uncover a method for knowledge assimilation within scientific pluralism is founded on the premise that a coherent, systematized body of knowledge will be reflected in improved client care. This assumption finds support within the epistemic analysis of the strategies. A meta-analysis of the knowledge generated within programs of research or expressed in clinician narratives heightens sensitivity to the substance of practice and the influences that shape the use of knowledge (tranformative and desiderative foci). There is no simple or shortcut approach to this process. Rather, it is an iterative endeavor moving between a meta-analysis to assimilate the products of science and uncovering the synthesis of knowledge inherent in practice. The author's current strategy, a *Chronic Illness Consortium*, comprised of scholars and practicing clinicians, provides a structure to facilitate this iterative process. Science has limits in addressing the complexities of the human condition, and clinicians are constrained and influenced by the historical and sociopolitical realities of practice. Yet, what else can one examine except science and practice to describe what is known about a substantive area? Each assimilation strategy, no matter how tentative, heightens an awareness of the knowledge available to the clinician. The issue remains how, in what form, and by what reasoning it is brought to the practice situation. In addition, how will we prepare nurses and create a curriculum that addresses the content of the science, the substance, and the practice? How too will we design a practice environment that will create expectations of nurses that reflect unity around knowledge that is used and practiced by all nurse providers? These questions require continued exploration and development as we advance nursing knowledge.

REFERENCES

Baker, C., Norton, S., Young, P., & Ward, S. (1998). An exploration of methodological pluralism in nursing research. *Research in Nursing & Health*, *21*, 545–555.

Baker, C., & Stern, P. N. (1993). Finding meaning in chronic illness as the key to self-care. *Canadian Journal of Nursing Research*, *25*, 23–36.

Benner, P. (1984). *From novice to expert: Excellence and power in clinical nursing practice.* Menlo Park, CA: Addison-Wesley.

Blalock, H. M., Jr. (1982). *Conceptualization and measurement in the social sciences.* Newbury Park, CA: Sage.

Blalock, H. M., Jr. (1984). *Basic dilemmas in the social sciences.* Newbury Park, CA: Sage.

Dluhy, N. M. (1995). Mapping knowledge in chronic illness. *Journal of Advanced Nursing*, *21*, 1051–1058.

Dressler, W. W. (2001). Medical anthropology: Toward a third moment in social science. *Medical Anthropology Quarterly*, *15*(4), 455–465.

Eulberg, J. R., Weekley, J. A., & Bhagat, R. S. (1988). Models of stress in organizational research: A metatheoretical perspective. *Human Relations*, *41*(4), 331–350.

Gergen, K. J. (2001). Psychological science in a postmodern context. *American Psychologist*, *56*(1), 803–813.

Hall, E. (1997). Four generations of nurse theorists in the U.S. *Veard i Norden* [Scandinavian Journal of Caring], *17*(2), 15–23.

Haworth, S., & Dluhy, N. M. (2001). Holistic symptom management: Modeling the interaction phase. *Journal of Advanced Nursing*, *36*(2), 302–310.

Kalmar, D. A., & Sternberg, R. J. (1988). Theory knitting: An integrative approach to theory development. *Philosophical Psychology*, *1*, 153–170.

Kim, H. S. (1989). Theoretical thinking in nursing: Problems and prospects. In J. Akinsamya (Ed.), *Recent advances in nursing: Models of nursing*, Edinburgh, Scotland: Churchhill Livinstone, 106–122.

Kim, H. S. (1993). Putting theories into practice: Problems and prospects. *Journal of Advanced Nursing*, *18*, 1632–1639.

Kim, H. S. (2000). An integrative framework for conceptualizing clients: A proposal for a nursing perspective in the new century. *Nursing Science Quarterly*, *13*(1), 37–44.

Kim, H. S. (2001). Directions for theory development—For an increased coherence in the new century. In N. Chaska (Ed.), *The nursing profession: Tomorrow and beyond.* (pp. 273–286). Thousand Oaks, CA: Sage.

Kuhn, T. S. (1970). Reflections on my critics. In I. Lakatos & A. Musgrave (Eds.), *Criticism and the growth of knowledge* (pp. 231–278). Cambridge, MA: Harvard University Press.

Lang, N. M. (1999). Discipline-based approaches to evidence-based practice: A view from nursing. *Journal of Quality Improvement*, *25*(1), 539–544.

Lazarus, R. S. (1966). *Psychological stress and the coping process.* New York: McGraw-Hill.

Litchfield, M. (1999). Practice wisdom. *Advances in Nursing Science, 22*(2), 62–73.

Meleis, A. F. (1987). Revisions in knowledge development: A passion for substance. *Scholarly Inquiry for Nursing Practice: An International Journal, 1*(1), 5–19.

Meleis, A. F. (1997). *Theoretical nursing: Development & progress* (3rd ed.). New York: Lippincott.

Mikulas, W. L. (1995). Conjunctive psychology: Issues of integration. *Journal of Psychotherapy Integration, 5*(4), 331–348.

Monti, E. J., & Tingen, M. S. (1999). Multiple paradigms of nursing science. *Advances in Nursing Science, 21*(4), 64–80.

Nagle, L. M., & Mitchell, G. J. (1991). Theoretic diversity: Evolving paradigmatic issues in research and practice. *Advances in Nursing Science, 14*(1), 17–25.

Selye, H. (1976). *The stress of life.* New York: McGraw-Hill.

Strauss, A. L., & Glaser, B. G. (1974). *Chronic illness and the quality of life.* St. Louis, MO: Mosby.

Thorne, S., & Hayes, V. E. (Eds.). (1997). *Nursing praxis: Knowledge and action.* Thousand Oaks, CA: Sage.

Thorne, S. E., & Patterson, B. L. (1998). Shifting images of chronic illness. *Image: Journal for Nursing Scholarship, 30*, 173–178.

Thorne, S. E., & Patterson, B. L. (2001). Focus on chronic illness: Two decades of insider research: What we know and don't know about chronic illness experience. *Annual Review of Nursing Research, 18*, 3–25.

Turner, J. (1989). *Theory building in sociology: Assessing theoretical cumulation.* Newbury Park, CA: Sage.

Upton, D. J. (1999). How can we achieve evidence-based practice if we have a theory–practice gap in nursing today? *Journal of Advanced Nursing, 29*(3), 549–555.

Winningham, M. L., Nail, L. M., Burke, M. B., Brophy, L., Cimprich, B., Jones, L.S., et al. (1994). Fatigue and the cancer experience: The state of the knowledge. *Oncology Nursing Forum, 21*, 23–36.

Unity, Diversity, Conformism, and Chaos: Applications of Roy's Epistemology of the Universal Cosmic Imperative

22

Debra R. Hanna

Roy's epistemology, *knowledge as universal cosmic imperative*, relates to the Roy adaptation model, and advances the idea that the stimuli we encounter as human beings are both internal and external (Roy & Andrews, 1999). As humans, we are interior people living within an exterior world. The cosmic imperative is universal because it permeates every aspect within the microcosm of our being, as well as the macrocosm of the expanding universe. Within the Roy adaptation model, Roy has always maintained that there is a type of stimuli, called residual, that might never be known consciously by anyone. Roy has described this as leaving room in her model for nursing practice, for human mystery, and this is important to me as a nurse. In her descriptions of the implications of knowledge as universal cosmic imperative, Roy (chapter 10, this volume) expands her epistemological stance to include a purposeful unity and a sense of promise, that again provides room for the mystery.

In previous writings, Roy speaks to mystery as including the mystery of God—this mystery of wonder and awe of a Creator of the cosmos—who attended not only to the big picture of galaxies and stars, the macrocosmos, but is also intimately involved in the microcosmos, the very center of my being. Roy showed this mystery in a most beautiful way with the slides from Young's book, *The Unfinished Universe* (1993).

Roy's Epistemology: The Universal Cosmic Imperative

Roy's epistemology of the universal *cosmic* imperative sounds very large, very out there, being that it's cosmic. And yet, how consistent with the rest of Roy's work that while telling us about the unity of humankind, she shows us an example of a butterfly's wings fluttering deep in the South American rain forest. This slight movement then has an impact on the entire universe. The interior, the exterior, and our own heartbeats are all a unity in Roy's epistemology.

We can ask if this is a bit too much. My response is, no, not at all. Not if we really understand what unity means in Roy's view of the philosophy of knowledge, in the epistemology of the universal cosmic imperative.

The Nature of Unity

Roy's earlier epistemological writings suggest that unity is not merely a quality of human existence. For example, the unity of purpose of human existence that Roy proposes as the second defining characteristic of her philosophical assumption of veritivity is not a quality (Roy, 1988, 1998, 1999, 2000a, 2000b, chapter 10, this volume). Neither is it an adjective or adverb that simply complements some other more important concept. Further, unity is not a noun. It is not a thing or an object. If we regard unity, especially the unity of purpose of human existence where unity is a quality or where unity is an object, a noun, then our thinking has not really advanced. And Roy is advancing our thinking.

Unity as a Verb

I propose that an interpretation of what Roy is suggesting when she speaks of the unity of purpose of human existence is that unity is a verb. What Roy means in her epistemology of the universal cosmic imperative is that unity is a way that we can characterize the actualization of human existence. But, unity is more than just any verb. More specifically, it is a transitive verb, or a verb that has an object. In the universal cosmic imperative, the object of unity, which is the purpose of human existence, shows us that "where unity acts, meaning unfolds" (Hanna, 2002, p. 48). It is, therefore, the inherent meaning of the purpose of human existence that is crucial to understanding Roy's epistemology of the universal cosmic imperative.

Action of Unity

To clarify the concept of unity as a verb rather that has an object, I would like to compare it with another word that, often thought of as a noun, even though it is best understood to be a verb. That word is peace. When people speak of peace, it is often viewed as an endpoint to be achieved, and that once achieved, peace will remain intact like a solid object without the need for any further effort. We know, too, that when some people speak of peace, what they actually mean is a cessation of open hostility or of actual war. But in order for true peace to be achieved, it must be viewed as an act, as an ongoing action of all parties so that peace is achieved as an act sustained. In order for the act of peace to ensue, all parties must seek a relationship of mutual benefit for the true good of self and other.

If it is true that where unity acts, meaning unfolds, I propose that the converse is also true. Where disunity acts, the meaning and purpose of human existence can be thwarted. Questions about the meaning and purpose of life itself arise for human beings when their lives are thrown into chaos by unexpected events or by tragedies. What restores meaning and gives purpose to the lives of those suffering from tragedy is the empathic outpouring of human actions that comfort and sustain people who can no longer act on their own behalf. As nurses, we are called in practical ways to engage in maintaining and restoring the action of unity to people who cannot manage independently. Although unity is not a concept unique to the discipline of nursing, as Roy reminds us, it is an essential property of the service we as professional nurses provide for society.

Unity Depends on Diversity

When we consider unity, we must also see that unity involves diversity, depends on diversity, and cannot exist without diversity. An analogy of how unity must have diversity to function would be to consider how the pieces of any puzzle will fit together best. This increased awareness will make the puzzle much more interesting, when every piece is slightly different from every other. Within this process, unity is achieved when the goodness of fit of some puzzle pieces with other pieces is understood and used to the advantage of the whole puzzle. Another analogy is found within the arrangement of the brickwork of a building. When viewing the building you notice that even though all the bricks are the same size, shape, and weight, they cannot be stacked in uniform vertical rows next to each other. Rather they must be stacked in an alternating, overlapping, interdependent pattern of support given and support received. If the bricks are not fit together in this way, the building's structure will lack the strength it needs to stand. The pieces to a puzzle usually have a variety of shapes, but put together, they make one coherent whole. The pieces of a building when standing alone lose their meaning until they are put into a proper relationship of good fit with each other. When Roy discusses unity she emphasizes the diversity of each person standing in relationality. Within this context, the unity of human existence means that we relate to one another in our sameness and in our differences. In this way, we reflect the interdependence of the universe in the significance of relationships to human existence.

When Unity Is Misunderstood as Conformism

There is the potential for unity not to be confused with the concept of conformism. Unity assumes the goodness of human and all created existence, the goodness of its meaning, and the fullness of its purpose. Conformism is inherently empty and purposeless, because it is an unnatural uniformity that oppresses the creativity and individuality of oneself and others. For example, an erroneous conclusion involves the belief that the active unity of groups of people cannot occur without a certain uniformity of thoughts, actions, and attributes of all members of the group. Therefore, we use the saying "birds of a feather flock together." If we understand unity as Roy intends it, we also understand that the feather that makes people flock together is the common purpose of human existence. In order to fulfill that purpose, people must retain their freedom of human creativity and activity, which enables them to reach their highest human potential.

Conformism is the antithesis of unity. It impoverishes people by stripping them of the meaning of their existence by inhibiting or denying human relationality, and by engendering a disinterest in others or in the world that is viewed as intrinsically evil. This type of thinking began in the 19th century with political philosophies about communistic social structures that led to 20th-century totalitarian government by oppression.

Conformist thinking is what enabled existentialist thought, such as that proposed by Jean Paul Sartre, to thrive throughout the mid-to-late 20th century. Sartre's philosophy centered on the meaninglessness of human existence, where one choice was viewed as good as any other, and where a dismal view of human life prevailed with no escape. In describing the universal cosmic imperative, Roy rejects this as a type of thinking. Rather, she speaks of subjectivity, relationality, meaning, and purpose. These are not new concepts in Roy's epistemology. Yet, these concepts are still being explicated in terms of their application to nursing science and clinical practice.

Simone Weil once said, "Nothing is so beautiful and wonderful, nothing is so continually fresh and surprising, so full of sweet and perpetual ecstasy, as the good. No desert is so dreary, monotonous, and boring as evil" (Weil, 1968, p. 160).

Weil's insight was beautifully and sensitively portrayed in the film, *Sophie's Choice* (Pakula & Barish, 1982). There is a moment in the film where the viewer is slightly above and outside the wall surrounding the concentration camp commander's own home. The director allows the viewer to see the flower garden inside the wall in full color while the camera slowly pans above, over, and inside the wall. The film changes to black and white just when the viewer is brought inside the wall of the concentration camp. In nursing, we have moved from the color, texture, and beauty of a noble profession where the unity of human purposefulness is an essential property of our knowledge development, to the evils of conformism being forced on us by some types of managed care with restriction on the growth and expression of the potential of nursing.

Clinical Relevance of Roy's Epistemology Today

Why is Roy's epistemology important now? Why bother developing new knowledge if the unity that gives meaning to human existence is not a noun, not a fact, but an act, and a human act at that? The reason Roy's epistemology is so important for our times and the future of the discipline of nursing is found in her understanding of subjectivity or the self-identity of human persons. Human consciousness is central to subjectivity and to the understanding of self and others.

Nurses view human consciousness in several ways, including the obvious cognitive component. We speak of the quality of life of individuals who can think, reflect, discuss ideas, reason, come to a judgment, make a decision, and appreciate the moments of their lives. However, some people question the quality of life of individuals who cannot reason well or who can no longer reflect or engage in meaningful conversation. If one posits cognition as central to human experience, then we can question the quality of life without this function intact. For this reason, people struggle over the right to life of individuals with dementia or who are in a persistent vegetative state. Questions are raised whether it is better to deny the ordinary care of food and fluids to these vulnerable people so as to spare them the supposed misery of their reduced quality of life.

As a neuroscience nurse who has worked with individuals in a persistent vegetative state or with dementia or whose quality of thinking and reasoning was impaired in some way, perhaps being due to a stroke, a brain tumor, or a trauma, I have a different perspective. I do not advocate the execution of other human beings who do not achieve some prescribed idea of a quality of life. To me, that is the response of conformists who seek to oppress the most vulnerable, and very possibly, the happiest, people in our society. When Roy speaks of the sacred depths of each individual in describing the concept of subjectivity and self-identity, I think that as nurses we are entrusted with treasuring others in our society so that they will be able to treasure themselves.

While working as a staff nurse on a neuroscience unit I was asked by a patient's daughter to end her mother's life, in the daughter's words, "as promptly as possible." The daughter used the expression "as promptly as possible" three times in the space of a few minutes. While I was listening to the daughter's rationale for asking me to withhold the ordinary nursing care, not just of food and fluids, but also taking her mother's vital signs, turning and repositioning her, and keeping her mother clean and dry, I felt very sad.

I realized that the daughter's response could have been influenced by many things. Since it seemed that her reaction went beyond not wanting her mother to suffer in a prolonged way, I considered the daughter's experience. She could have suffered from the mother's denial of care and love for her all her life. The daughter's individuality, the daughter's sacred depths of being, could not have been very much appreciated by her mother, or the daughter could not have asked me to withhold ordinary care to the extent she proposed and to encourage administering massive doses of unneeded pain medications to help her mother die "as promptly as possible." I could not assent to that daughter's request. In fact, I saw the need to involve the bioethics committee to advocate for the mother, who seemed depressed, a depression exacerbated—in my opinion—by the mother's realization that she was too healthy to die as promptly as her daughter would have wished.

If we look at the unity of the purpose of human existence as a consideration in producing new nursing knowledge, we see the importance of the meaning of each human life in relationship to the whole of humanity. This knowledge reshapes how we approach our moral-ethical challenges and thus guides nursing care. Do I condemn the daughter who asked me to withhold ordinary care from her mother? Certainly not. Do I obey the daughter's request for a hastened death? Certainly not. What do I do with this information? As an illustrative example, I point out now that neither the daughter who could not tolerate her mother, nor the mother who may not have a strong relationship with her daughter is at fault. As the nurse, I am not the judge, nor do I have all the facts. I would not ascribe fault or blame or penalty or punishment.

As the nurse, I am able to use knowledge about the common purpose of human existence and recognize that something had gone very wrong in this family relationship. I could see that the mother needed protection at that moment, and the daughter needed care, love, and attention. Could I provide that? It is not so easily done in today's health care systems. With the constraints of managed care, these goals are difficult to accomplish. We have planned points for achieving goals to be reached along critical pathways. In some cases, where the level of care is task oriented and simple, critical pathways work well to keep things in a large hospital system moving along. But there are too many cases where the problems of family life or of individual circumstances militate against that kind of conformist view of health care. The system dictates that we do just what is absolutely necessary without attention to the human situation. As nurses, we need to be aware of how quickly conformism leads to evil premises and evil actions. We need to safeguard the unity of human existence, which is tied to the meaning of human existence.

Doesn't Diversity Lead to Chaos?

Some could challenge what I have said about how important diversity is to the unity of human existence by claiming that too much diversity can lead to chaos, that is, complete confusion. My view is that chaos does not result from people having different cultures, religions, genders, or ages. Rather, the diversity of human attributes and the variety of natural endowments in our universe contribute to a very beautiful world, especially when we energetically work together in acts of peace. When Roy addresses the diversity needed for unity, she does not imply a type of pallid respect called tolerance, but rather an enthusiastic interest eager to include all for a greater good.

Chaos, as used in this discussion, results from a certain type of self-centeredness that impairs social relationality. We usually think of self-centeredness as an attribute belonging to individual people, not to whole societies. Yet, history has recorded eras where self-centeredness manifested in different forms of self-indulgence was an endemic, sociocultural pattern that led to the decline and fall of empires.

As noted earlier, where unity acts, meaning unfolds, and conversely, where disunity acts, meaning is lost. When the tragic events of September 11, 2001, were unfolding in New York City, Pennsylvania, and at the Pentagon, the suddenness of the attack and its large scale seemed to lead to chaos. Yet, what we witnessed repeatedly, were acts of unity that restored relatedness and averted chaos as confusion. That is, the heroic, other-centered, prompt and focused attention of ordinary people for and toward others turned the sources of possible chaos (the large crashes of two tall buildings, one plane, and an attack on the center of our military operations) into an exemplar of the unity of humankind. From this example, we see that it isn't the largeness, suddenness, or even the type of event we encounter that plunges people into chaos but, rather, the way we respond socially in the midst of threatening events.

We can apply the same observations in our nursing practice. As nurses, we often encounter patients whose lives appear to be in complete confusion. They are unable to climb out of the quagmire within their own lives. Instinctively, nurses know that these patients need our help and our attention. Very often, they need the neighborly love of the nurse as well as scientific knowledge, to effect their lives, especially during illness. Yet sometimes, when we meet their family members, we may see that the family members care very much about the patient but that the caring may not be mutual. The patient is not able to return affection or share effectively in familial concerns. Likewise, we also see patients concerned about their family, but the family is not well-connected to the patient. If we understand the relationship of unity to meaning and purpose, we know that nurses can help foster the healthy interdependence of all family members and help restore a sense of meaning and purpose and, thereby, eliminate familial chaos.

It is not the variety of human attributes that undermine the unity of human existence because that variety enriches humankind. It is the constriction of authentically relational interactions between and among people that can lead to the disruption, fear, and chaos that undermines the unity of human existence. As nurses, we act most usually in an other-directed service to people and society. Therefore, it is nurses who can articulate clearly the importance of unity, that is, unity understood as a verb, in order to advance contemporary nursing science.

Conclusion

Sr. Callista Roy has pursued a previously uncharted territory and given us the richness of the epistemology of the *universal cosmic imperative*. It is an innovative epistemology, a new way of developing knowledge. The approach can effect change and improve life across diverse populations. The universal cosmic imperative calls for a new response to today's challenges in human health care. It directs us away from the emptiness of postmodernism and the positivist prescriptions that immediately preceded postmodern thinking. In her position on knowledge development, Roy makes the concepts of inherent purposefulness, the unity of human existence, and the promise of meaning and value important to future knowledge development. By linking this conceptualization to the trust that nurses have to treasure life in all forms, Roy has developed, possibly for the first time in history, an epistemology that includes and makes room for mystery: the mystery of the human person, the mystery of the universe, and in my opinion, the mystery of God.

REFERENCES

Hanna, D. R. (2002). *Moral distress redefined: The lived experience of moral distress of nurses who participated in legal, elective, surgically induced abortions.* Unpublished Doctoral Dissertation, Boston College, Chestnut Hill, MA.

Pakula, A. J., & Barish, K. (Producers). (1982). *Sophie's choice* [motion picture]. Burbank, CA: Universal Pictures.

Roy, C. (1988). An explication of the philosophical assumptions of the Roy adaptation model. *Nursing Science Quarterly, 1*(1), 26–34.

Roy, C. (1998). Future of the Roy model: Challenge to redefine adaptation. *Nursing Science Quarterly, 10*(1), 42–48.

Roy, C. (1999). State of the art: Discussion and utilization of nursing literature in practice. *Biological Research for Nursing, 1*(2), 147–155.

Roy, C. (2000a). A theorist envisions the future and speaks to nursing administration. *Nursing Administration Quarterly*, *24*(2), 1–12.

Roy, C. (2000b). The visible and invisible fields that shape the future of the nursing care system. *Nursing Administration Quarterly*, *25*(1), 119–131.

Roy, C., & Andrews, H. A. (1999). *The Roy adaptation model* (2nd ed.). Norwalk, CT: Appleton & Lange.

Weil, S. (1968). *On science, necessity, and the love of God* (R. Rees, Ed., Trans.). London: Oxford University Press.

Young, L. B. (1993). *The unfinished universe*. New York: Oxford University Press.

Global Applications of the Cosmic Imperative for Nursing Knowledge Development

23

Donna J. Perry
Katherine E. Gregory

n her discussion of knowledge as a cosmic imperative, Roy states that "Nursing as a profession carries a social mandate to contribute to the common good" (2001a, p. 1). This chapter will discuss two global applications of nursing knowledge related to the Cosmic Imperative: transcendent pluralism and the global ecosystem.

The epistemology of nursing has gone through many phases that have been analyzed and classified by nursing scholars (Meleis, 1997; Stevenson & Woods, 1986). It seems useful to consider three historical phases of evolution of nursing epistemology (see Fig. 23.1). The first phase was the *receptive phase* in which nursing knowledge was received from other disciplines such as medicine. The last few decades have seen a move into the *self-generative phase* in which nurses have begun to develop their own knowledge for nursing practice. The third phase holds the future for nursing knowledge, the *transformative phase*. This phase calls for the development of nursing knowledge that influences not only nursing practice but other disciplines and society as a whole. The transformative phase encompasses true engagement and exchange of knowledge between nursing and other professions in order to transform society. It is in this transformative

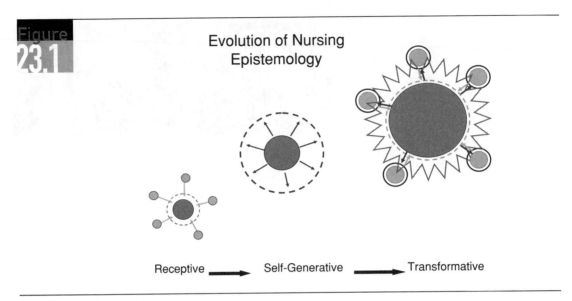

Figure 23.1

Evolution of Nursing Epistemology

Receptive ⟶ Self-Generative ⟶ Transformative

Evolution of Nursing Epistemology.

phase that nursing knowledge of both transcendent pluralism and the global ecosystem can play a role.

Transcendent Pluralism as a Foundation for Global Understanding and Social Justice

Within contemporary society, advances in communication and transportation have brought together diverse groups of people in a way that has never been experienced before. Innovations in technology and high speed Internet connections have dramatically united the world. Events in distant places are communicated across the globe instantaneously. Unfortunately, ongoing conflicts threaten globalization with discord and destruction. For the peaceful evolution of an increasingly globalized society, we must consider how to build understanding between people of diverse backgrounds. Transcendent pluralism will be discussed as an ethical framework to support transcultural understanding and social justice.

Nursing as a discipline is in a central position to promote global understanding because of its primary focus on the human person. The Consensus Statement on Emerging Nursing Knowledge (chapter 1, this volume) affirms that nursing views personhood on the individual, family, and community levels. Nurses have a moral obligation to transcend ethnocentrism. The work of nursing includes raising global consciousness about the intrinsic worth of each human being. The discipline of nursing has a social mandate to transform society. The American Nurses Association (2003) Code of Ethics for Nurses maintains that nursing has a commitment to social reform and that health goes beyond health care delivery systems to include broader issues such as human rights. This commitment is grounded in human dignity, the foundational principle of nursing ethics.

In a *Position Statement: Towards Elimination of Weapons of War and Conflict (1999)*, the International Council of Nursing called for the promotion of world peace as an essential foundation for human health and development.

Roy (2001a) views the social mandate for nursing as a moral imperative. Knowledge as a cosmic universal imperative (see chapter 10, this volume) describes the expectation that nurses will be leaders in the transformation of society. Roy's principles of veritivity and cosmic unity (Roy & Andrews, 1999) speak to the integration of knowledge as a unified truth and a strategy toward global understanding. The concept of transcendent pluralism (Perry, 2005) as a component of global understanding is consistent with the cosmic imperative in that it brings pluralism into unity without losing the richness of diversity or drifting into relativism. This common goal is achieved through self-transcendence based on universal human dignity.

Pluralism

Diane Eck, founder of The Pluralism Project, describes *pluralism* as a commitment to shaping society through dialogue and engagement (Eck, 1993). According to Eck, pluralism goes beyond mere tolerance as a strategy to learn about each other and reach understanding. It goes beyond relativism in that pluralism allows individuals to remain committed to the relationships that bind society.

The word *pluralism*, however, as it is commonly understood today, often does imply a certain relativity. An overemphasis on diversity itself as an ultimate value can undermine relationships. Sometimes pluralism implies that in striving for the goal to embrace diverse types of behavior, anything is acceptable in the name of culture. We can avoid this sort of relativism by focusing on the foundational value that grounds pluralism. This foundational value is the underlying dignity of each human being that we identified earlier as the core value of nursing. The value of universal human dignity means that we cannot have complete *relativism* because our behavior must be consistent with that which affirms the value of each human being. For example, in the *United Nations Background Note*, Ayton-Shenker (1995) states that,

> Cultural rights are not unlimited . . . There are legitimate, substantive limitations on cultural practices, even on well-entrenched traditions. For example, no culture today can legitimately claim a right to practice slavery. Despite its practice in many cultures throughout history . . . all forms of slavery, including contemporary slavery-like practices, are a gross violation of human rights under international law. (p. xx)

Self-Transcendence

The word *transcendent* in the position we are proposing is meant to evoke a sense of going beyond relativism toward universal values. This connotation is based on the work of Bernard Lonergan (1972), a 20th-century philosopher. Lonergan used the term *self-transcendence* to indicate a goal or direction of human action that carries one beyond one's individual horizon to the universal horizon based on a progressive realization of truth. Moral self-transcendence is the achievement of actions of benevolence that are consistent with God's love in the world. Such actions lead to becoming an authentic person. Lonergan's understanding of God was informed by his vocation as a Jesuit priest, and he also acknowledged the significance of diverse beliefs. He described religion as the word of God that enters the world and is interpreted differently by people of different cultures and historical periods. Different interpretations lead to diverse beliefs, but there is a deeper unity that underlies these differences. Lonergan warned that religion must be directed toward the good, love of one's neighbor, and self-denial. If not, differences in belief will result in societal decay leading to hatred and violence. It is self-sacrificing love based on charity that will lead people to self-transcendence and out of social decline (Lonergan, 1972).

Transcendent Pluralism

Transcendent pluralism is being developed as a framework to support the evolution of a social consciousness that is grounded in human dignity, leading to understanding and justice (Perry, 2005). In a recent study, Perry (2006) has defined transcendent pluralism as "the evolution of the human spirit through mutually transformative relationships between diverse peoples leading to a loving human community through the development of human dignity" (p. 53).

Transcendent pluralism is pluralistic in that it recognizes the diverse manifestations of the good within each person. It is transcendent in that to achieve it we must transcend our own particular horizon or beliefs to reach a broader horizon of love. Lonergan said that for us to move into the practical pattern of individual experience without contracting the universal horizon requires charity, or love (2000). By using self-transcendent love, we can meet people in the concrete experience of their daily living. As nurses, we are accustomed to caring for people in the practical horizon of their daily lives even though their beliefs and practices might be quite different from our own. Through self-transcendence, nurses can go beyond the boundaries of difference by grounding nursing care in the intrinsic value of each and every person (Perry, 2004). The ability to transcend differences, so central to good nursing care, is what society needs. Nurses are able to do this in each caring interaction with patients, families, and communities. The humanity of the person emerges in all encounters with the goal of helping and caring for others, regardless of what some would consider status or potential based on cultural, ethnic, social, or financial conditions. By building a pluralistic culture that is grounded in the value of human dignity, humankind can learn to transcend differences. Nursing, whose core value is human dignity, has much to contribute toward achieving global understanding.

Lonergan described the *dialectic* as a tension that exists between our current horizon and the universal horizon of truth (2001). It is the difference between where we are and where we need to be, both as individuals and as a community. Through the dialectic, each person considers the current situation, reflects on the situation, and develops ideas for change. Within the technical, social, and cultural fields, humanity's ideas about humanity will determine the transformation of human living. Thus, the effects of the dialectic should be to point out the defects in the current situation and establish strategies that will help us move toward self-transcendence. The essence of this dialectic is not a conflict between different philosophies or schools of thought. It is the opposition between "the self as transcending and the self as transcended" (Lonergan, 1972, p. 111).

The significance of the dialectic for transcendent pluralism is to help us realize the gap between the current global situation and the potential for universal human dignity. Recognition of this gap helps us to realize the need to move as a community toward the common goal of realizing human dignity. Social justice involves narrowing the gap. Narrowing the gap begins in the encounter between people of diverse horizons. As people of diverse horizons encounter one another, the goal should not be to impose one's own beliefs on the other, but to engage in a process of openness and dialogue leading to shared meanings and mutual transformation. This is the path to peace. However, this process takes time. It requires reflection and discernment both as an individual and as a community. It also requires the courage to ask the hard questions about what is truly good and a willingness to make changes based on the answers to those questions.

Lonergan (1957/2000) connected knowing with doing. Ethical behavior develops from a reflective and critical process of understanding based on asking questions and then translating one's understanding into action. An authentic person is one whose actions are consistent with transcendent love. Thus, transcendent pluralism goes beyond sentimental feelings of good will toward others or the so-called celebration of diversity. Authenticity demands that this understanding be followed by concrete actions that truly promote human dignity. As long as we live in a world with striking social, economic, and health disparities, an awareness of the dialectic should inspire us to take actions that promote human dignity leading to social justice.

Transcendent pluralism can be seen in the so-called Righteous Gentiles or people who risked their own lives to help Jews escape the Nazis during the Holocaust. Oliner and Oliner (1988) studied the characteristics of these rescuers. The rescuers, as compared to nonrescuers, were more likely to believe that ethical values should be applied universally to all people. One Dutch rescuer hid a Jewish woman and helped the Jewish woman to maintain her traditions by getting her Yom Kippur candles even though they were difficult to obtain. She stated, "What did I know about Yom Kippur? I just respected it" (p. 88).

Transcendent pluralism goes beyond any single religious tradition to a higher spiritual realm. This higher spirit can serve as a foundation for relationships with any group of "others." I witnessed a moving example of this during a recent visit to Cuba where, despite the countries' hardships caused in part by the U.S. embargo, the Cuban people were able to transcend geopolitical boundaries and reach out to Americans in warmth and friendship. In a visit to the national director of nursing to present her with a copy of *The Roy Adaptation Model* she said,

> This is a very meaningful day, especially considering the U.S. embargo, because it shows that, in spite of the difficulties our governments have, we have come to foster friendship. It is the spirit of humanity which is important. This is an example of friendship, solidarity, and the human spirit. (B. Escalona, personal communication, February 19, 2003)

Transcendent Pluralism and the Cosmic Imperative

The concept of transcendent pluralism is consistent with Roy's call for knowledge as a *universal cosmic imperative* and human participation in the transformation of the future.

This position (see chapter 10, this volume) is based in the principles of unity, or universal knowledge, purposefulness, or an orderly unfolding of the universe in accordance with God, and promise, which involves the participation of human consciousness in the transformation toward a common destiny for mankind. We propose that transcendent pluralism is an important step toward the worthy goal of achieving global understanding.

In the transformative phase of nursing knowledge, we have the knowledge, opportunity, social responsibility, and underlying value system to accomplish the task. We now look at a second perspective that can contribute to the transformative phase of nursing knowledge.

Nursing Knowledge of the Global Ecosystem and Human Health

Life and nursing are products of all conditions, event and actions of yesterday. Life and nursing tomorrow will relate to today. (Johnson, 1965, p. 38)

Dorothy Johnson's prophetic words of 1965 are important in grounding nursing knowledge of the global ecosystem, environmental conservation, and physiologic sustainability. More than 40 years after these words were published, Johnson's thoughts provide inspiration as we reflect on yesterday's conditions, events, and actions of ourselves as nurses, significantly influenced by changing conditions. One might consider yesterday's history and its influence on today's nursing and life patterns from a number of important vantage points: globalization, human rights, economic trends, and the biotechnology boom are just a few of the stimuli that create the need for transcendent pluralism leading to global understanding.

The crisis in our global ecosystem and the associated health ramifications is perhaps the most significant context in which nurses are called to contemplate the influence of yesterday on today. By developing knowledge for practice through research that is based on the relationship between the ecosystem and health today, nurses will demonstrate the use of yesterday's challenges while seeking to improve life for all people and nursing for tomorrow. Contemporary nursing knowledge development of the global ecosystem can benefit greatly from using the philosophical underpinnings of views such as the universal cosmic imperative as proposed by Roy to guide our evolution (see chapter 10, this volume).

Professional nursing has a social responsibility to promote the health and wellness of people worldwide. "As a profession, nursing utilizes specialized knowledge to contribute to the needs of society for health and well-being" (Roy, 2001b, p. 6). This specialized knowledge is rooted in an understanding of people and their environment, which has been central to the discipline since Florence Nightingale documented her findings on the physical environment and the soldier's recovery in military hospitals during the Crimea War. "A woman far beyond her time, her broad conceptualization of the environment included recognition of the effect of social, economic, and political forces on the health of British soldiers during the Crimean War" (Salazar & Primomo, 1994, p. 317). As a result of her work in the Crimea, Nightingale honed in on "five essential points in securing the health of houses: pure air, pure water, efficient drainage, cleanliness, and light" (Nightingale, 1869).

This conceptualization of environment was revolutionary at the time. The ideals promoted by Nightingale remain part of the foundation of nursing practice today, however the "conceptualization of environment she typified represents a myopic view" (Butterfield, 2000, p. 385). With the environment as a primary determinant of health and environmental health hazards affecting all aspects of life and all areas of nursing practice (Pope, Snyder, & Mood, 1995), it is essential that nursing's knowledge of the dynamic relationship between person and environment be recognized. Nightingale was a visionary, and her focus on the relationship between environment and health was historic. But "nurses today are challenged to shift paradigms and to embrace a broader understanding and new way of thinking about the person and environment interaction" (Salazar & Primomo, 1994, p. 318). It is proposed that nurses develop a broader, more contemporary knowledge of environment defined as the global ecosystem and person defined in the context of physiologic integrity and sustainability. This focus has the potential to alter the conceptual approach and philosophical underpinning of current nursing practice.

The paradigm shift that is needed is inevitable as the intertwining of our natural world and health has become increasingly evident over the past 50 years. Unfortunately, this evidence has come as a result of disasters such as Love Canal, Chernobyl, and Bhopal (Salazar & Primomo, 1994). In his book *Earth in the Balance*, former Vice President Gore (1993) describes this situation as a collision between worldwide civilization and the ecological system of the Earth. Gore points to the population explosion, the technology revolution, and individual apathy and indifference about one's personal relationship with the environment as factors that have played a role in this collision.

The Cosmic Imperative as a Framework for Nursing Knowledge of the Global Ecosystem

Nurses have unique ways of knowing how one's physical environment might be manipulated to improve health or alleviate suffering. Knowledge about person and environment is not only the core of nursing practice, it is what differentiates it from other health science professions. Nursing knowledge development that focuses on the environment on a global scale will contribute to the next generation of strategies needed to prevent further planetary damage and world health decline. An increasingly expansive and contemporary framework in which to structure thought is required to contemplate the concepts of person and environment on this scale. The universal cosmic imperative and associated Earth principls introduced by Roy (see chapter 10, this volume) offers such a framework.

Unity

The universal cosmic imperative core characteristics of unity, purposefulness, and promise are central to this perspective. These characteristics have been expanded by Roy in her articulation of the three Earth principles of unity, diversity, and subjectivity (Roy, 2001a). Although not predominant in the nursing literature, the attributes of the

Earth principles lend themselves to the broad thinking that is necessary to view the big picture relationships between global ecosystems and human sustainability. These components provide a structure in which to consider nursing knowledge development through research on the interdependence between the global ecosystem and sustainability of the human species.

The universal cosmic imperative is characterized by *unity* among all living things that stems from the scientific reality that "everything we know is made of the same kind of stuff. Our chemical nature is literally the same as the stars" (Roy, 2001a, p. 2). Swimme and Berry have contributed a great deal to the development of this train of thought in their writing on cosmology (1992). The aspect of unity within the universal cosmic imperative hinges on the following set of premises:

- To be is to be related; relationship is the essence of existence.
- Nothing is itself without everything else.
- We are one with our universe and one with each other.

Berry writes that "the entire universe is bonded together in such a way that the presence of each individual is felt throughout its entire spatial and temporal range" (1999, p. 163). Integrating the components of the universe with one another enables the vast variety of beings to come into existence and form a comprehensive unity with one another. It is the need for unity among the components of the universe and for synthesis between the individual person and the natural environment that will enable nurses to "encounter a world in transition that is like no other time in history. In this encounter nursing care makes decisions that create visions and actions to promote the future good of humankind integrated with the environment" (Roy, 2001a, p. 6). In summary, the Earth principle of unity describes that although we are unique human persons, we must be cognizant of our evolutionary biology, which reminds us on a molecular level that we are much like the millions of other living species with whom we share this planet. This thesis is integral to the universal cosmic imperative.

Diversity

Even as we reflect on unity, we can ask: What would it be like if everything on Earth were the same? What would life be like without seasons, a range of plants and animals to inhabit different landscapes and climates, a variety of nourishment and culture to enrich the globe? How are we going to survive without clean drinking water; how are the 1 billion people in developing nations surviving right now? The crises that face our natural world as it moves toward what Berry (1999) calls a *monoculture* underscore the importance of the second Earth principle, that is, *diversity*.

This second principle complements the principle of unity by suggesting that though the Earth is a single community that shares similar molecular history as well as extensive amounts of natural resources, impending global sameness is contrary to evolutionary processes that naturally move toward constant differentiation (Roy, 2001a). Reduction in biodiversity toward a monoculture is perhaps the greatest threat to our human survival. With each species that becomes extinct, so does a potential antidote for any number of ailments that plague other species. Several human and plant diseases might be eradicated by currently unknown natural elements that are at risk within Earth's biology. The universal cosmic imperative is contingent on unity among a vast *diversity* of populations of species. Nursing knowledge of this highly complex unity and diversity within the natural world promises to lead to the development of unique solutions in which the Earth's species will live in a more harmonious and sustainable manner than they do today.

Subjectivity

Subjectivity, the third component of the universal cosmic imperative, focuses on the true treasure of each individual being. To quote Roy (2001a), "This principal provides us with a deep sense of individuality and of the sacred depth of each person" (p. 4). The essence of subjectivity is seen in the unique beauty and mystery of human creation in the natural world and the universe around us. All life is sacred; the depth of humanity and the wonder of natural events are captured in subjectivity. Kindnesses seen among strangers, the affinity between those of different cultures, the magnificence of mountain waterfalls in springtime, or the brilliant rainbow after a summer thunderstorm might best be explained by subjectivity. Being wholly who we are contributes to both the unity of people and creation as well as to its diversity. Roy eloquently summarizes "the whole universe or community emerges into being from expression of the unique properties of the individual" (Roy, 2001a, p. 4).

Nursing has a professional social responsibility to improve health. This requires the use of current knowledge and the development of new knowledge that will contribute solutions needed by global communities whose health has been compromised by changes in their natural world. This responsibility stems from nursing's unique understanding of how the environment has an impact on human health and disease. The consequences of the current gap in nursing knowledge and a proactive approach to the global ecosystem and human sustainability have become painfully obvious in today's world. The economic and political turmoil over the utilization of natural resources continues to escalate, the crisis of millions who lack clean drinking water and sanitation is far from a resolution, and the staggering increase in obesity and comorbid conditions have overrun the American health care system. Nursing knowledge development that recognizes the global ecosystem will not be the fix-all of the complex issues facing the health of communities worldwide. Nonetheless, nurses taking responsibility to articulate new knowledge related to the changing ecosystem and sustainability of global populations, as defined in the context of the universal cosmic imperative, have the potential to contribute to solutions that will reconcile the environmental and social issues that wrap themselves around the health and well-being of human beings around the globe.

Recommendations for Nursing Knowledge Development Based on the Universal Cosmic Imperative

The universal cosmic imperative serves as a philosophical underpinning for a myriad of recommendations for nursing knowledge development. These recommendations stem from the responsibility of nursing as a profession to contribute to solutions that promote social and environmental justice in communities around the globe. Nursing knowledge that serves this purpose has the potential to influence decisions that currently lack nursing insight. Future nurse leaders who champion the findings of nursing research and disseminate knowledge in forums where the nursing voice has not been heard before will contribute to the transformation of global societies.

Recommendations for nursing in relation to transcendent pluralism reflect the connection between knowing and doing that is grounded in Lonergan's ethics. Nurses will become actively engaged in learning about cultural and religious beliefs of people with diverse backgrounds. Education will be grounded in uncovering the underlying value of each individual and will emphasize each person's uniqueness linked to their ethnic or religious background. As a society, we will avoid cultural reductionism, or simply labeling someone with a *cultural diagnosis*. Culley (1996) pointed out that current practices in nursing cultural education may actually reinforce ethnic categories that lead to stereotypes. Approaching the topic from universal values can help avoid this pitfall.

Nursing research continues to strive toward answering questions that will contribute to global understanding. What are the qualities that lead to transcendent pluralism? How can we foster such an attitude in society? How can nursing address social injustices such as health disparities? Once we answer these questions, knowing will be followed by doing. Knowledge alone is insufficient. We will translate nursing knowledge into actions that are consistent with the universal values of transcendent love. Nursing knowledge will be brought to bear beyond the health care system in advocating for public policy that meets the needs of the voiceless and oppressed. As political powers wage the war on terrorism, nurses will be a voice to heal the roots of terrorism that are fueled by poverty and despair. Nurses will work to promote a peaceful and just society where the needs of all are met equitably. Nursing, guided by transcendent pluralism, could help to transform the world into a true global community where understanding and social justice prevail.

The universal cosmic imperative and Earth principles underpin recommendations for nursing research and knowledge development related to the interconnected nature of the global ecosystem and human health. Whereas the concepts of environment and health should be broadened and redefined for the 21st century using the tenets of the universal cosmic imperative, nurses will acknowledge that they are in a position to take the lead in global ecosystem protections and related health research. Recommendations include nursing theory and scientific development of environmental conservation activities that are correlated to enhanced human health. Nurse researchers can focus on generating and disseminating knowledge that will reduce current threats to the global ecosystem and enhance the physiologic integrity of all humans. As a discipline founded on an understanding of person, environment, and health, nurses will take a leading role in educating individuals on the importance of the environmental influences on health and in developing strategies that empower persons in all communities to respect the unity, diversity, and subjectivity of each other and of the natural world. In doing so, our profession will ensure the health and well-being of individuals and foster the sustainability of the global ecosystem.

REFERENCES

American Nurses Association (2003). *Code of ethics for nurses with interpretive statements*. Retrieved July 17, 2003, from http://nursingworld.org/ethics/code/ethicscode150.htm.

Ayton-Shenker, D. (1995). The challenge of human rights and cultural diversity. In *United Nations Background Note*. Retrieved August 24, 2000, from United Nations Department of Public Information Web site: http://www.un.org/rights/dpi1627e.htm.

Berry, T. (1999). *The great work: Our way into the future*. New York: Bell Tower.

Butterfield, P. (2000). Recovering a lost legacy: Nurses' leadership in environmental health. *Journal of Nursing Education, 39*(9), 385–386.

Culley, L. (1996). A critique of multiculturalism in health care: The challenge for nurse education. *Journal of Advanced Nursing, 23*(3), 564–570.

Eck, D. L. (1993). The challenge of pluralism. *Nielman Reports "God in the Newsroom," 47*(2), 7. Retrieved December, 26, 2002, from http://www.pluralism.org/research/articles/cop.php?from=articles_index

Gore, A. (1993). *Earth in the balance: Ecology and the human spirit*. New York: Plume.

International Council of Nursing. (1999). *Position statements 1999: Towards elimination of weapons of war and conflict*. Retrieved July 17, 2003, from http://www.icn.ch/pswar.htm.

Johnson, D. E. (1965). Today's action will determine tomorrow's nursing. *Nursing Outlook, 13*, 38.

Lonergan, B. (2001). Horizon, history, philosophy. In P. H. McShane (Ed.), *Phenomenology and logic* (pp. 298–365). Toronto, Ontario, Canada: University of Toronto Press.

Lonergan, B. (2000a). The possibility of ethics. In F. E. Crowe & R. M. Doran (Eds.), *Collected works of Bernard Lonergan: Insight: A study of human understanding* (pp. 196–231). Toronto, Ontario, Canada: University of Toronto Press. (Original work published 1957)

Lonergan, B. (2000b). The human good as the developing subject. In F. E. Crowe & R. M. Doran (Eds.), *Collected works of Bernard Lonergan: Topics in education* (pp. 79–106). Toronto, Ontario, Canada: University of Toronto Press. (Original work published 1959)

Lonergan, B. (1972). Religion. In *Method in theology* (pp. 101–124). New York: Herder & Herder.

Meleis, A. I. (1997). *Theoretical nursing: Development and progress*. Philadelphia: Lippincott.

Nightingale, F. (1869). *Notes on nursing: What it is and what it is not*. New York: Dover.

Oliner, S. P., & Oliner, P. M. (1988). *The altruistic personality: Rescuers of Jews in Nazi Europe*. New York: The Free Press.

Perry, D. (2004). Self-transcendence: Lonergan's key to integration of nursing theory, research and practice. *Nursing Philosophy, 5*, 67–74.

Perry, D. (2005, February). Transcendent pluralism and the influence of nursing testimony on environmental justice legislation. *Policy, Politics & Nursing Practice, 6*(1), 60–71.

Perry, D. (2006). *The role of transcendent pluralism in the evolution of human consciousness*. Unpublished doctoral dissertation, Boston College, Chestnut Hill, MA. p. 53.

Pope, A. M., Snyder, M., & Mood, L. H. (Eds.). (1995). *Nursing, health and the environment: Strengthening the relationship to improve the public's health*. Washington, DC: National Academy Press.

Roy, C. (2001a, October 25–27). *Knowledge as cosmic imperative and impact on the health care system*. Paper presented at the Knowledge Impact Conference 2001, Newton, MA.

Roy, C. (2001b). Reflections on nursing: A time of challenge and change. *Australian Journal of Advanced Nursing, 19*(1), 6–7.

Roy, C., & Andrews, H. A. (1999). *The Roy adaptation model* (2nd ed.). Stamford, CT: Appleton & Lange.

Salazar, M. K., & Primomo, J. (1994). Taking the lead in environmental health: Defining a model for practice. *American Association of Occupational Health Nurses, 42*(7), 317–324.

Stevenson, J. S., & Woods, N. F. (1986). Nursing science and contemporary science: Emerging paradigms. In G. E. Sorensen (E.d), *Setting the Agenda for the Year 2000: Knowledge Development in Nursing* (pp. 6–20). Kansas City, Missouri: American Academy of Nursing.

Swimme, B., & Berry, T. (1992). *The universe story: From the primordial flaring forth to the Ecozoic era—A celebration of the unfolding cosmos.* San Francisco: Harper.

History of New England Knowledge Conferences

Boston University School of Nursing, 1984–1987

In 1984, Boston University initiated a series called the *Annual Nursing Science Colloquia*. These colloquia were developed by doctoral students from the graduate program, notably Bianca Chambers and Christine Bridges, at the School of Nursing in collaboration with Margaret Hardy and other faculty. Conferences focused on strategies for theory development and included presentations by nursing leaders such as Margaret Hardy, Ada Sue Hinshaw, Afaf Meleis, Glenys Hamilton, Shake Ketefian, Hesook Suzie Kim, Jean Johnson, Donna Swartz-Barcott, and Jeanie Quint Benoliel. The first colloquia focused on modes of inquiry to develop theory and inductive and qualitative strategies used to develop and test knowledge. These strategies were further explored at subsequent conferences with specific attention to concept formation and theory testing. The colloquia started at Boston University were noteworthy for two reasons; first, they served as a forum to discuss the development of knowledge for nursing science; and second, they created an opportunity for doctoral students to be mentored into the discipline and associate with leaders in the field.

University of Rhode Island College of Nursing, 1990–1994

The University of Rhode Island made the decision in 1990 to continue with the well-received conferences at Boston University and to run a series of five symposia devoted to knowledge development in nursing. The emphasis of these symposia was on the interconnectedness among philosophy, theory, research, and practice and the influence on the development of nursing knowledge. The first symposium examined the linkages among philosophy, theory, methods of inquiry, and practice. The second addressed the conceptualization and philosophy of nursing practice within the philosophies of realism, interpretivism, humanism, and praxis. The focus of the third symposium was on the nature of nursing practice theories and their relationship to research and practice, and the fourth symposium emphasized pluralism in theories and its influence on the application of theory into practice. The final symposium examined domain, theory, substantive area, and method primacy as paths to synthesize knowledge for nursing in the face of pluralism. Throughout the series, speakers included Susan Gortner, Frederick Suppe, Robert Putnam, Margaret Newman, Marilyn Rawnsley, David Allen, Nancy Fulgate Woods, Sr. Callista Roy, Hesook Suzie Kim, John Phillips, Lorraine Walker, Sue Donaldson, and Nancy Dluhy.

Boston College School of Nursing, 1996–1998 (with Eastern Nursing Research Society and Sigma Theta Tau, Alpha Chi Chapter)

The theme of these conferences hosted by Boston College in the later 1990s focused on the impact of nursing knowledge and began by exploring linkages of philosophy, theory, and research as the basis for outcomes for practice. At the first of the series, main speakers, Beth Rodgers, Margaret Newman, and Sr. Callista Roy, explored three perspectives: problem solving, process, and cosmic imperative. Panels of specialists addressed implications of the perspectives for nursing language, clinical reasoning, and health policy. For the second of the series, a case analysis approach was used to link nursing knowledge to practice outcomes from three philosophical perspectives. Betty Lenz used a postpositivistic problem-solving perspective to analyze the case about end-of-life decisions and Jacqueline Fortin acted as respondent. Patricia Winstead-Fry approached the case from the perspective of knowledge as process and Sarah Jo Brown was the respondent. Janice Thompson provided a poststructuralist feminist analysis and Peggy Chinn responded. Other main contributors were Lorraine Walker as keynote and Dorothy Jones who spoke on an integrated perspective of nursing knowledge and outcomes for the closing address. The spirit of participant involvement and dialogue, established at the earlier series, was maintained in this series, culminating in an entirely participatory conference in 1998. The aim was to build on the work of nurse scholars and their perspectives on developments within nursing science. Consensus builders, Janice Brencick, Glenn Webster, Peggy Chinn, Dorothy Hones, Hesook Suzie Kim, Margaret Newman, Beth Rodgers, Sr. Callista Roy, and Janice Thompson, were provided for each table of participants. After a day and a half of dialogue, in both small and large groups, the outline of a value-based position paper linking nursing knowledge and practice outcomes was generated. The paper addressed the ontology of person and of nursing, nursing theory, and nursing practice and was offered as a guide to future knowledge development for nursing education, practice, and research. This position paper was then placed on the World Wide Web to become the stimulus for a larger international conference.

Boston Circle for Emerging Nursing Knowledge, Boston College School of Nursing, in collaboration with Sigma Theta Tau International, Alpha Chi Chapter; School of Nursing and Midwifery, University of Dublin, Ireland; and Institute of Nursing Science, University of Oslo, Norway, 2000

For Emerging Nursing Knowledge 2000, planners from eight countries (Brazil, Canada, Ireland, Japan, The Netherlands, Norway, United Kingdom, and the United States) created a program to expand the dialogue on the emerging perspectives of nursing knowledge to a global arena and to link the focused view of nursing knowledge derived in the 1998 consensus paper to effective practice outcomes. Peggy Chinn presented a challenging keynote and scholars from seven other countries addressed issues from the consensus paper from the richness of their cultural and ethnic diversity. For the first time in the Knowledge Conference series, concurrent and poster sessions were used to highlight efforts to create an impact on quality of health care, particularly for women, vulnerable populations, elders, infants, and children. Throughout the conference, dialogue among participants from 15 countries sought to address global health issues and discuss knowledge and collaborative research needed to create an impact on practice outcomes. The co-chairs summarized the conference as follows: "The clear message from participants is that there must be linguistic and semantic clarity in our language for nurses to communicate the knowledge of the discipline globally," said Dorothy Jones. Sr. Callista Roy added, "It is rare that every paper at a conference is excellent and that participants so totally immerse themselves in the process of dialogue."

Boston Circle for Emerging Nursing Knowledge, Boston College William F. Connell School of Nursing, 2001

The final conference of the series aimed to expand discussion of philosophical perspectives and to explore further links of given perspectives to change in practice. Pamela Reed gave the keynote address; Hesook Suzie Kim presented on critical narrative epistemology, Betty Lenz on middle range theory, Dorothy Jones on process knowledge and integration in practice, and Sr. Callista Roy on knowledge development from a cosmic imperative as it affects health systems. A panel of reactors to each of the four perspectives provided exemplars of links to practice. Posters on practice applications of knowledge were presented. It is noteworthy that the conference was held in Boston, MA, within 6 weeks of the defining event of the terrorist attacks of September 11, 2001. Yet conference participants were a focused and dedicated group of scholars who were all the more intent on finding ways to make a difference in our changing world. No speaker cancelled from the program and the number of participants equaled the number at conferences earlier in the series. The dialogue was rich and the energy stimulated the immediate goal of developing a book on knowledge development and practice and the long-range plan of another series of Knowledge Development Conferences.

Index

Nursing Theories, 2nd Edition
Conceptual and Philosophical Foundations

Hesook Suzie Kim, PhD, RN
Ingrid Kollak, PhD, Editors

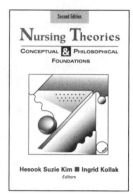

"The breadth and scope of this valuable book produces a unique and much-needed totality of nursing theory that will enhance nursing students' understanding...Highly recommended for all levels." —**Choice Magazine**

This book is designed to help readers gain a deeper understanding of nursing theories, through examining them in their conceptual and philosophical context. It is organized around major themes in nursing and health care, into which information on specific nursing theories is integrated. In this new edition, the authors have added discussion on middle-range theories as well as the "grand" theories of nursing. New chapters are included on pragmatism, evidence-based nursing, and biography.

Partial Contents:
- Human Needs and Nursing Theory, *J. Fortin*
- Adaptation as a Basic Conceptual Focus in Nursing Theories, *D. Schwartz-Barcott*
- The Concept of Self-Care, *I. Kollak*
- The Concept of Interaction in Theory and Practice, *S. Wied*
- The Concept of Need in Nursing Theory, *P. Powers*
- The Concept of Holism, *H.S. Kim*
- Systems Theory and Nursing Theories, *H. Kleve*
- Existentialism anad Phenomenology in Nursing Theories, *H.S. Kim*
- Humanism in Nursing Theory: A Focus on Caring, *M.S. Fagermoen*
- Pragmatism, Nursing, and Nursing Knowledge Development, *H.S. Kim and B. Sjöström*
- Biography and Biographical Work: An Approach for Nursing, *B. Schulte-Steinicke*
- Evidence-based Nursing for Practice and Science, *M. Hasseler*
- Transculturality and Nursing, *B. Rommelspacher*
- Illness as Risk, *F. Balke*

Springer Series on Rehabilitation
2005 · 309pp · 0-8261-4005-X · hardcover

11 West 42nd Street, New York, NY 10036-8002 • Fax: 212-941-7842
Order Toll-Free: 877-687-7476 • Order On-line: www.springerpub.com